Mayo Clinic Cardiology

Board Review Questions and Answers

Mayo Clinic Cardiology

Board Review Questions and Answers

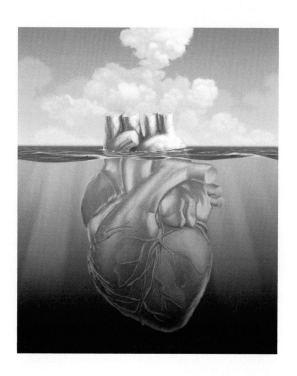

Written by

Mayo Clinic Cardiovascular Fellows

Editors

Margaret A. Lloyd, MD

Joseph G. Murphy, MD

MAYO CLINIC SCIENTIFIC PRESS

AND INFORMA HEALTHCARE USA, INC.

ISBN 1-4200-6746-X / 978-1-4200-6746-0

The triple-shield Mayo logo and the words MAYO, MAYO CLINIC, and MAYO CLINIC SCIENTIFIC PRESS are marks of Mayo Foundation for Medical Education and Research.

For order inquiries, contact Informa Healthcare, Kentucky Distribution Center, 7625 Empire Drive, Florence, KY 41042 USA.

E-mail: orders@taylorandfrancis.com
www.informahealthcare.com

Library of Congress Cataloging-in-Publication Data

Mayo Clinic cardiology: board review questions and answers / edited by Margaret A. Lloyd, Joseph G. Murphy.
    p. ; cm.
  ISBN-13: 978-1-4200-6746-0 (pb : alk. paper)
  ISBN-10: 1-4200-6746-X (pb : alk. paper) 1. Cardiology—Examinations, questions, etc. 2. Heart—Diseases—Examinations, questions, etc. I. Lloyd, Margaret A. II. Murphy, Joseph G. III. Mayo Clinic. IV. Title: Cardiology.
  [DNLM: 1. Heart Diseases—Examination Questions. WG 18.2 M4725 2007]
RC669.2.M37 2007
616.1'20076–dc22   2007035216

Care has been taken to confirm the accuracy of the information presented and to describe generally accepted practices. However, the authors, editors, and publisher are not responsible for errors or omissions or for any consequences from application of the information in this book and make no warranty, express or implied, with respect to the contents of the publication. This book should not be relied on apart from the advice of a qualified health care provider.

The authors, editors, and publisher have exerted efforts to ensure that drug selection and dosage set forth in this text are in accordance with current recommendations and practice at the time of publication. However, in view of ongoing research, changes in government regulations, and the constant flow of information relating to drug therapy and drug reactions, the reader is urged to check the package insert for each drug for any change in indications and dosage and for added warnings and precautions. This is particularly important when the recommended agent is a new or infrequently employed drug.

Some drugs and medical devices presented in this publication have Food and Drug Administration (FDA) clearance for limited use in restricted research settings. It is the responsibility of the health care providers to ascertain the FDA status of each drug or device planned for use in their clinical practice.

Printed in Canada
10 9 8 7 6 5 4 3 2 1

PREFACE

This publication, organized in a question-and-answer multiple-choice format, is a companion to *Mayo Clinic Cardiology: Concise Textbook*, 3rd edition. It was written by cardiology fellows, primarily for fellows in training, and focuses on hot topics in cardiology and likely board examination areas. It will also be useful for practicing cardiologists preparing for recertification in cardiology.

It was an honor for us to edit the work of five talented cardiovascular fellows training at Mayo Clinic in Rochester, Minnesota. They are the heart and soul of this project, and this book would not have been successfully completed without them.

Busy clinical demands mean that preparation time for the certification examination in cardiology be used judiciously. The topics and question format were developed to help trainees and recertifying physicians focus their preparation for the American Board of Internal Medicine cardiology examination. The book is designed to allow readers to self-test before the examination and to identify areas that need further review. We strongly encourage trainees to read beyond the multiple-choice answers and develop a deeper understanding of the science that underpins cardiovascular medicine.

As always, thanks are due to the many persons involved in the production of this book. Rick A. Nishimura, MD, and Steve R. Ommen, MD, directors of the annual Mayo Clinic Cardiovascular Review Course, provided encouragement for this book and *Mayo Clinic Cardiology: Concise Textbook*. Patra A. Baker assisted with typing the manuscripts. Roberta J. Schwartz (production editor), Traci J. H. Post (scientific publications specialist), and LeAnn M. Stee and Randall J. Fritz, DVM (editors), all staff in Mayo Clinic Scientific Publications, were of tremendous assistance. Karen Barrie (art director) provided guidance on the design. Sandra Beberman, Vice President, Informa Healthcare, provided valuable advice.

Every effort was made to ensure that the answers and discussion are timely and accurate. If errors are noted, please contact us so that corrections can be made in future editions. We are also interested in additional topics you would like to have included in future editions of this review book.

Margaret A. Lloyd, MD
Consultant, Division of Cardiovascular Diseases,
    Mayo Clinic, Rochester, Minnesota
Assistant Professor of Medicine,
    College of Medicine, Mayo Clinic
lloyd.margaret@mayo.edu

Joseph G. Murphy, MD
Consultant, Division of Cardiovascular
    Diseases, and Chair, Section of Scientific
    Publications, Mayo Clinic,
    Rochester, Minnesota
Professor of Medicine, College of Medicine,
    Mayo Clinic

AFFILIATIONS

EDITORS

Margaret A. Lloyd, MD, Consultant, Division of Cardiovascular Diseases, Mayo Clinic, Rochester, Minnesota; Assistant Professor of Medicine, College of Medicine, Mayo Clinic

Joseph G. Murphy, MD, Consultant, Division of Cardiovascular Diseases, and Chair, Section of Scientific Publications, Mayo Clinic, Rochester, Minnesota; Professor of Medicine, College of Medicine, Mayo Clinic

AUTHORS

T. Jared Bunch, MD, is from Logan, Utah. He graduated from Utah State University with undergraduate degrees in chemistry, liberal arts, and sciences. He received his MD from the University of Utah. He completed a residency in internal medicine and a fellowship in cardiovascular diseases and is currently a fellow in electrophysiology at Mayo School of Graduate Medical Education, College of Medicine, Mayo Clinic.

Garvan C. Kane, MD, PhD, is from Dublin, Ireland, and received his MD and PhD from University College Dublin, Ireland. He completed his internal medicine residency and clinical pharmacology and cardiovascular diseases fellowships at Mayo School of Graduate Medical Education, College of Medicine, Mayo Clinic. He is completing his cardiovascular fellowship, and he is an Assistant Professor of Medicine, College of Medicine, Mayo Clinic. His clinical focus will include echocardiography and pulmonary vascular diseases.

Charles X. Kim, MD, is from Chicago, Illinois. He received dual BS degrees in cellular biology and chemistry from the University of Illinois, Urbana-Champaign, and his MD from the University of Chicago. He completed his residency in internal medicine at Northwestern University in Chicago. He is a fellow in cardiovascular diseases at Mayo School of Graduate Medical Education, College of Medicine, Mayo Clinic, and his areas of expertise are coronary care and interventional cardiology.

Matthew W. Martinez, MD, is from Wading River, New York. He attended Longwood University in Farmville, Virginia, and received his BS in biological sciences from Wright State University in Dayton, Ohio. He received his MD at Mayo Medical School and completed his residency in internal medicine at Mayo School of Graduate Medical Education, College of Medicine, Mayo Clinic. He is a fellow in cardiovascular diseases at Mayo School of Graduate Medical Education and an Instructor in Medicine, College of Medicine, Mayo Clinic. His area of expertise is advanced cardiac imaging in MRI, CT, echocardiography, and nuclear cardiology. His clinical interests include cardiomyopathies and cardiac assessment in athletes.

Brian P. Shapiro, MD, is from Miami, Florida. He received his undergraduate degree from the University of Florida in history, and his MD from the University of Miami. He completed his residency in internal medicine and a clinical investigator research fellowship (in heart failure) and he is currently a cardiovascular fellow at Mayo School of Graduate Medical Education, College of Medicine, Mayo Clinic, with expertise in imaging (MRI, CT, echocardiography, nuclear cardiology).

TABLE OF CONTENTS

ABBREVIATIONS

5-HIAA	5-Hydroxyindoleacetic acid
AAA	Abdominal aortic aneurysm
ACC	American College of Cardiology
ACE	Angiotensin-converting enzyme
ACS	Acute coronary syndrome
ACUITY	Acute Catheterization and Urgent Intervention Triage Strategy
ADMIRAL	Abciximab Before Direct Angioplasty and Stenting in Myocardial Infarction Regarding Acute and Long-Term Follow-up
AF	Atrial fibrillation
AFFIRM	Atrial Fibrillation Follow-up Investigation of Rhythm
AHA	American Heart Association
AMI	Acute myocardial infarction
ANP	Atrial natriuretic peptides
Ao	Aorta
AR	Aortic regurgitation
ARB	Angiotensin receptor blocker
ARDS	Acute respiratory distress syndrome
AS	Aortic stenosis
ASA	Aminosalicylic acid
ASD	Atrial septal defect
AV	Aortic valve
AVA	Aortic valve area
AVNRT	Atrioventricular node reentry tachycardia
AVR	Aortic valve replacement
AVRT	Atrioventricular reentrant tachycardia
BARI	Bypass Angioplasty Revascularization Investigation
BARI 2D	Bypass Angioplasty Revascularization 2—Diabetes
BENESTENT	Belgium Netherlands Stent Study Group
BID	Twice daily
BIV-ICD	Biventricular implantable cardioverter defibrillator
BMI	Body mass index
BNP	Brain natriuretic peptide
BP	Blood pressure
bpm	Beats per minute
BSA	Body surface area
CABG	Coronary artery bypass graft/Coronary artery bypass grafting
CAD	Coronary artery disease
CARE-HF	Cardiac Resynchronization in Heart Failure
CASS	Coronary Artery Surgery Study
CBC	Complete blood count
CCS	Canadian Cardiovascular Society
CCU	Critical care unit
CHF	Congestive heart failure
CK	Creatine kinase
CK-MB	Creatine kinase myocardial fraction
CNS	Central nervous system
CO	Cardiac output

COMPANION	Comparison of Medical Therapy, Pacing, and Defibrillation in Heart Failure
COPD	Chronic obstructive pulmonary disease
COURAGE	Clinical Outcomes Utilizing Revascularization and Aggressive Drug Evaluation
CPR	Cardiopulmonary resuscitation
CREDO	Clopidogrel For Reduction of Events During Observation
CRP	C-reactive protein
CRT	Cardiac resynchronization therapy
CS	Coronary sinus
CT	Computed tomography
CURE	Clopidogrel in Unstable Angina to Prevent Recurrent Events
CV	Cardiovascular
CVA	Cerebrovascular accident
DANAMI	Danish Multicenter Randomized Study on Fibrinolytic Therapy Versus Acute Coronary Angioplasty in Acute Myocardial Infarction
DC	Direct current
DES	Drug-eluting stent
DINAMIT	Defibrillator in Acute Myocardial Infarction Trial
DM	Diabetes mellitus
DOE	Dyspnea on exertion
E/A	E:A wave ratio
EBCT	Electron beam computed tomography
ECG	Electrocardiographic/Electrocardiogram/Electrocardiography
ECSS	European Cooperative Surgery Study
ED	Emergency department/Emergency room
EECP	Enhanced external counterpulsation
EF	Ejection fraction
EOA	Effective orifice area
EP	Electrophysiology
ERASER	Evaluation of ReoPro and Stenting to Eliminate Restenosis
ET-A	Endothelin-A
ET-B	Endothelin-B
FA	Femoral artery
FAA	Federal Aviation Administration
FDA	Food and Drug Administration
FDG	Fluorodeoxyglucose
FFV	Forward flow volume
FMD	Fibromuscular dysplasia
FREEDOM	Future Revascularization Evaluation in Patients with Diabetes
GISSI	Gruppo Italiano per lo Studio della Streptochinasi nell'Infarto Miocardico
GUSTO-I	Global Utilization of Streptokinase and Tissue Plasminogen Activator for Occluded Coronary Artery
Hgb	Hemoglobin
HCM	Hypertrophic cardiomyopathy/Hypertrophic obstructive cardiomyopathy
HCTZ	Hydrochlorothiazide
HDL	High-density lipoprotein
HIT	Heparin-induced thrombocytopenia
HR	Heart rate
HRA	High right atrium
HTN	Hypertension
ICD	Implantable cardioverter defibrillator
ICH	Intracerebral hemorrhage

ICU	Intensive care unit
IE	Infective endocarditis
INR	International normalization ratio
ISHLT	International Society for Heart and Lung Transplantation
IU	International units
IV	Intravenous
IVC	Inferior vena cava
IVUS	Intravascular ultrasound
JVD	Jugular venous distention
JVP	Jugular venous pressure
LA	Left atrium
LAD	Left anterior descending
LAO	Left anterior oblique
LBBB	Left bundle branch block
LCA	Left coronary artery
LCX	Left circumflex
LDL	Low-density lipoprotien
LIMA	Left internal mammary artery
Lp(a)	Lipoprotein a
LSB	Left sternal border
L-TGA	Levo transposition of the great arteries
LV	Left ventricle/Left ventricular
LVAD	Left ventricular assist device
LVEDP	Left ventricular end diastolic pressure
LVH	Left ventricular hypertrophy
LVOT	Left ventricular outflow tract
MACE	Major adverse cardiac event
MADIT-II	Multicenter Automatic Defibrillator Implantation Trial II
MASS	Medicine, Angioplasty, or Surgery Study
MCA	Middle cerebral artery
mCi	milli Curies
MELLITUS	Optimal Management of Multivessel Disease
MET	Metabolic equivalent
MI	Myocardial infarction
MIRACLE	Multicenter InSync Randomized Clinical Evaluation
MPI	Myocardial perfusion imaging
MR	Mitral regurgitation
MRI	Magnetic resonance imaging
MS	Mitral stenosis
MUGA	Multiple gated acquisition/Multigated image acquisition analysis
MUSTT	Multicenter Unsustained Tachycardia Trial
MV	Mixed venous
MVA	Mitral valve area
MVR	Mitral valve replacement
NCEP	National Cholesterol Education Panel
NO	Nitrous oxide/Nitric oxide
NOS	Nitric oxide synthetase
NPH	Neutral Protamine Hagedorn
NRAF	National Registry of Atrial Fibrillation
NSAID	Nonsteroidal anti-inflammatory medication
NSTEMI	Non-ST elevation myocardial infarction

NTG	Nitroglycerine
NYHA	New York Heart Association
OM	Obtuse marginal
PA	Pulmonary artery
PABV	Percutaneous aortic balloon valvulotomy
PAF	Paroxysmal atrial fibrillation
PAH	Pulmonary artery hypertension
PAI-1	Plasminogen activator inhibitor 1
PAP	Pulmonary artery pressure
PCI	Percutaneous coronary intervention
PCWP	Pulmonary capillary wedge pressure
PET	Positron emission tomography
PFO	Patent foramen ovale
PMBV	Percutaneous mitral balloon valvotomy
PTCA	Percutaneous transluminal coronary balloon angioplasty/Percutaneous transluminal coronary angioplasty
PVC	Premature ventricular contraction
QTc	Corrected QT interval
RA	Right atrium
RAO	Right anterior oblique
RCA	Right coronary artery
REACT	Rescue Angioplasty Versus Conservative Treatment or Repeat Thrombolysis
REM	Rapid eye movement sleep
RF	Regurgitant fraction
RV	Right ventricle/Right ventricular
RVOT	Right ventricular outflow tract
RVSP	Right ventricular systolic pressure
SCD-HeFT	Sudden Cardiac Death in Heart Failure Trial
SEM	Systolic ejection murmur
SEP	Systolic ejection period
SHOCK	Should We Emergently Revascularize Occluded Coronaries for Cardiogenic Shock
SIRIUS	Sirolimus-coated stent in treatment of de novo coronary artery lesions
SISR	Sirolimus Eluting Stents Versus Vascular Brachy Therapy for In-Stent Restenosis
SL NTG	Sublingual nitroglycerine
SR	Sarcoplasmic reticulum
STEMI	ST elevation myocardial infarction
SV	Stroke volume
SVC	Superior vena cava
SVT	Supraventricular Tachycardia
TD CO	Thermodilution cardiac output
TEE	Transesophageal echocardiogram/Transesophageal echocardiography
TGA	Transposition of the great arteries
TICM	Tachycardia-induced cardiomyopathy
TID	Three times daily
TIMI	Thrombolysis in myocardial infarction
TMET	Treadmill exercise test
TnI	Troponin I
TnT	Troponin T
tPA	Tissue plasminogen activator
TR	Tricuspid regurgitation
TTE	Transthoracic echocardiogram/Transthoracic echocardiography

TTP	Thrombotic thrombocytopenic purpura
TV	Total volume
TVI	Time-velocity integral
TVR	Tricuspid valve replacement
US	Ultrasound
VA	Veterans Administration
VANQWISH	Veterans Affairs Non-Q-Wave Infarction Strategies in Hospital
VF	Ventricular fibrillation
VLDL	Very low-density lipoprotein
VSD	Ventricular septal defect
VT	Ventricular tachycardia
vWF	von Willebrand factor
WBC	White blood cell count
XRT	Radiation therapy

MAYO CLINIC NORMAL BLOOD VALUES

Acid base balance

pH, venous	7.32–7.42
pCO_2, venous	41–51 torr
Std bicarbonate	21.3–24.8 mEq/L
pO_2, arterial	80–90 torr

Activated partial thromboplastin time   21–33 sec

Amiodarone   1.5–2.5 µg/mL (therapeutic range)
Desethylamiodarone   1.5–2.5 µg/mL (therapeutic range)

Angiotensin-converting enzyme   7.0–46.0 U/L

Atrial natriuretic factor   ≥2 M: 20–77 pg/mL

C-reactive protein, high sensitivity   ≤3 mg/L

Calcium, total
Male:
≥22 Y: 8.9–10.1 mg/dL
Female:
≥19 Y: 8.9–10.1 mg/dL

Catecholamines, fractionation

Norepinephrine	Supine: 70–750 pg/mL
	Standing: 200–1700 pg/mL
Epinephrine	Supine: 0–110 pg/mL
	Standing: 0–140 pg/mL
Dopamine	Supine: <30 pg/mL
	Standing: <30 pg/mL

Chemistry group

Sodium	135–145 mEq/L (same in children age 1 and older)
Potassium	3.6–4.8 mEq/L (higher in children age 1–16)
Calcium	8.9–10.1 mg/dL (higher in children age 1 and older)
Phosphorus	2.5–4.5 mg/dL (higher in children age 1 and older)
Protein, total	6.3–7.9 g/dL (same in children age 1 and older)
Glucose	70–100 mg/dL (same in children age 1 and older)
Alkaline phosphatase	Male:
	98–251 U/L (higher in children)
	Female:
	17 Y–23 Y: 114–312 U/L
	24 Y–45 Y: 81–213 U/L
	46 Y–50 Y: 84–218 U/L
	51 Y–55 Y: 90–234 U/L
	56 Y–60 Y: 99–257 U/L

	61 Y–65 Y:	108–282 U/L
	≥66 Y:	119–309 U/L
	(higher in children)	

AST (GOT)
Male:
12–31 U/L (higher in children)
Female:
≥14 Y: 12–31 U/L (higher in children)

Bilirubin, total	0.1–1.0 mg/dL (lower in children)
Bilirubin, direct	0–0.3 mg/dL
Uric acid	Male: 4.3–8.0 mg/dL
	Female: 2.3–6.0 mg/dL
Creatinine	Male: 0.9–1.4 mg/dL
	Female: 0.7–1.2 mg/dL
Albumin	3.5–5.0 g/dL (same in children age 1 and older)

Cholesterol

Total	Desirable:	<200 mg/dL
	Borderline high:	200–239 mg/dL
	High:	≥240 mg/dL
Low-density cholesterol (LDL)	Optimal:	<100 mg/dL
	Low Risk:	100–129 mg/dL
	Borderline high:	130–159 mg/dL
	High:	160–189 mg/dL
	Very high:	≥190 mg/dL
High-density cholesterol (HDL)	Low HDL:	<40 mg/dL
	Normal:	40–60 mg/dL
	Desirable:	>60 mg/dL

CK-MB

≤6.2 ng/mL

Cyclosporine

100–400 ng/mL

D-dimer

D-dimer, P	<301 ng/mL
D-dimer, P, manual	<250 µg/L

Digoxin

0.5–2.0 ng/mL

Hematology group (adult)

	Male	Female	Units
Hemoglobin	13.5–17.5	12.0–15.5	g/dL
Hematocrit	38.8–50.0	34.9–44.5	%
Erythrocytes	4.32–5.72	3.90–5.03	$\times 10^{12}$/L
MCV	81.2–95.1	81.6–98.3	fL
Leukocytes	3.5–10.5	3.5–10.5	$\times 10^9$/L
Neutrophils	1.7–7.0	1.7–7.0	$\times 10^9$/L
Lymphocytes	0.9–2.9	0.9–2.9	$\times 10^9$/L
Monocytes	0.3–0.9	0.3–0.9	$\times 10^9$/L
Eosinophils	0.05–0.50	0.05–0.50	$\times 10^9$/L
Basophils	0–0.3	0–0.3	$\times 10^9$/L
Platelet count	150–450	150–450	$\times 10^9$/L

Homocysteine
    Total   ≤13 µmol/L

Lidocaine   2–5 µg/mL (therapeutic range)

Metanephrine, fractionated, free
    Normetanephrine, free   <0.90 nmol/L
    Metanephrine, free   <0.50 nmol/L

Mexiletine   0.75–2.00 µg/mL (therapeutic range)

Procainamide
    Procainamide   4–8 µg/mL (therapeutic range)
    N-Acetyl procainamide   <30 µg/mL (therapeutic range)
    Procainamide + NAPA   ≤30 µg/mL (therapeutic range)

Propafenone   0.5–2.0 µg/mL (therapeutic range)

Propranolol   50–100 ng/mL (therapeutic range)

Prothrombin time   8.4–12.0 sec
    INR   INR = International Normalized Ratio for monitoring stable warfarin
                            anticoagulation
                   Suggested INR therapeutic ranges*

	Intensity	
Standard	Higher**	
2.0–3.0	2.5–3.5	

                   *Target INR should be individualized.
                   Occasionally, INR range 3.0–4.5 may be appropriate.
                   **Higher intensity INR: Mechanical heart valve, etc.

Quinidine   2.0–5.0 µg/mL (therapeutic range)

Renin
    Sodium depleted upright   18–39 Y: Mean = 10.8
                                     Range = 2.9–24.0 ng/mL/h
                         ≥40 Y: Mean = 5.9
                                     Range = 2.9–10.9 ng/mL/h
    Sodium replete upright   18–39 Y: Mean = 1.9
                                     Range = ≤0.6–4.3 ng/mL/h
                         ≥40 Y: Mean = 1.0
                                     Range = <0.6–3.0 ng/mL/h

Sedimentation rate   <u>Male:</u>   0–22 mm/1h
                        <u>Female:</u>   0–29 mm/1h

Sirolimus   4.0–20.0 ng/mL

Thyroid-stimulating hormone (sTSH)   0.30–5.0 mIU/L

Thyroxine, total

<u>Male</u>:   5.0–12.5 μg/dL
<u>Female</u>:   5.0–12.5 μg/dL

Triiodothyronine (T3)   80–180 ng/dL

Troponin T   ≤0.03 ng/mL

Mayo Clinic Cardiology

Board Review Questions and Answers

SECTION I

Cardiac Electrophysiology

T. Jared Bunch, MD

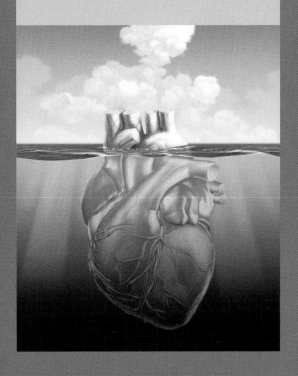

Questions

1. A 16-year-old female was admitted to the coronary care unit after an aborted sudden cardiac death. The patient was awakened to answer a telephone call and suddenly collapsed. The fall was witnessed and a rapid 911 call allowed the paramedics to arrive within 5 minutes. The patient was in VF and was successfully defibrillated with one shock. She remained comatose and was intubated and transported to the hospital.

   On physical exam she was intubated and withdrew to painful stimuli. Her pupils were dilated, but reactive to light symmetrically. Her past medical history is remarkable for 3 brief fainting episodes. She was not using any prescription medication. The mother denied knowledge of substance abuse. Her family history is notable for a sister who died suddenly at the age of 20.

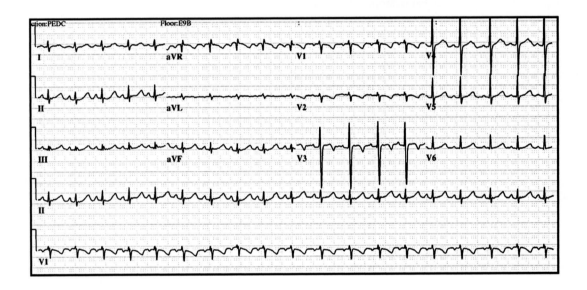

   What is the most likely diagnosis at this time?

   a. HCM
   b. Brugada syndrome
   c. Idiopathic VF
   d. RVOT tachycardia
   e. Long QT syndrome

2. Based upon the above patient presentation what subtype of long QT syndrome is expected?

   a. Long QT syndrome 1
   b. Long QT syndrome 2
   c. Long QT syndrome 3
   d. Jervell and Lange-Nielsen syndrome
   e. Timothy syndrome

Answers to this section start on page 35.

3. Within the first 24 hours of hospitalization the patient recovers quickly until there are no apparent neurologic deficits. She provides no additional history and reports no symptoms prior to the cardiac arrest. What is the next step in her management?

    a. Left cardiac sympathetic denervation
    b. Dual-chamber permanent pacemaker
    c. Amiodarone
    d. Single-chamber ICD
    e. Atenolol

4. What is the most common mechanism involved in clinically important cardiac arrhythmias?

    a. Triggered activity
    b. Abnormal automaticity
    c. Reentry
    d. Early afterdepolarizations
    e. Parasystole

5. Torsades de pointes is characterized by all of the following **except:**

    a. Results from triggered activity (early afterdepolarizations) that occurs during phase 2 or 3 of the cardiac action potential
    b. Prolonged QT interval
    c. Exacerbation by bradycardia with short-long coupling intervals
    d. Polymorphic VT
    e. Often provoked during amiodarone administration

6. Which one of the following currents is responsible for maintaining stable resting membrane potential in the atrial and ventricular cells?

    a. I_f
    b. I_{Na}
    c. I_{Kl}
    d. I_K
    e. I_{Ca}

7. The I_{KATP} is a potassium channel that is inhibited by physiologic intracellular concentrations of ATP. How is this channel activated?

    a. A consequence of I_f activation that enhances pacemaker activity
    b. Physical opening of the channel pore by the N-terminal portion of the channel
    c. Chemical ligand binding in response to depletion of ATP from ischemia
    d. Conformational changes in channel structure
    e. The channel is only inhibitory and is not activated

8. The sinus node is predominantly characterized by depolarization in which phase of the action potential?

    a. Phase 0
    b. Phase 1
    c. Phase 2
    d. Phase 3
    e. Phase 4

9. A 26-year-old man is referred to the arrhythmia clinic for evaluation of exercise-induced palpitations. He denies presyncope or syncope during these episodes. He had no other significant medical history. He has no family history of cardiomyopathy, arrhythmia, or sudden death. An ECG, echocardiogram, and 24 hour ambulatory Holter monitor were all within normal limits.

During TMET, the wide complex tachycardia was induced. The 12 lead ECG is shown. The patient reports palpitations without lightheadedness.

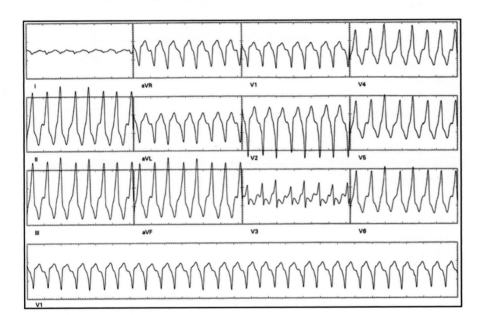

ECG provided by Dr. John D. Day

What is the most likely clinical diagnosis?

a. RVOT tachycardia
b. Wolff-Parkinson-White syndrome
c. Atrial flutter with rapid ventricular response
d. Sinus tachycardia with aberrancy
e. Scar-mediated VT

10. What treatment should be considered for this patient?

a. ICD
b. Beta blocker
c. Digoxin
d. Referral for catheter ablation of a ventricular arrhythmogenic focus
e. Referral for catheter ablation of the caval-tricuspid isthmus

11. Which one of the following antiarrhythmic agents does **not** prolong the QT interval?

a. Quinidine
b. Lidocaine
c. Sotalol
d. Procainamide
e. Ibutilide

12. Which one of the following antiarrhythmic agents has the **least** effect on slowing conduction through the AV node?

    a. Calcium channel blockers
    b. Beta blockers
    c. Amiodarone
    d. Lidocaine
    e. Sotalol

13. Which of the following antiarrhythmic agents may promote AF?

    a. Adenosine
    b. Quinidine
    c. Propafenone
    d. Amiodarone
    e. Atenolol

14. Which one of the following antiarrhythmic agents is **least** likely to cause torsades de pointes?

    a. Quinidine
    b. Procainamide
    c. Flecainide
    d. Ibutilide
    e. Sotalol

15. All of the following statements regarding the AV node are true **except:**

    a. Conduction through the node displays decremental behavior
    b. It is positioned in the subendocardium at the base of the triangle of Koch
    c. It is composed of nodal cells and transitional cells
    d. It is a right atrial structure

16. In which of the following tissues is the upstroke of the action potential generated by ingoing calcium currents?

    a. Atrial
    b. AV node
    c. His-Purkinje
    d. Ventricular

17. Conduction velocity is most rapid in which tissue?

    a. Atrial
    b. AV node
    c. His-Purkinje
    d. Ventricular

18. Repolarization of the myocardial cells is determined mostly by which current?

    a. Outgoing sodium
    b. Ingoing calcium
    c. Outgoing potassium
    d. Ingoing chloride
    e. Ingoing sodium

19. All of the following statements regarding AV nodal cells are true **except:**

   a. The resting membrane potential is typically −80 to −90 mV
   b. The activation threshold ranges between −30 and −40 mV
   c. The upstroke of the action potential is carried by inward calcium current
   d. Conduction in the AV node proceeds at a velocity of 0.01 to 0.1 m/sec

20. Vagal stimulation in each of the following tissue types changes the action potential duration **except** in which cardiac structure?

   a. AV node
   b. His-Purkinje system
   c. Ventricular myocardium
   d. Atrial myocardium

21. Early afterdepolarizations are favored by:

   a. High potassium concentrations
   b. Type III antiarrhythmic drugs
   c. Fast underlying HR
   d. Increased magnesium concentrations

22. The underlying arrhythmia mechanism most likely present in digitalis toxicity is:

   a. Reentry
   b. Delayed afterdepolarizations
   c. Enhanced automaticity
   d. Early afterdepolarizations

23. Which of the following contain the normal A–H and H–V intervals?

   a. 40–80 msec, 35–60 msec
   b. 60–120 msec, 35–60 msec
   c. 60–120 msec, 25–50 msec
   d. 60–100 msec, 60–80 msec

24. Patients with the Wolff-Parkinson-White syndrome typically show each of the following features **except:**

   a. A wide QRS complex during normal sinus rhythm
   b. A narrow complex SVT
   c. A delta wave on the surface QRS
   d. A long H–V interval on the His-bundle recording

25. Prerequisite conditions of the reentrant arrhythmia include all of the following **except:**

   a. Two functionally distinct conducting pathways
   b. An anatomical obstacle around which the impulse reenters
   c. Unidirectional block in one pathway
   d. Slow conduction via one pathway with return via the second

26. Antidromic reciprocating tachycardia in a patient with Wolff-Parkinson-White refers to:

    a. AV conduction proceeding via the normal AV conduction system with return via the accessory pathway
    b. AV conduction via the accessory pathway with return via the normal ventriculoatrial conduction system
    c. AVNRT with additional conduction via the accessory pathway
    d. None of the above

27. A 24-year-old female presents with recurrent palpitations. There is no pattern to what triggers the arrhythmia, but she is typically able to terminate it by performing a Valsalva-type maneuver. She has no significant past medical history. She denies alcohol or illicit drug use. There is no family history of arrhythmia, sudden death, or cardiomyopathy. The baseline ECG and echocardiogram are normal. The following ECG was obtained when the patient presented to the ED with persistent palpitations.

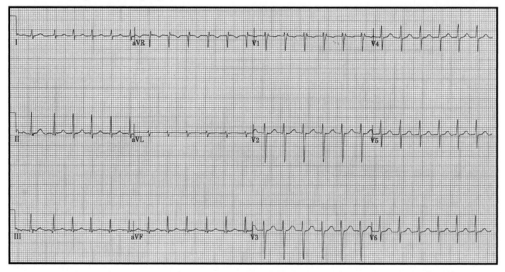

    What is the most likely diagnosis based upon the clinical history and ECG?

    a. Antidromic reciprocating tachycardia
    b. Atrial flutter with rapid ventricular response
    c. Inappropriate sinus tachycardia
    d. AVNRT
    e. His-Purkinje extrasystoles

28. Patients with the tachycardia in Question 27 usually have:

    a. Dual AV nodal physiology
    b. A concealed accessory pathway
    c. Retrograde atrial activation spreading from the free wall of the AV groove to the septum
    d. A wide QRS complex during tachycardia that narrows at lower HR
    e. Structural heart disease

29. The most common mechanism of arrhythmia in sustained VT is:

    a. Sympathetically facilitated enhanced automaticity
    b. Reentry involving ventricular myocardium
    c. Triggered automaticity arising from early afterdepolarizations
    d. Reflection of propagated impulses

30. A 54-year-old man is referred to you due to an enlarged cardiac silhouette discovered on routine chest X-ray as part of his employment physical exam. He reports no known past medical history. Although he denies symptoms of overt heart failure, he states that he tends to become short of breath with strenuous activity—a symptom that he felt was due to lack of exercise.

    On physical examination he has a displaced apical impulse and a third heart sound. An ECG shows sinus rhythm with a LBBB. An echocardiogram discloses global LV dysfunction with an EF of 25% and mild functional mitral valve regurgitation. Coronary angiography is normal. A 24-hour Holter monitor shows 35,000 PVCs and 85 runs of nonsustained VT, 3 to 9 beats in duration.

    What is the next appropriate test?

    a. EP study
    b. RV biopsy
    c. Serum ferritin
    d. Signal average ECG
    e. No further testing is required; schedule the patient to receive an ICD

31. All of the following clinical characteristics are associated with cardiogenic syncope and should prompt referral for an invasive EP study **except:**

    a. Age >65 years
    b. History of CHF
    c. Bundle branch block
    d. History of ventricular arrhythmias
    e. Recurrent unexplained falls in a 70-year-old patient

32. A 38-year-old man underwent radiofrequency ablation in the RA for medically refractive symptomatic atrial tachycardia. He was dismissed on aspirin 325 mg/day. Six days following the procedure he developed left-sided persistent chest pain and mild dyspnea. His exam is notable only for tachycardia with a HR of 110 bpm. An ECG discloses sinus tachycardia. What is the next most appropriate test to request?

    a. Echocardiogram
    b. CT scan
    c. Coronary angiography
    d. Arterial blood gas, D-Dimer
    e. Ventilation perfusion scan

33. All the following are true about head-up tilt testing **except:**

    a. The test should be performed at 60 to 80 degrees
    b. Sensitivity and specificity of the test are approximately 80%
    c. A vasodepressor response occurs most often in patients younger than 60
    d. In patients without structural heart disease, it can provide a diagnosis in approximately 60% of them
    e. A cardioinhibitory response tends to be infrequent in older patients

34. The arrhythmic substrate **least** likely to be definitely ruled out with a negative EP study is:

    a. Sinus node dysfunction
    b. Severe His-Purkinje disease
    c. Accessory bypass tract
    d. VT in a patient with ischemic cardiomyopathy
    e. AVNRT

35. An active 78-year-old woman with recurrent syncope has an EP study. With atrial pacing at 150 bpm for 30 sec, a 7-sec atrial pause occurs when the pacing ceases. Her baseline examination and echocardiogram are all within normal limits. ECG shows sinus rhythm with first degree AV block. What is the next appropriate management step?

    a. Implant a VVI single-chamber permanent pacemaker

    b. Implant a dual-chamber ICD

    c. Implant a DDDR dual-chamber rate responsive pacemaker

    d. Implant an AAI single-chamber permanent pacemaker

    e. Medical management with atropine

36. Programmed ventricular stimulation is an important tool in risk assessment in patients with CAD for which of the following patient subsets?

    a. An EF of 30% to 35% and the presence of nonsustained VT

    b. An EF of 35% to 40% and the presence of nonsustained VT

    c. An EF of 30% to 35% and an abnormal signal averaged ECG

    d. An EF of 35% to 40% and a history of cardiac arrest

37. All of the following examples are considered positive responses to a drug in a patient with an expected cardiac channelopathy **except:**

    a. A decreased QT interval with lidocaine in a patient suspected to have long QT3

    b. An increased QT interval with epinephrine in a patient suspected to have long QT1

    c. Abnormal ST-T changes in leads V1–V2 with procainamide in a patient suspected to have Brugada syndrome

    d. An increased QT interval with notched T waves with epinephrine in a patient suspected to have long QT2

    e. An increased QT interval with ajmaline in a patient suspected to have long QT4

38. Acute success rates for ablation of accessory pathways could be stated as:

    a. 50% to 70%

    b. 75%

    c. 85%

    d. 90% to 95%

    e. Virtually 100%

39. A 69-year-old woman presents to the ED with palpitations, lightheadedness, and no other symptoms. She denies syncope. She had no additional past medical history. The following rhythm strip is obtained. Her BP is 110/70 mmHg, she is mildly uncomfortable with her palpitations, but otherwise her exam is within normal limits.

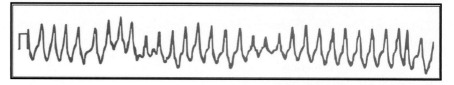

Telemetry strip provided by Dr. Paul A. Friedman

What is the next step in her acute and then chronic management?

   a. Adenosine and then radiofrequency ablation
   b. Lidocaine and then coronary angiogram and EP testing
   c. DC cardioversion and then ICD implantation without further testing
   d. Procainamide and then radiofrequency ablation
   e. Procainamide and then amiodarone

40. The following findings are considered positive results during EP testing **except:**

   a. A >3 sec pause, a fall in BP >50 mmHg with symptoms, or syncope with carotid sinus massage
   b. A >3 sec asystole, hypotension <60 mmHg, syncope with head up tilt
   c. Sinus node recovery time >2 sec
   d. A corrected sinus node recovery time >525 sec
   e. An H–V interval 55 to 75 msec

41. A patient has a loss of function mutation in KCNQ1. This patient is most likely to have events triggered by:

   a. Swimming
   b. Doorbells
   c. The postpartum period
   d. Sleeping

42. Efforts to identify patients with concealed long QT syndrome (genotype positive and resting ECG negative) are improved by which testing and response?

   a. Exercise testing with failure to lengthen the QT interval appropriately
   b. Paradoxical lengthening of the QT interval with low-dose epinephrine infusion
   c. EP testing with induction of polymorphic VT with ventricular extra stimuli
   d. No further testing is required in these patients unless they experience syncope

43. Which of the following sports can be played in patients with long QT syndrome?

   a. Golf
   b. Cricket
   c. Bowling
   d. Billiards
   e. All of the above

44. Each of the following statements about Romano-Ward syndrome is true, **except:**

   a. It is a heterogeneous disorder involving mutations in different ion channels
   b. It is inherited as an autosomal recessive disorder
   c. It is associated with sudden cardiac death in young patients
   d. It is not associated with congenital deafness
   e. It is more frequent than the Jervell and Lange-Nielsen syndrome

45. Treatments of drug-induced prolongation of QT interval and torsades de pointes include all of the following **except:**

    a. Withdrawal of the offending agent
    b. Correction of electrolyte and acid-base disturbance
    c. IV magnesium
    d. IV isoproterenol infusion or temporary pacing
    e. IV beta blocker

46. A 23-year-old male with no known medical history suddenly collapsed while playing a vigorous game of ultimate Frisbee. His friends immediately started CPR and called 911. The paramedics arrived within 5 minutes and found him in VF. He was defibrillated successfully with one shock with return of spontaneous circulation. He was transported to the hospital for subsequent care.

    The following ECG was obtained upon arrival to the hospital:

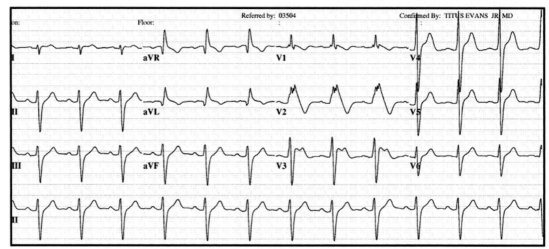

    What is the most likely diagnosis?

    a. Short QT syndrome
    b. Long QT syndrome
    c. Brugada syndrome
    d. Catecholaminergic polymorphic VT
    e. Timothy syndrome

47. The patient in Question 46 makes a complete neurologic recovery. An echocardiogram is within normal limits. What is the next appropriate step in management?

    a. Start a beta blocker and restrict him from participation in competitive sports
    b. EP testing with administration of a class 1 antiarrhythmic (flecainide and procainamide) to determine risk of sudden death
    c. Exercise testing to assess if his QT shortens appropriately
    d. Implant an ICD
    e. Implant a dual-chamber pacemaker

48. The channelopathy underlying the clinical presentation in the patient in Question 46 is:

   a. Gain of function in the sodium channel
   b. Loss of function in the sodium channel
   c. Gain of function in the potassium channel
   d. Loss of function in the potassium channel
   e. Gain of function in the calcium channel

49. All of the following medications are known to prolong the QT interval and potentially cause torsades de pointes **except:**

   a. Amiodarone
   b. Erythromycin
   c. Haloperidol
   d. Sotalol
   e. None of the above

50. Which of the following disorders results from alterations of intracellular calcium release from the sacroplasmic reticulum?

   a. Catecholaminergic polymorphic VT
   b. Short QT syndrome
   c. Long QT syndrome
   d. Andersen-Tawil syndrome
   e. Romano-Ward syndrome

51. Symptomatic patients diagnosed with mutations in the RyR2-encoded cardiac ryanodine receptor should receive what first line therapy?

   a. Calcium channel blocker
   b. Beta blocker
   c. ICD
   d. Amiodarone
   e. Surgical myectomy

52. A 16-year-old male presents to you after a screening ECG was performed for a sports physical that demonstrated pre-excitation. What is the next step in his evaluation?

   a. EP testing and ablation of the accessory pathway
   b. Echocardiogram
   c. No further evaluation is required
   d. Empiric treatment with a beta blocker
   e. None of the above

53. A common form of SVT in teenagers is:

   a. Atrial ectopic tachycardia
   b. Atrial flutter
   c. Junctional ectopic tachycardia
   d. AVNRT
   e. Familial AF

54. In the pediatric population, which of the following cardiac diseases is associated with second degree AV block?

    a. Tumor (rhabdomyoma)
    b. Myopathy (Duchenne muscular dystrophy)
    c. Immunologic (maternal systemic lupus erythematosus)
    d. Long QT syndrome
    e. All of the above

55. A 17-year-old female presents for a routine gynecologic appointment. She reports no complaints. She has no known medical history other than a "low HR" shortly after she was born. She is not using any medications and denies illicit drug use. Her examination was within normal limits with exception of a low pulse rate at 36 bpm. The following ECG was obtained.

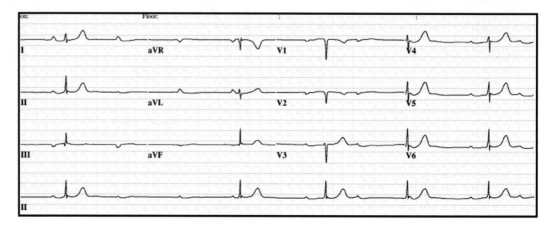

What is the most likely diagnosis?

    a. Third degree AV block
    b. Second degree AV block
    c. Ectopic atrial tachycardia with variable AV conduction
    d. Accelerated junction tachycardia with variable atrial conduction
    e. AVNRT

56. An echocardiogram was normal in the patient outlined in Question 55. What is the most common cause of her rhythm abnormality?

    a. Medications
    b. Duchenne muscular dystrophy
    c. Maternal systemic lupus erythematosus
    d. L-TGA
    e. Kearns-Sayre syndrome

57. What is the next step in the evaluation of the patient in Question 55?

    a. Holter monitor
    b. Reassurance and repeat ECG in 6 months
    c. Exercise testing to assess for myocardial ischemia
    d. Genetic testing of the patient and her first degree relatives
    e. Muscle biopsy

58. The following rhythm strip was recorded during Holter monitoring. She reported no symptoms in her diary.

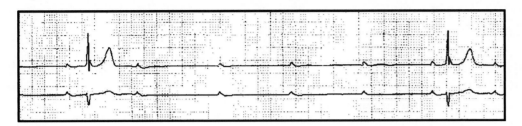

What is the next step in her care?

a. ICD

b. Implantable loop recorder

c. Reassurance and return in 6 months for repeat Holter monitoring and clinical evaluation

d. Dual-chamber permanent pacemaker implantation

e. Single-chamber permanent pacemaker implantation

59. All of the following are reasons to consider implanting a permanent pacemaker in a patient with congenital third degree AV block **except:**

a. Declining exercise performance

b. Junctional instability or wide QRS escape rhythm

c. Progressive cardiomyopathy with declining ventricular performance

d. QT prolongation

e. Persistent third degree AV block after isoproterenol infusion

60. Typical mechanisms associated with the initiation and maintenance of AF include all of the following **except:**

a. Substrate abnormalities that permit and promote wavelet reentry

b. Autonomic nervous system

c. Focal rapidly discharging triggers

d. Dual AV node physiology

61. Risk factors associated with AF include all of the following **except:**

a. HTN

b. Sick sinus syndrome

c. Obstructive sleep apnea

d. Wolff-Parkinson-White syndrome

e. None of the above

62. The major finding of the AFFIRM trial was which of the following?

a. Rhythm control patients were more likely to live longer and experience an improved quality of life

b. Rate control patients were less likely to develop heart failure

c. Patients >65 years of age assigned to rhythm control were likely to be in sinus rhythm

d. Patients <65 years of age assigned to rate control were more likely to be in sinus rhythm

e. Rhythm control patients were less likely to develop heart failure

63. AFFIRM trial type patients that are placed on an antiarrhythmic agent and are maintained in sinus rhythm can stop their anticoagulation. True or false?

   a. True
   b. False

64. Risk factors for stroke in patients with AF include all of the following **except:**

   a. Age >75 years
   b. Dyslipidemia
   c. HTN
   d. Heart failure
   e. Stroke or transient ischemic attack

65. Adequate rate control in a patient with AF is defined as:

   a. Resting HR < 80, maximal HR < 110 during a 6-minute walk
   b. Resting HR < 60, maximal HR < 110 during a 6-minute walk
   c. Resting HR < 80, maximal HR < 140 during a 6-minute walk
   d. Resting HR < 60, maximal HR < 140 during a 6-minute walk
   e. Resting HR < 100, maximal HR < 140 during a 6-minute walk

66. In patients with heart failure, the following antiarrhythmic drug options are acceptable:

   a. Amiodarone
   b. Flecainide
   c. Dofetilide
   d. Both a and c
   e. All of the above

67. On the ECG shown below, all of the following are present **except:**

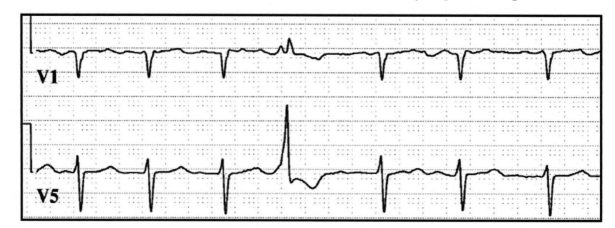

   a. AF
   b. PVC
   c. Ashman phenomenon
   d. None of the above

68. A 42-year-old man walks into the ED complaining of dizziness and the sensation of a racing heart. He takes no medications and has a systolic BP of 100 mmHg. An ECG is obtained and shown below. Which of the following medications would be an appropriate initial therapy?

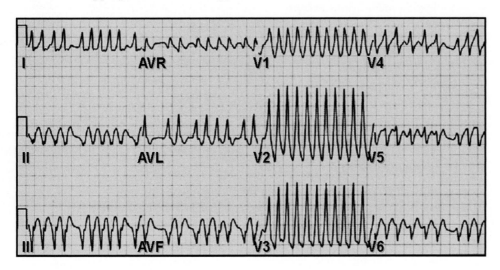

ECG provided by Dr. Paul A. Friedman

    a. Lidocaine
    b. Adenosine
    c. Metoprolol
    d. Procainamide
    e. Diltiazem

69. A 56-year-old male with HTN presented with palpitations and dyspnea with exertion. He is unsure when the symptoms started, but feels he has had a gradual decline over a one week period. He takes HCTZ for his HTN. He has no other known medical history. His systolic BP is 170 mmHg and the diastolic pressure is 80 mmHg. An ECG reveals AF with a rapid ventricular rate at 120 bpm.

All of the following are acceptable options in his subsequent care **except:**

    a. Initiate anticoagulation, add a rate control medication, and return for cardioversion in 3 weeks
    b. Initiate anticoagulation, perform a TEE, and, if negative for an intracardiac thrombus, proceed with DC cardioversion
    c. Initiate anticoagulation, start amiodarone
    d. Initiate anticoagulation, add a rate control medication, and aggressively improve his BP treatment

70. PAF is associated with a decreased risk of stroke compared with chronic AF. True or false?

    a. True
    b. False

71. A 56-year-old man presents with an 8-day history of palpitations. He has known PAF and takes warfarin. His INR levels have been consistently therapeutic. His systolic BP is 128 mmHg. His exam is normal. An ECG shows AF with rapid ventricular rate of 115 bpm. It is appropriate to initiate therapy with all the following medications **except:**

    a. Digoxin
    b. Diltiazem
    c. Procainamide
    d. Metoprolol

72. A relatively healthy 60-year-old patient presents with persistent PAF despite, first, a trial of propafenone, and now amiodarone. All of the following approaches are appropriate **except:**

    a. Left atrial ablation to isolate the pulmonary veins
    b. AV node ablation with implantation of a permanent pacemaker
    c. Rate control only if relatively asymptomatic during the episodes of AF
    d. Investigate for obstructive sleep apnea and treat if present
    e. None of the above

73. Radiofrequency catheter ablation of AF is characterized by all of the following **except:**

    a. The approach is more successful in patients with PAF in comparison to chronic AF
    b. Risks include pulmonary vein stenosis, cardiac perforation, atrial esophageal fistula formation, and stroke
    c. In the majority of patients, the procedure is successful in restoring sinus rhythm and improving quality of life
    d. Anticoagulation can be stopped in these patients after 3 months if they remain in sinus rhythm

74. Atrial flutter is characterized by which of the following:

    a. It accounts for 10% of patients presenting with SVT
    b. It is 2.5 times more common in men than women
    c. Overall mortality is similar in comparison to patients with AF
    d. Intra-atrial macroreentrant tachycardia involving a critical slow conduction zone
    e. All of the above

75. A 45-year-old male with no known cardiac history presents to the ED with palpitations, dyspnea, and mild chest discomfort. An ECG is obtained as shown. Due to respiratory distress and mild hypotension, the patient underwent DC cardioversion, which was successful in restoring his rhythm to sinus and alleviating his symptoms. He reports frequent episodes of palpitations with associated dyspnea, although less severe than what prompted his ED presentation.

An echocardiogram is normal. The ECG is shown below:

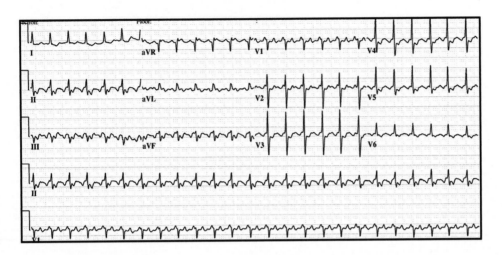

All of the following are reasonable pharmacologic approaches for his long-term care **except:**

a. Flecainide with metoprolol
b. Flecainide with diltiazem
c. Flecainide
d. Metoprolol
e. Dofetilide

76. All of the following are contraindications for use of Ibutilide to chemically terminate atrial flutter with rapid ventricular rates **except:**

a. A prolonged QT interval
b. A history of polymorphic VT with class 1 or 3 antiarrhythmic drugs
c. Severe hypokalemia
d. Hemodynamic instability
e. Structural heart disease

77. All of the following are factors that are associated with atrial flutter **except:**

a. HTN
b. Valvular heart disease
c. Prior cardiac surgery
d. Pericardial disease
e. Sarcoidosis

78. Which of the following summarizes the best approach for anticoagulation in a patient with persistent cavo-tricuspid isthmus dependent atrial flutter?

a. Aspirin 325 mg daily
b. Plavix 75 mg daily
c. Warfarin therapy with a goal INR of 2.0 to 3.0 when risk factors for thromboembolic events are present
d. Aspirin 81 mg daily and warfarin therapy with a goal INR of 2.0 to 3.0 when risk factors for thromboembolic events are present
e. Anticoagulation is not necessary in patients with flutters that originate from the RA since they are not associated the a high risk of arterial thromboembolism

79. The following ECG is suggestive of which type of atrial flutter?

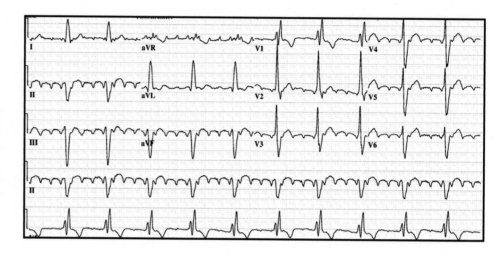

    a. Cavotricuspid isthmus-dependent counterclockwise atrial flutter
    b. Cavotricuspid isthmus-dependent clockwise atrial flutter
    c. Left atrial flutter along a surgical scar
    d. Left atrial flutter along the mitral annulus

80. A clinical history of a gradual onset of palpitations that become more rapid over time favors which diagnosis?

    a. AVNRT
    b. AVRT
    c. Atrial tachycardia
    d. AF

81. A useful general approach for the assessment of a supraventricular arrhythmias includes all of the following **except:**

    a. AVNRT: short RP tachycardia with P waves seen within or just after the QRS complex
    b. AVRT: short RP tachycardia with P waves 110 msec or more after the QRS complex
    c. Atrial tachycardia: long RP tachycardia
    d. AVNRT: termination with a P wave
    e. Atrial tachycardia: P-wave variation with subsequent beats during the tachycardia acceleration (warm up)

82. Which of the following situations can result in SVT with a wide QRS in the absence of a preexisting or rate-related bundle branch block?

    a. Orthodromic AVRT
    b. Antidromic AVRT
    c. Atypical AVNRT
    d. Typical AVNRT

83. An 18-year-old male presents to his primary care provider with a complaint of episodic palpitations that tend to start abruptly. There is not a consistent triggering event. After these episodes, he often senses the urge to micturate. The following ECG was obtained.

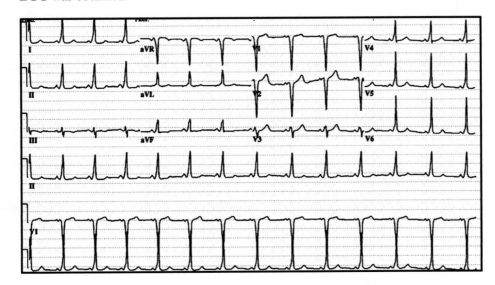

The most likely diagnosis based upon the clinical symptoms and ECG is:

a. AVNRT
b. AVRT
c. Atrial tachycardia
d. PAF
e. Paroxysmal atrial flutter

84. All of the following are characteristics of atrial tachycardia **except:**

a. Long RP tachycardia associated with exertion
b. Incessant atrial tachycardia associated with tachycardia-related cardiomyopathy
c. May appear to be inappropriate sinus tachycardia
d. Valsalva-like maneuvers terminate the tachycardia

85. Which of the following characteristics are associated with the permanent form of junction reciprocating tachycardia?

a. Mild tachycardia with rates from 100 to 130 bpm
b. Inverted P waves in II, III, AVF
c. Dilated cardiomyopathy
d. All of the above
e. None of the above

86. It is an acceptable approach to treat a tachycardia associated with QRS morphologic variation with an AV nodal blocking agent if there is proper hemodynamic monitoring. True or false?

a. True
b. False

87. Where is the most likely site of the accessory pathway based upon the following ECG?

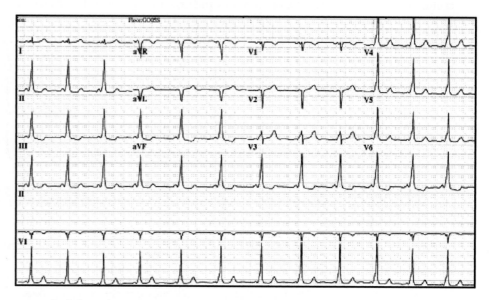

    a. Left lateral
    b. Left posterior/septal
    c. Right posterior/septal
    d. Right lateral/anterior

88. A 21-year-old female was referred for an EP study due to recurrent palpitations that gradually increased in frequency and duration. The following intracardiac electrograms were obtained during the study when the patient spontaneously developed a tachyarrhythmia.

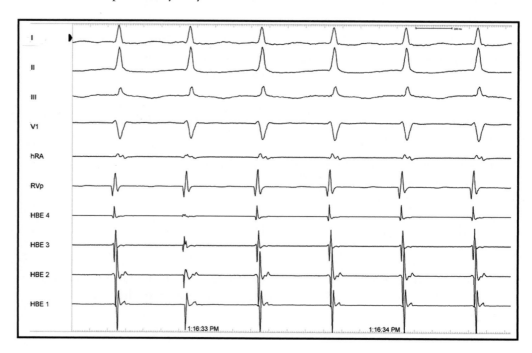

The arrhythmia present is best characterized as:

a. VT
b. AF
c. Long RP atrial tachycardia
d. Short RP atrial tachycardia
e. Atrial flutter

89. What is the most likely arrhythmia present in this patient?

a. Antidromic reciprocating tachycardia
b. Atrial flutter with rapid ventricular response
c. VT
d. AVNRT
e. AF with rapid ventricular response

90. A 62-year-old female presents to the ED with a 2-hour history of severe chest pain, dyspnea, and diaphoresis. An initial ECG shows ST elevation in leads V2–V6. She proceeds immediately to coronary angiography where a 100% proximal LAD artery stenosis is discovered. The lesion is successfully opened with angioplasty followed by stent implantation, with resultant normal TIMI flow.

An echocardiogram shows a LV EF of 30% with regional wall motion abnormalities along the anterior and lateral walls. In hospital telemetry reveals frequent PVCs and infrequent episodes on nonsustained VT (3–5 beats). What is the next step in her care?

a. Medical therapy and implantation of an ICD
b. Medical therapy and implantation of an ICD if VT is induced
c. Medical therapy and implantation of an ICD if a signal averaged ECG is abnormal
d. Medical therapy and defer implantation of an ICD
e. Medical therapy and refer for radiofrequency ablation of the VT

91. A 32-year-old male is referred to you by his primary care provider after an episode of syncope. The patient was briskly walking with friends when he suddenly passed out with recovery after falling to the ground. The patient takes no medication and does not use illicit drugs. A family history is notable for a father who died suddenly while shoveling snow at the age of 45. The physical examination is consistent with a healthy male with no distinct abnormalities. His ECG is displayed on the next page. An echocardiogram shows mild-to-moderate RV enlargement with a mild reduction in systolic function.

91. (continued)

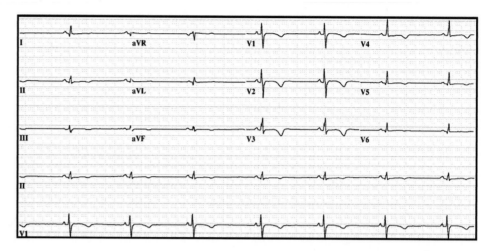

The history, examination, and tests are most suggestive of what disease process?

   a. Arrhythmogenic RV dysplasia
   b. RVOT tachycardia
   c. HCM
   d. Long QT syndrome
   e. Vasovagal syncope

92. What is the next step in the evaluation and care of the patient in Question 91?

   a. Signal-average ECG
   b. Exercise testing
   c. Radiofrequency ablation
   d. ICD
   e. Event monitor to look for occult ventricular arrhythmias

93. A 14-year-old male presents for what is described as seizure-like activity with participation in athletics. The patient's parents describe an episode that occurred while playing soccer in which he suddenly collapsed with what appeared to be tonic-clonic seizure activity and loss of urine. Outside of these discrete episodes the patient is otherwise healthy, takes no medications, and denies illicit drug use. There is no family history of arrhythmia, CV disease, or sudden death. What is the next step in his care?

   a. Referral to a neurologist for an EEG
   b. Empiric treatment with an antiepileptic medication
   c. ECG and additional testing if necessary for long QT syndrome
   d. Beta blockade and exercise restrictions
   e. EP test

94. A 62-year-old male presents with gradual onset fatigue, DOE, and lower extremity edema. He also reports intermittent palpitations with presyncope that occur 1 to 2 times a month and last 2 to 4 minutes. He has a history of CAD and underwent three-vessel coronary artery bypass surgery 10 years ago.

   His examination is remarkable for a JVP of approximately 10 mmHg, an S3 gallop and displaced apical impulse, crackles in the base of the lungs bilaterally, and 1+ pedal edema bilaterally.

An ECG shows sinus rhythm with evidence of a previous anterior MI. An echocardiogram reveals a LV EF of 40% with anterior akinesis from the base of the heart to the apex. A myocardial perfusion study showed no reversible ischemia. A 24-hour ambulatory Holter shows frequent PVCs and 20 episodes of nonsustained VT ranging from 3 to 5 beats. He reported no symptoms in his diary. What is the next step in his care?

a. Maximize his medical therapy for heart failure

b. Maximize his medical therapy for heart failure and refer for ICD based upon the Holter results

c. Maximize his medical therapy for heart failure and refer for an EP study

d. Maximize his medical therapy for heart failure and start amiodarone to suppress the ventricular ectopy

e. Refer for coronary angiography followed by optimization of his medical therapy

95. The following statements in regard to inclusion criteria for the ICD trials are correct **except:**

a. MADIT II: prior MI (>1 month), EF ≤ 0.30, decreased HR variability

b. ScD-HeFT: history of CHF (NYHA class II, III), EF ≤ 0.35, ischemic and nonischemic disease

c. MUSTT: ischemic heart disease, nonsustained VT, EF ≤ 0.40, and inducible VT

d. DINAMIT: recent MI (6–40 days) prior to trial entry, EF ≤ 0.35, and decreased HR variability

e. MADIT I: nonsustained VT, CHF (NYHA class I, II, or III), Q-wave or enzyme-positive MI > 3 weeks prior to enrollment

96. A 34-year-old man presents to the ED with sustained palpitations and mild dyspnea. He has no history of syncope, cardiac arrhythmia, or structural heart disease. He takes no medications and denies illicit drug use. Other than tachycardia his examination is normal. The following ECG was obtained.

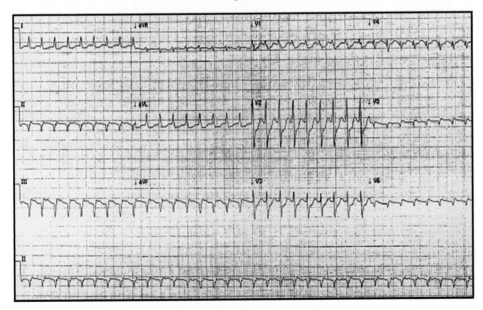

96. (*continued*)

What is the likely appropriate treatment?

a. Verapamil
b. Adenosine
c. Amiodarone
d. Sotalol
e. Vagal maneuvers

97. All of the following favor VT over paroxysmal SVT **except:**

a. AV dissociation
b. Fusion beats
c. Precordial nonconcordance
d. Lead V1 RBBB with larger left peak (Rsr')
e. Lead V6 QRS with rS or S morphology

98. The following ECG was obtained in a 16-year-old female referred for evaluation of palpitations.

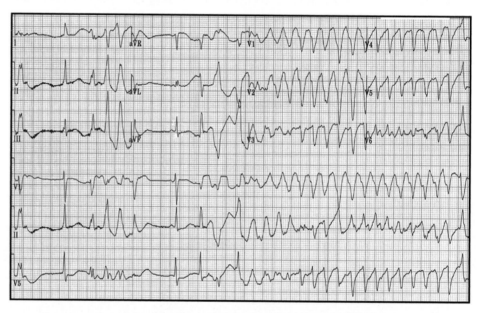

All of the following are characteristic of this tachyarrhythmia **except:**

a. Patients often have structurally normal hearts
b. Early afterdepolarizations can produce polymorphic VT
c. Pacing to increase the HR can decrease the early afterdepolarizations
d. Lidocaine increases the number of early afterdepolarizations, but does not confer risk of VT
e. The disorder can be both inherited and drug-induced

99. Patients with repaired tetralogy of Fallot have frequent ventricular arrhythmias. All of the following are risk factors for VT **except:**

a. Number of years post operatively
b. RV failure
c. Pulmonary HTN
d. ASD resulting in RV overload

100. A 46-year-old female presents with episodic palpitations that once were controlled with rate control medications and now have increased in frequency and duration. Her palpitations are associated with mild lightheadedness. She had no known medical history of cardiac disease or arrhythmias. She takes no medication. Her baseline ECG is normal. The following intracardiac electrograms were obtained during an EP study.

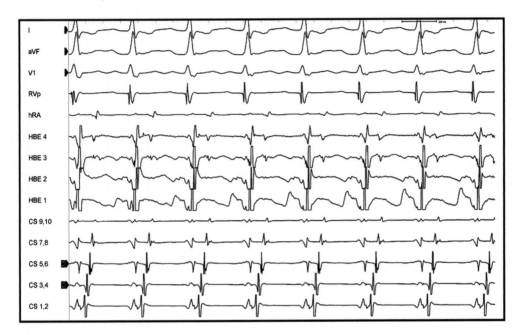

What is the most likely diagnosis?

a. RVOT tachycardia
b. AVNRT
c. Antidromic reciprocating reentrant tachycardia
d. Orthodromic reciprocating reentrant tachycardia
e. LVOT tachycardia

101. All of the following are congenital heart defects associated with an increased risk of an accessory pathway **except:**

a. Shone's syndrome
b. Ebstein's anomaly
c. Congenitally corrected transposition of the great vessels
d. Atrio-VSD
e. HCM

102. A 16-year-old male with no known cardiac or other medical history presents with infrequent palpitations. He has no family history of cardiac disease, arrhythmia, or sudden death. He uses no medication or illicit drugs. His examination is normal with the exception of a split S2. The following ECG is obtained.

102. (*continued*)

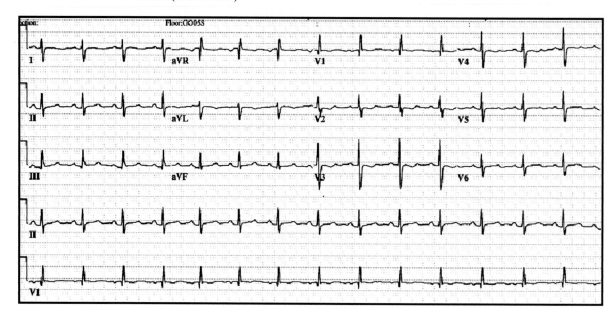

What is the most likely diagnosis?

a. Arrhythmogenic RV dysplasia
b. Secundum ASD
c. Pulmonary stenosis
d. Ebstein's anomaly
e. Bicuspid aortic valve

103. Which of the following arrhythmias are associated with the likely congenital abnormality of the patient in Question 102?

a. VT
b. Atrial flutter
c. Sinus node dysfunction
d. b and c
e. All of the above

104. Which of the following is true in regard to patients with Ebstein's anomaly of the tricuspid valve?

a. Loss of a typical LBBB is suggestive of a right-sided pathway
b. Accessory pathway mediated tachycardia is the most common atrial arrhythmia
c. Atrial flutter and fibrillation are common after the age of 35 years
d. Patients without a history of Wolff-Parkinson-White do not require a preoperative EP study to assess for an accessory pathway

105. A 32-year-old female with a history of congenital heart disease presents with a history of progressive weakness and fatigue. The following ECG is obtained.

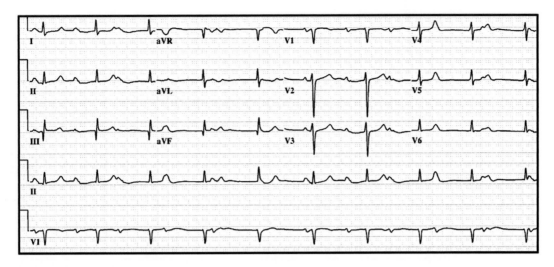

What is the most likely congenital abnormality?

a. VSD
b. ASD
c. Hypoplastic LV
d. Congenitally corrected L-TGA
e. Ebstein's anomaly

106. The patient in Question 105 is at high risk for which complication?

a. Complete AV block
b. LV failure
c. High risk of congenital birth defects in her children
d. Mitral valve regurgitation

107. A 65-year-old male with a history of symptomatic sinus node dysfunction recently underwent dual-chamber permanent pacemaker implantation. Two weeks following implantation he presented to the ED with sustained palpitations, dyspnea, and lightheadedness. The following telemetry strip was obtained in the ED.

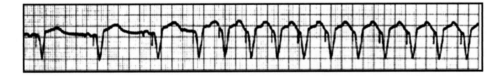

What is the most likely diagnosis?

a. VT
b. AF with a rapid ventricular rate
c. Ventricular lead oversensing
d. Pacemaker-mediated tachycardia
e. Sinus tachycardia with appropriate ventricular pacing

108. A 45-year-old obese male is referred for a formal sleep study due to a history of severe snoring with daytime somnolence and fatigue. He reports no history of palpitations, lightheadedness, or syncope. He is taking no medications. The following tracing is obtained during the sleep study.

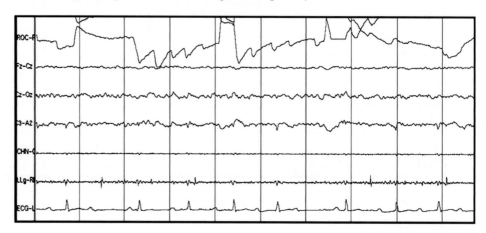

Courtesy of Dr. Apoor S. Gami and Dr. Sean M. Caples

What is the next step in his care?

   a. Continuous positive airway pressure
   b. Dual-chamber permanent pacemaker implantation
   c. Single-chamber permanent pacemaker implantation
   d. EP study to further assess the sinus and AV node function

109. All of the following are neurally mediated reflex syncopal syndromes **except:**

   a. Vasovagal
   b. Postmicturition
   c. Gastrointestinal stimulation (swallow, defecation, visceral pain)
   d. Carotid sinus
   e. Parkinson disease with autonomic failure

110. The following factors are associated with noncardiogenic syncope **except:**

   a. Young age
   b. Isolated syncope without underlying CV disease
   c. Normal examination and ECG
   d. Abrupt onset
   e. Symptoms consistent with a vasovagal cause

111. All of the following are class I indications for pacing **except:**

   a. Symptomatic acquired complete (third degree) and advanced second degree AV block
   b. Asymptomatic acquired complete (third degree) and advanced second degree AV block with asystole (>3 sec) or a HR < 40 bpm
   c. Complete (third degree) AV block in a patient with an acute inferior MI
   d. Symptomatic sinus bradycardia (<40 bpm)
   e. Symptomatic sinus bradycardia secondary to drug treatment only for which there is no acceptable alternative

112. A 72-year-old male received a dual chamber permanent pacemaker for complete heart block. He had a previous system explanted on the left side due to a lead erosion with a externalized "temporary" PM via the right internal jugular vein. Shortly after the new system was placed on the right he noted chest pain, palpitations, and dyspnea. The following chest X-ray was obtained.

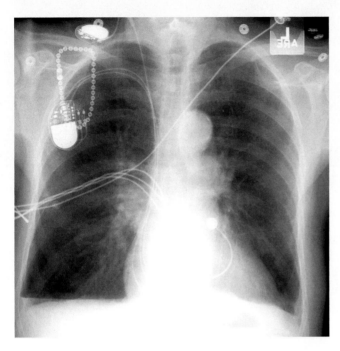

Chest X-ray courtesy of Dr. Apoor S. Gami

What is the most likely diagnosis for his symptoms?

a. Pacemaker lead dislodgement
b. Recurrent infection in the new right-sided system
c. Pneumothorax
d. Pulmonary embolus
e. CHF

113. Pacemaker syndrome is a hemodynamic abnormality that results from which of the following abnormalities?

a. The delay between the right and LV pacing leads is too long to allow a synchronous contraction
b. Ventricular pacing is uncoupled from the atrial contraction
c. Cross talk that results in inappropriate inhibition of the pacing stimulus
d. Endless-loop tachycardia that results from retrograde P waves that trigger another ventricular stimulation

114. A 72-year-old female with a history of ischemic dilated cardiomyopathy presents after receiving a shock from her ICD. This was her first shock and she had no symptoms prior to the therapy. The ICD was implanted 3 years ago due to her reduced LV function with underlying ischemic heart disease. The device was interrogated and the following information obtained.

114. (*continued*)

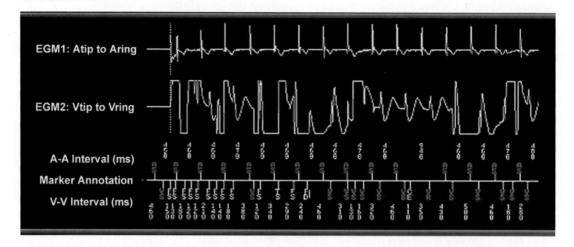

Device interrogation electrogram courtesy of Medtronic

What is the most likely diagnosis?

  a. Inappropriate therapy for AF
  b. Ventricular lead undersensing
  c. Appropriate therapy for VF
  d. Appropriate therapy for VT
  e. Lead fracture

115. The following stored electrogram was obtained from a permanent pacemaker in a patient that presented with general malaise.

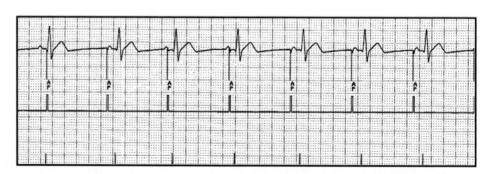

Device interrogation electrogram courtesy of Medtronic

What is the potential cause of the patient's symptom?

  a. Atrial lead oversensing
  b. Atrial lead undersensing
  c. Ventricular lead oversensing
  d. Ventricular lead undersensing
  e. Pacemaker syndrome

116. Which of the following statements is **incorrect** regarding the intraoperative assessment of a pacing system?

a. Wire fracture: high voltage threshold, high-normal-low current threshold, high impedance

b. Insulation break: low voltage threshold, high current threshold, low lead impedance

c. Lead dislodgement: high voltage threshold, high current threshold, high lead impedance

d. Exit block: high voltage threshold, high current threshold, normal lead impedance

117. A 34-year-old female underwent dual-chamber ICD implantation. She had a history of a VSD closure at birth with a persistent nonischemic dilated cardiomyopathy with a reduced LV EF. After the device was implanted the following chest X-ray was obtained.

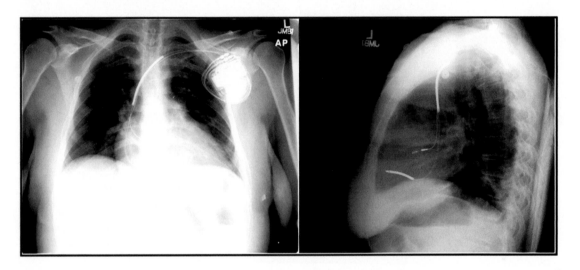

What is the complication with this device implantation?

a. Lead dislodgement
b. Pneumothorax
c. Cardiac perforation
d. Lead fracture
e. Poor connection at the connector block

118. The following statements regarding CRT are true **except:**

a. It is a class IIa indication in patients with symptomatic medically refractory NYHA class III or IV failure with idiopathic or ischemic cardiomyopathy, prolonged QRS interval ($\geq$130 msec), EF $<$ 0.35, and a LV end-diastolic diameter $\geq$ 55 mm

b. It improves distance in 6-minute walk tests

c. In general, it improves NYHA functional class and quality of life

d. It reduces death and hospitalization for any cause

e. It is technically not feasible in patients with AF with rapid ventricular rates

Answers

1. Answer e.

The most likely diagnosis is long QT syndrome. The prolonged QT > 480 msec, history of syncope, and family history of sudden death in a relative < 30 years of age yield a Moss and Schwartz score of 4.5 (see Table for scoring criteria), which places her at high risk of long QT syndrome. Although both Brugada syndrome and idiopathic VF present with sudden death, the clinical circumstance surrounding the arrest, gender of the patient, and ECG make these diseases less likely. RVOT tachycardia is typically not associated with sudden death. HCM often presents with exertional symptoms.

Table Point system for the diagnosis of congential long QT syndrome (Circulation 1993; 88:782–4)

Variable	Points
ECG	
QTc	
>480 msec	3
460–470 msec	2
450 msec (males)	1
Torsades de pointes	2
T-wave alternans	1
Notched T wave in 3 leads	1
Low HR for age	0.5
Clinical History	
Syncope	
with stress	2
without stress	1
Congenital deafness	0.5
Family History	
Family member with long QT syndrome	1
Sudden death in a family member <30 years of age with no other identifiable cause	0.5

Cumulative point score for risk of having congential long QT syndrome:
  ≤1 low risk
  2–3 intermediate risk
  ≥ 4 high risk

2. Answer b.

The most likely genotype for the presented phenotype is long QT2 syndrome. This is supported by the family gender and the auditory stimuli. Exertion related triggers are more common with long QT1 syndrome. Sleep-related events are more common in long QT3 syndrome. Jervell and Lange-Nielsen long QT syndrome is rare, autosomal recessive, and associated with congenital deafness. Timothy syndrome (long QT8 syndrome) is associated with other phenotypic manifestations, such as syndactyly, and significant learning disabilities.

3. Answer d.

The patient suffered an aborted sudden death and thereby has a class I indication for an ICD. There is little role for a permanent pacemaker. If pacing is required, the implantation of a dual-chamber ICD should be considered. Amiodarone often further prolongs the QT interval. Left cardiac sympathetic denervation can be considered in patients with recurrent appropriate ICD shocks. Beta blockers (preferably nadolol or propranolol) should be considered as standard therapy in all patients with long QT1 or 2 syndromes.

4. Answer c.

Reentry is the most common mechanism underlying cardiac tachyarrhythmias, including AVNRT, atrial flutter, AVRT with an accessory pathway, and VT in a diseased heart.

5. Answer e.

Torsades de pointes is characterized by prolonged QT intervals, exacerbation by bradycardia, short-long couple intervals, "salvos" of nonsustained polymorphic VT before degeneration into a sustained ventricular arrhythmia, and polymorphic VT with characteristic "twisting around the axis" morphology. Although amiodarone often prolongs the QT interval, it rarely causes torsades de pointes.

6. Answer c.

I_{K1} (inward rectifier) is crucial for maintaining the resting potential near -90 mV. It is also responsible for the rapid terminal repolarization in phase 3.

7. Answer c.

The I_{KATP} potassium channel is inactivated by chemical ligand binding in response to ischemia and depletion of ATP. Ventricular myocytes have high densities of these channels and their activation accounts for the ST elevation on the ECG seen during a MI.

8. Answer e.

The sinus node is predominantly characterized by its phase 4 depolarization, which accounts for the pacemaker activities. There are few sodium channels and the upstroke is primarily mediated by $I_{Ca,L}$. There is no discernible phase 1. The lack of I_{K1}, which is active in phase 3, accounts for the relative depolarized state of the tissue.

9. Answer a.

The ECG showed a wide complex tachycardia, with a left bundle branch morphology, inferior axis, and negative deflections in AVL and AVR. The clinical scenario, provocation with exercise, and ECG are consistent with exercise-mediated VT originating from RVOT. The arrhythmia is catecholamine-sensitive with calcium-mediated triggered activity from delayed depolarizations.

10. Answer b.

The treatment decision for this type of VT depends on the symptoms. If the symptoms are infrequent and mild, then no treatment is necessary. However, if the symptoms are severe, such as presyncope or syncope or extrasystoles that impact the patient's quality of life, then catheter ablation of the focus is the treatment of choice. Pharmacologic therapy improves symptoms in up to 50% of patients. The initial choice for therapy is usually a beta blocker. Although first line referral for catheter ablation is an option, since the patient is only mildly symptomatic, a trial of medications is warranted. Digoxin increases intracellular calcium and can potentially promote triggered activity.

11. Answer b.

Lidocaine is a weak sodium channel blocker and does not have significant potassium channel blockade. It does not prolong the QT and it is the one antiarrhythmic that may actually shorten it.

12. Answer d.

Lidocaine is a rather specific sodium channel blocker. The AV node conduction is mediated by $I_{Ca,L}$. The AV node is similar to the sinoatrial node in its lack of I_{Na}. Lidocaine does not have a significant effect on AV nodal conduction.

13. Answer a.

Adenosine activates the $I_{K,Ach}$ channel in atrial tissue. Activation of the $I_{K,Ach}$ channel shortens the action potential duration, thereby shortening the refractoriness of the atrial tissue and promoting the induction of AF.

14. Answer c.

Of the answer choices given, class 1A agents (quinidine and procainamide) and class 3 agents (ibutilide and sotalol) have a significant potassium channel blocking effect, therefore prolonging the QT interval and potentially causing torsades de pointes. Flecainide (a class 1C agent) is a fairly specific sodium channel blocker without a significant potassium channel blocking effect. Prolongation of the QT interval is not associated with flecainide.

15. Answer b.

The AV node is positioned in the low RA at the apex, rather than the base, of the triangle of Koch. The triangle of Koch is comprised of the ostium of the CS, tendon of Todaro, and septal attachment of the tricuspid valve leaflet. The region within the triangle is comprised of nodal and transitional cells.

16. Answer b.

Both the AV and sinoatrial nodal cells lack I_{Na}. Conduction is mediated in these tissues by $I_{Ca,L}$.

17. Answer c.

The conduction velocity is the most rapid in the His-Purkinje tissue.

18. Answer c.

The outgoing potassium current is the principal determinant of repolarization of myocardial cells.

19. Answer a.

The resting membrane potential of AV nodal cells is -40 to -70 mV.

20. Answer c.

Vagal stimulation has little effect on the ventricular myocardial action potential, whereas it increases the action potential in the AV node and reduces it in the atrial myocardium.

21. Answer b.

Early afterdepolarizations are depolarizations that occur in phases 2 and 3 of the action potential. Conditions that prolong the action potential duration promote the development of early afterdepolarizations. They are facilitated by a low potassium level, low magnesium level, and class I or III antiarrhythmic drugs, and are typically pause-dependent.

22. Answer b.

The mechanism that underlies the development of delayed afterdepolarizations is intracellular calcium overload. Digoxin increases intracellular calcium that can promote delayed afterdepolarization-triggered activity. Delayed afterdepolarizations have also been implicated in ischemic reperfusion arrhythmias and ryanodine receptor dysfunction.

23. Answer b.

24. Answer d.

The H–V interval in Wolff-Parkinson-White syndrome can be negative or very short with antidromic tachycardia because the ventricle is activated prematurely by the accessory pathway or normal in orthodromic tachycardia since conduction proceeds down the AV node to the ventricle and returns retrograde through an accessory pathway. The more typical form of Wolff-Parkinson-White syndrome is orthodromic and the QRS is narrow, even in tachycardia, unless functional bundle branch block occurs since the antegrade conduction proceeds through the AV node and His-Purkinje system.

25. Answer b.

An anatomical obstacle is not necessary for reentrant arrhythmia. Recent studies have shown that reentry can occur in the absence of an obstacle as a consequence of conduction and refractoriness in the atrial or ventricular tissue.

26. Answer b.

In antidromic reciprocating tachycardia, conduction is "anti" the normal path through the AV node. Thus there is AV conduction via the accessory pathway with the return ventriculoatrial conduction via His-Purkinje system followed by the AV node.

27. Answer d.

AVNRT tends to occur in younger patients (average 20–35 years), is slightly more common in women (ratio 1.2:1), may terminate with Valsalva or other vagotonic maneuvers, and typically is not associated with structural heart disease. This rhythm typically has a short H–A interval (usually 25–90 msec) measured with the His-bundle catheter. The short interval usually results in a P wave superimposing the QRS on the ECG. However, the terminal portion of the P wave may be distinguishable from the QRS with a late positive component of V1 (pseudo-r′, asterisks) or a pseudo-s in the inferior leads.

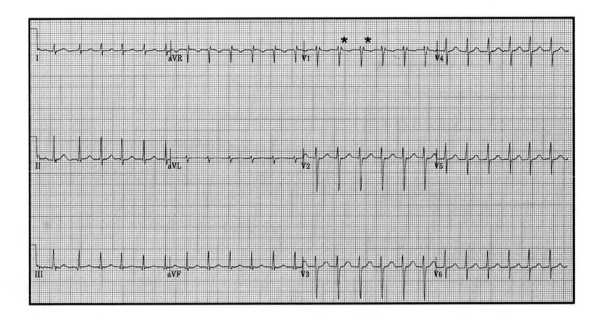

28. Answer a.

Patients with AVNRT usually have dual nodal physiology. In the most common form of this arrhythmia, conduction proceeds antegrade through the slow pathway and then retrograde over the fast pathway (slow–fast AVNRT). Variations such as slow–slow and fast–slow conduction are also variants of this reentrant tachycardia.

29. Answer b.

The most common mechanism of arrhythmias in sustained VT is reentry involving ventricular myocardium, most often from scars due to underlying CAD.

30. Answer c.

The patient has nonischemic cardiomyopathy and a search for potential secondary causes is warranted. Noninvasive testing, such as obtaining a serum ferritin to assess for hemochromatosis, should be performed prior to invasive studies, such as RV biopsy. In a minimally symptomatic patient, an EP study is not a first line test. Nonetheless, if the PVCs are monomorphic and other causes of cardiomyopathy are excluded, the patient may be considered for an EP study and attempted ablation of the focus. Prior to considering an ICD in this patient who has no other significant symptoms, medical therapy needs to be started and titrated to therapeutic doses.

31. Answer e.

Answers **a** to **d** are all considered high risk characteristics for cardiogenic syncope. If any of these are present, the rate of spontaneous ventricular tachyarrhythmia or death is between 4% and 7% in 1 year. If 3 or more are present, this rate increases to 58% to 80%. Recurrent unexplained falls in an elderly patient should first be assessed with tilt table testing unless other high risk features are present.

32. Answer d.

The temporal presentation and symptoms of the patients are consistent with pulmonary embolism, complicating the EP study he had 6 days before. The next step is to assess for this complication with screening tests, such as an arterial blood gas and D-Dimer, followed by an imaging modality, such as a ventilation perfusion scan or CT scan. If the evaluation for a pulmonary embolus is negative, a next step is to consider pericarditis.

33. Answer c.

Vasodepressor response characterized by a profound drop in BP with minimal change in HR is more common in patients more than 60 years old. In contrast, cardioinhibitory response characterized by asystole and profound bradycardia that coincides with a decrease in BP, or a mixed-type event that is a combination of HR and BP reduction, is the initial event occurring more often in younger patients.

34. Answer a.

The sensitivity of EP testing for sinus node disease is <50%. For all other diagnoses listed, detection rates of EP tests are typically >90%.

35. Answer c.

The patient has recurrent syncope with evidence of significant sinus node dysfunction. In this patient a pacemaker is indicated. The choices of therapy include an AAI versus a DDDR permanent pacemaker. AAI is indicated in a patient when AV conduction is completely normal. If there is evidence of dysfunction, such as this patient with first degree AV block, DDDR is the generally agreed upon treatment.

36. Answer b.

MUSTT showed that patients with an EF < 40%, CAD, and the presence of non-sustained VT who underwent an EP study and had inducible VT benefited from implantation of an ICD. Patients with an EF < 35% and CAD benefit from implantation of an ICD independent of an EP study or other provocative tests, such as a signal averaged ECG. Patients that suffer a VF cardiac arrest that is not from reversible causes (perimyocardial infarction, abnormal electrolytes, etc.) should receive an ICD.

37. Answer e.

Answers **a** to **d** are all considered a positive response to pharmacologic stress in patients suspected to have a cardiac channelopathy. Ajmaline is a sodium channel blocking agent used in patients suspected to have Brugada syndrome.

38. Answer d.

Acute success rates for accessory pathway ablation in Wolff-Parkinson-White syndrome are approximately 90% to 95%. Right-sided pathways tend to have lower acute success rates in comparison to left-sided pathways.

39. Answer d.

The patient has pre-excited AF due to Wolff-Parkinson-White and a shortest R–R interval during AF near 240 msec; thus, she is at risk of sudden death in the future and should receive radiofrequency ablation of the accessory pathway to cure the Wolff-Parkinson-White. Acutely, procainamide is the drug of choice for termination (or DC cardioversion if she is hemodynamically unstable). AV nodal blocking agents such as adenosine are contraindicated in this situation.

40. Answer e.

An H–V interval from 55 to 99 msec is considered an intermediate result and requires either the presence of additional symptoms or other findings to direct therapy. An H–V interval >100 msec is considered a positive result, as well as infra-His block.

41. Answer a.

The vast majority of long QT cases are due to mutations in the KCNQ1 gene that encodes the slow component of the delayed rectifier potassium current (long QT1).

During exercise these patients fail to shorten their QT. The gene-specific triggers of patients with long QT1 are exertion-related activities, in particular swimming. In long QT2 auditory stimuli and the postpartum period are important triggers. In long QT3 the most common trigger is sleep.

42. Answer b.

Paradoxical lengthening of the QT with low-dose epinephrine ($\leq 0.1\,\mu g/kg/min$) and the presence of paradoxical lengthening ($>30\,msec$) with exercise of the absolute QT interval is suggestive of concealed long QT1 (75% positive predictive value). Identifying those with concealed long QT is important for counseling regarding activities and therapy.

43. Answer e.

According to the 2005 Bethesda Conference guidelines, competitive sports are restricted with the exception of class IA activities. These activities include: golf, cricket, bowling, billiards, and riflery.

44. Answer b.

All of the above statements are true except **b.** Romano-Ward syndrome is a heterogeneous disorder associated with prolonged QT interval and recurrent syncope, cardiac arrest, or sudden death. It is inherited in an autosomal dominant pattern and several mutations involving sodium and potassium channels have been recognized. Jervell and Lange-Nielsen syndrome is inherited in an autosomal recessive pattern. It is associated with prolonged QT interval, history of recurrent syncope or sudden death, and congenital neural deafness. The Romano-Ward syndrome is more frequent than the Jervell and Lange-Nielsen syndrome.

45. Answer e.

All of the given statements, except **e**, are true in the management of drug-induced QT prolongation. Both isoproterenol infusion and temporary pacing can be used to increase the baseline HR. Beta blockers, which have a role in reducing arrhythmias in long QT1 and 2, are not effective in drug-induced tachyarrhythmia, and could worsen the condition by promoting bradyarrhythmia and pauses.

46. Answer c.

Brugada syndrome is characterized by ECG findings of ST elevation in the right precordial leads V1 through V3, in the presence or absence of incomplete or complete right bundle branch block, and an increased risk of sudden death. Patients are more often male and present with sudden death due to VF. Although both long QT and short QT syndromes can present with sudden death, the ECG is not consistent with these channelopathies.

47. Answer d.

The patient sustained a VF cardiac arrest from an underlying channelopathy (Brugada syndrome). He should receive an ICD without further testing for risk assessment. Provocative testing with class 1 agents is used strictly for diagnosis and has little prognostic value, in particular is this patient that has already experienced a sudden cardiac arrest.

48. Answer b.

Brugada syndrome is due to a loss of function mutation involving the SCN5A-encoded cardiac sodium channel. This is in contrast to long QT3, which is due to a gain of function mutation involving the SCN5A-encoded cardiac sodium channel.

49. Answer e.

All the medications listed in answers **a** to **d** have been shown to increase the QT interval. Although Amiodarone is on the list of agents that prolong the QT interval, it rarely causes torsades de pointes. Nonetheless, this potential complication must be considered. For a complete list of drugs that are known to cause this complication see www.torsades.org or www.qtdrugs.org

50. Answer a.

Mutations in the RyR2-encoded cardiac ryanodine receptor or the calcium release channel account for the majority of catecholaminergic polymorphic VT cases. These mutations result in increased calcium leak during sympathetic stimulation, particularly during diastole.

51. Answer c.

Patients with symptomatic catecholaminergic polymorphic VT should receive an ICD as first line therapy since other therapies, such as calcium channel and beta blockers, have not been shown to be sufficiently protective.

52. Answer b.

In patients with manifest pre-excitation, an echocardiogram should be performed since the incidence of associated congenital heart disease can be a high as 30% in some series. The most common associated congenital heart disease is Ebstein anomaly. Furthermore, an echocardiogram allows assessment of LV function, which is often depressed after conversion from a SVT. Finally, exercise testing can be considered as a further means to assess risk. Exercise provides information regarding the accessory pathway and its conduction at higher HRs. Disappearance of the delta wave with exercise has been reported to coincide with a low risk of sudden death.

53. Answer d.

AVNRT is a rare form of SVT in infants, but gradually increases with time. In teenagers, this rhythm and accessory-pathway mediated tachycardia account for nearly 95% of the SVT cases. AVNRT is more common in females. All the other arrhythmias listed are uncommon in this age group.

54. Answer e.

All of the answer choices **a** to **d** are associated with second degree AV block. Regarding long QT syndrome, a subgroup of infants with this channelopathy present with 2:1 AV block due to His-Purkinje system or ventricular myocardial refractoriness. Other causes of second degree AV block include mechanical trauma during catheterization, metabolic, and drug induced etiologies.

55. Answer a.

The ECG shows sinus rhythm with third degree AV block.

56. Answer c.

Although all the answers are associated with AV block, maternal systemic lupus erythematosus is the most likely diagnosis in this patient. Her history suggests longstanding rhythm disease. Her echocardiogram is normal, which rules out L-TGA. Her clinical history is not consistent with answers **b** and **e**. In mothers with systemic lupus erythematosus, antibodies (anti-Ro) can pass the placenta and affect the fetal AV conduction system.

57. Answer a.

The patient is asymptomatic but in complete heart block. The next step in her care is to determine if she requires implantation of a dual-chamber permanent pacemaker. A Holter monitor will show if the patient has pauses >3 sec, which would be a reason to implant a pacemaker. Exercise testing is also important to assess exercise performance, but in this patient ischemia is not the cause of her rhythm disturbance.

58. Answer d.

The patient has third degree AV block and has pauses in excess of 3 sec. These findings suggest the need for a pacemaker implantation. Since the patient is in sinus rhythm, a dual-chamber device is required to prevent pacemaker syndrome.

59. Answer e.

Answers **a** to **d** are all reasons to implant a permanent pacemaker in a patient with congenital AV block. An additional reason is >3 sec pauses during Holter monitoring. Isoproterenol infusion has no role in risk assessment in these patients.

60. Answer d.

Dual AV node physiology provides the substrate for typical AVNRT. Answers **a** to **c** are proposed mechanisms underlying the initiation and maintenance of AF.

61. Answer e.

Each of answers **a** to **d** has been shown to be a risk factor for AF. Other established causes include advancing age, valvular heart disease, excessive alcohol intake, thyrotoxicosis, pericarditis, cardiac surgery, acute pulmonary disease, and MI.

62. Answer c.

The AFFIRM trial studied 4,060 patients older than 65 years with a history of AF and additional risk factors for stroke or death. They were randomized to either rate control or rhythm control. Patients in the rhythm control group were more likely to be in sinus rhythm. However, there was no statistically significant difference in mortality, stroke, quality of life, or development of heart failure between the rate and rhythm control groups.

63. Answer b.

False. One of the most important findings in the AFFIRM trial was that anticoagulation should be strongly considered in these patients even in the presence of sinus rhythm. One reason is that these patients often have silent or subclinical AF. The second reason is that AF is often associated with many other medical comorbidities that increase stroke risk, such as HTN, diabetes, CAD, heart failure, etc.

64. Answer b.

Risk factors with AF can be remembered with the CHADS2 mnemonic, which stands for: C, cardiac failure; H, hypertension; A, age >75 years; D, diabetes mellitus; and S2, stroke or transient ischemic attack. From data based upon a long-term study of the NRAF participants, the risk of stroke increases incrementally as patients accumulate more of these risk factors.

65. Answer a.

Adequate rate control in patients with AF is defined as a resting HR < 80 bpm and maximal HR < 110 bpm during a 6-minute walk. Rate control can be achieved with a variety of medications. Digoxin alone is often insufficient to control HR during exercise.

66. Answer d.

Dofetilide and amiodarone are acceptable drug choices in patients with AF and heart failure.

67. Answer b.

This tracing demonstrates AF with Ashman phenomenon. The long–short interval and classic right bundle branch morphology with a "right rabbit ear taller than left" and R–R interval variability demonstrate that this is aberrant conduction. A premature ventricular complex is not present.

68. Answer d.

The ECG shows AF in a patient with Wolff-Parkinson-White syndrome. The widest complexes represent activation down the accessory pathway, whereas narrower ones represent fusion beats in which the ventricles are activated in part by conduction down the AV node and in part by the accessory pathway. Adenosine shortens atrial refractory periods, causes AV block, and could accelerate the ventricular rate, resulting in degeneration to VF. Lidocaine has no effect on atrial tissue and is not effective in this setting. Both metoprolol and diltiazem also slow the AV node, possibly limiting concealed conduction from the node to the accessory pathway and accelerating conduction down the pathway. Procainamide is the agent of choice in this setting. If this fails to control the rhythm, or the patient becomes hemodynamically unstable, cardioversion is appropriate.

69. Answer c.

Direct interventions to restore sinus rhythm, such as DC cardioversion or starting an antiarrhythmic, should be avoided in this patient with AF >24 hours unless a TEE reveals no evidence of intracardiac thrombus or anticoagulation has been used for a minimum of 3 weeks at documented therapeutic levels (INR 2.0–3.0). Regardless of the treatment choice, his BP requires aggressive control.

70. Answer b.

False. Randomized studies of nonrheumatic AF in patients with paroxysmal and chronic AF have shown no difference in the rate of stroke between the subgroups. First, patients with AF often have other comorbidities that are associated with a higher risk of stroke. Also, recent studies of different therapies have documented that patients typically experience multiple subclinical or asymptomatic episodes of AF. These patient characteristics may account in part for why there is little difference in stroke risk between these arrhythmia subtypes.

71. Answer c.

Digoxin, diltiazem, and metoprolol will slow the AV node conduction and control the ventricular rate. Although procainamide can be used to restore normal sinus rhythm, it enhances AV node conduction and may result in an increase in ventricular rate. Therefore, rate control should be achieved before initiating procainamide.

72. Answer e.

Answers **a** to **d** are all appropriate for a patient who presents with persistent AF despite the use of an antiarrhythmic agent. The patient requires anticoagulation and needs treatment of HTN and obstructive sleep apnea if present. AV node ablation remains a highly successful means of long-term rate control, but the patient requires long-term pacemaker dependency with RV pacing. Left atrial ablation has emerged as a highly successful alternative to drug therapy for rhythm control.

73. Answer d.

In patients who have failed a trial of antiarrhythmic drugs, left atrial ablation has emerged as a highly successful alternative nonpharmacologic therapy. The technique is more successful in patients with PAF. Despite AF subtype, the approach is successful in the majority of patients. It is unclear when and if anticoagulation can be stopped, and a standardized approach is difficult to adapt to variable patient comorbidities and persistent asymptomatic episodes of AF. One study has shown that, in patients <65 years of age and without HTN, if sinus rhythm is restored, the long-term stroke risk is low. Recent guidelines suggest for those patients in sinus rhythm, the decision to continue anticoagulation should be based on the presence of known risk factors for stoke.

74. Answer e.

Answers **a** to **d** are all associated with atrial flutter.

75. Answer c.

Class 1C agents used in the treatment of atrial flutter may slow the ventricular rate; however, they may also result in 1:1 AV conduction, and should be used in combination with a beta blocker or calcium channel blocker. Dofetilide has a 1 year efficacy of 73% in maintaining sinus rhythm in patients with atrial flutter.

76. Answer e.

Patients with prolonged QT and a history of polymorphic VT with class I or III antiarrhythmic agents should not received ibutilide due to an increased risk of torsades de pointes. Likewise, significant hypokalemia can increase the risk of torsades de pointes. In patients with hemodynamic instability, emergency DC cardioversion is necessary. Patients with a structurally normal heart have a very low risk of torsades de pointes (1%) although lack of a normal heart in itself is not a contraindication (risk of torsades de pointes up to 4%).

77. Answer e.

Sarcoidosis is not a commonly recognized cause of atrial flutter. Answers **a** to **d** are all factors that predispose to atrial flutter. Other factors include dilated or HCM, CHF, sick sinus syndrome, thyrotoxicosis, chronic lung disease, and alcohol.

78. Answer c.

The risk of thromboembolism in patients with atrial flutter ranges from 1.7% to 7%. The guidelines for anticoagulation for patients with AF are extended to those with atrial flutter. For example, chronic warfarin therapy with a goal INR from 2.0 to 3.0 is recommended in those individuals with recurrent or persistent atrial flutter when risk factors for a thromboembolic event are present.

79. Answer a.

Typical atrial flutter is dependent on the cavo-tricuspid isthmus. In counterclockwise cavo-tricuspid isthmus-dependent atrial flutter there is a cranial-caudal activation sequence along the right atrial lateral wall, across the cavo-triscupid isthmus, and then superiorly in the right atrial septum. On a 12-lead ECG this is characterized as negative sawtooth flutter waves in leads II, III, and AVF; and a positive wave in lead V1 with a transition to a negative deflection in V6.

80. Answer c.

Patients with automatic atrial tachycardia often report a gradual onset of symptoms that become more rapid (warm-up). In contrast, patients with AVNRT and AVRT tend to paroxysms of palpitations with an abrupt onset and offset.

81. Answer e.

All of the answers are correct with the exception of **e**. In atrial tachycardia, the P wave morphologic features of the initial and subsequent beats are typically identical.

82. Answer b.

In antidromic AVRT, antegrade conduction is through an accessory pathway, with retrograde conduction through the AV node (anti-against the normal AV node conduction). An important exception to other forms of SVT is that a bystander accessory pathway, not involved in the tachycardia, may conduct to the ventricle and cause a pre-excited wide QRS.

83. Answer b.

It is important to remember that, although an accessory pathway is present, it is not necessarily a part of the tachycardia. Nonetheless, the history of abrupt onset, no clear triggering event, and urge to micturate with tachycardia termination are most consistent with AVNRT and AVRT. The ECG is consistent with pre-excitation and with his history suggest a preliminary diagnosis of AVRT.

84. Answer d.

Valsalva-like maneuvers that terminate the tachycardia is a characteristic of AVNRT rather than atrial tachycardia.

85. Answer d.

Answers **a** to **c** are all features that should prompt suspicion of the permanent form of junctional reciprocating tachycardia. The tachycardia is an AVRT utilizing a retrograde posterior septal accessory pathway and is often incessant resulting in a tachycardia-mediated cardiomyopathy.

86. Answer b.

False. QRS morphologic variation is an important clue to the presence of a pre-excited arrhythmia. With any pre-excited tachycardia, if AV node conduction is slowed, the degree of pre-excitation increases. With AV node slowing with blocking agents the ventricular response can paradoxically increase and predispose the patient to VF.

87. Answer a.

The initial deflection in V1 is positive. This becomes more apparent when looking at where the delta wave begins as seen in V3. AVL is negative. AVF is positive. These electrocardiographic characteristics suggest a left lateral pathway.

88. Answer d.

There is an equal number of ventricular (V) and atrial (A) electrograms (labeled) present. The A measured in the HRA falls nearly simultaneously with the V measure at the RV apex. These electrograms correspond with a P wave that falls within the QRS, thereby, in general, characterizing this arrhythmia as a short RP atrial tachycardia.

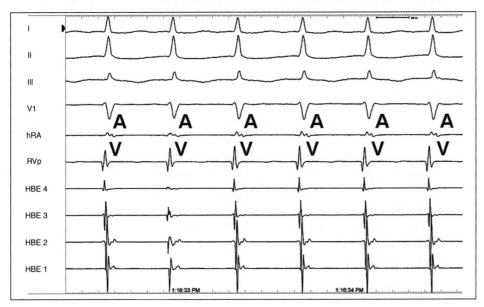

89. Answer d.

The patient is a young female presenting with a very short RP tachycardia. The most common atrial arrhythmia in this clinical scenario is AVNRT. The V–A interval on the intracardiac electrograms is <70 msec, which makes an accessory pathway mediated tachycardia unlikely. In atrial flutter the A should come before the V as it is driving the arrhythmia. There is no chaotic activity in the atrium to suggest AF.

90. Answer d.

The patient described had a large MI that was treated with percutaneous revascularization. PVCs and nonsustained VT are common. This type of patient was studied in DINAMIT. Although these patients are at relatively high risk of both sudden and total mortality, implantation of an ICD did not improve outcomes. If the patient has periods of sustained VT, an antiarrhythmic should be considered. Otherwise, medical therapy alone is appropriate, with follow-up assessment of her EF to determine if any functional recovery results from the revascularization.

91. Answer a.

The patient's early presentation, family history of sudden death, ECG suggestive of RV disease (T wave inversion in leads V2–V4), and echocardiogram consistent with RV abnormalities are consistent with arrhythmogenic RV dysplasia. The echocardiogram is not consistent with HCM. The RV structural disease is more consistent with arrhythmogenic RV dysplasia in comparison to RVOT tachycardia.

92. Answer d.

The patient most likely has arrhythmogenic RV dysplasia. Although late potentials on a signal-average ECG may suggest a higher risk patient, the absence of findings is not sensitive enough to not proceed with other assessment or treatment. Exercise testing likewise is helpful if exercise-induced arrhythmias develop. In this patient, the episode of syncope

92. (*continued*)

with activity is concerning for a cardiac source. Furthermore, there is a family history of sudden death and there are notable changes on both the ECG and echocardiogram. ICD placement is the best current therapy to decrease sudden death. Additional imaging that may further characterize the tissue, such as a MRI, should be considered prior to implantation of the device. Radiofrequency ablation has been reported to successfully treat VT in 40% of these patients, although recurrence is common as the cardiomyopathy process progresses.

93. Answer c.

Exercise-induced seizures in this young patient require careful investigation for a cardiac tachyarrhythmia. Although such a patient may have a primary neurologic disorder, the temporal correlation with activity is concerning for a primary cardiac disorder with a second neurologic manifestation. Long QT1 patients often present with exertion-related symptoms. The presence of long QT can be sought on the baseline ECG and, if needed, with exercise testing and an epinephrine challenge. Beta blockade and exercise restrictions are premature in this patient without a clear diagnosis, as HCM and other channelopathies may also cause a similar presentation. For this latter reason, although not offered as a choice in the question, an echocardiogram is appropriate to screen for structural heart disease.

94. Answer c.

The patient may benefit from treatment with an ICD due to his ischemic heart disease and reduced LV EF. He is not a candidate based upon the MADIT I or II nor the ScD-HeFT due to his EF. The MUSTT examined patient with ischemic heart disease and a reduction LV EF (≤ 0.40). In this patient cohort, those with inducible VT benefited from an ICD. Also, in the MUSTT trial the ICD was superior to antiarrhythmic therapy, primarily with amiodarone. The patient had no evidence of ischemia to suggest need for coronary angiography.

95. Answer a.

The MADIT II did not require evidence of decreased HR variability for study enrollment.

96. Answer a.

The patient is a young male who presents with probable idiopathic VT with a narrow R–S interval. At EP testing this patient was found to have a left posterior fascicular VT. Careful inspection of lead II shows occasional QRS complexes not followed by a P wave. This type of arrhythmia is sensitive to verapamil, but generally unresponsive to vagal maneuvers or adenosine. The morphology is not consistent with an outflow tract tachycardia in which adenosine characteristically terminates the arrhythmia.

97. Answer c

Precordial concordance is suggestive of VT. All the other answer choices are more consistent with SVT. In addition, clinical findings, such as a history of CAD, cannon a waves, and variable first heart sound on auscultation, favor VT.

98. Answer d.

Lidocaine suppresses early afterdepolarizations, as does acetylcholine, magnesium, beta blockers, pacing, and potassium channel openers. Patients with long QT syndrome often have structurally normal hearts.

99. Answer d.

Answers **a** to **c** are all associated with the development of VT late after repair for tetralogy of Fallot. An ASD is not associated with risk of VT, although the presence of a significant residual shunt is associated with an increased risk of sudden death.

100. Answer d.

The patient has an orthodromic reciprocating tachycardia. In this tachycardia, conduction from the atrium proceeds through the AV node to the ventricle and then back up to the atrium through an accessory pathway. In the tracing there are equal numbers of ventricular (V) and atrial (A) electrograms (below). The antegrade Vs preceed the retrograde As activated through the accessory pathway. A close inspection of the CS electrograms shows the V–A interval to be very small along (CS 1,2), which is in the distal CS, suggestive that the accessory pathway is along the left lateral ventricle.

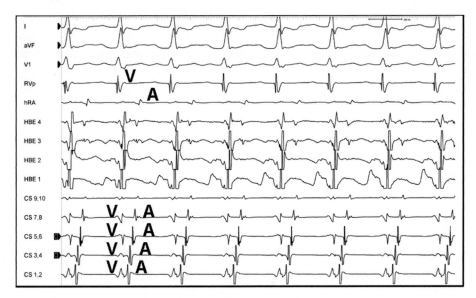

101. Answer a.

Shone's syndrome, which is manifest by multiple LV outflow obstructions, is not associated with an increased risk of an accessory pathway. All of the other conditions convey an increased risk, in particular Ebstein's anomaly.

102. Answer b.

The ECG shows sinus rhythm with right axis deviation. The ECG and physical examination with a fixed split S2 are suggestive of a secundum ASD. The ECG is not consistent with significant RV disease that would suggest arrhythmogenic RV dysplasia, pulmonary stenosis, or Ebstein's anomaly.

103. Answer d.

In patients with an ostium secundum ASD, both atrial arrhythmias and late sinus node dysfunction are complications. In the absence of surgical repair, isthmus dependent atrial flutter is the most common atrial arrhythmia.

104. Answer c.

Atrial flutter and fibrillation are more common in patients more than 35 years of age. These two atrial arrhythmias combined exceed in prevalence accessory pathway mediated tachycardia in this age group. Loss of a typical right bundle branch block is suggestive of

104. (*continued*)

a right-sided pathway. Finally, patients with a history of palpitations or a documented tachycardia should undergo preoperative EP study, regardless of the presence or absence of pre-excitation on ECG.

105. Answer d.

In congenitally corrected TGA, the right and left bundles are inverted, which causes the septal activation to proceed from right-to-left. This can cause Q waves in leads II and III, but not in V5 and V6. The second clue is the complete AV block. Patients with congenitally corrected transposition are at high risk of AV block from progressive fibrosis to the conduction system over time.

106. Answer a.

The patient has congenitally corrected TGA. In these patients, both the AV node and His bundle have an atypical course and position and are vulnerable to fibrosis with age, with a risk of complete block of approximately 2% per year. These patients are at risk for systemic ventricular failure (morphologic RV) and TR. In one series of 50 pregnancies, 40 (83%) resulted in live births and none had congenital heart disease.

107. Answer d.

The tracing initially shows dual-chamber pacing. At onset of the tachycardia, a retrograde P wave can be seen in the T wave. This P wave is sensed and the ventricle is subsequently paced. The tachycardia persists as this paced beat results in a retrograde P wave that is sensed triggering a subsequent ventricular-paced beat. The P wave morphology argues against sinus tachycardia and AF. Ventricular lead oversensing results in failure to pace the ventricle.

108. Answer a.

In patients with obstructive sleep apnea, multiple cardiac rhythm disturbances have been reported, such as AF, bradyarrhythmias, heart block, and ventricular ectopy. The most common are severe sinus bradycardia and AV block that are reflex responses to the apnea and hypoxia. Treatment of these rhythm disturbances is directed at the sleep apnea rather than the secondary rhythm disturbance.

109. Answer e.

Parkinson disease with autonomic failure typically results in orthostatic syncope. Answers **a** to **d** are all neurally mediated reflex syncopal syndromes. Others causes of neurally mediated reflex syncope include: acute hemorrhage, cough, sneeze, postexercise glossopharyngeal and trigeminal neuralgia, and a situational faint.

110. Answer d.

An abrupt onset of syncope, particularly with exertion or while supine, is more consistent with a cardiogenic mechanism. All the other factors other than the correct answer **d** are more suggestive of a noncardiac mechanism. Factors suggestive of a cardiac mechanism include: CAD, CHF, older age, abrupt onset, serious injuries, abnormal cardiac examination, structural heart disease, and an abnormal ECG (presence of a Q wave, bundle branch block, sinus bradycardia).

111. Answer c.

Patients with an acute inferior infarction can develop multiple types of electrical abnormalities, including sinoatrial node dysfunction, first-degree AV block, second-degree block, and third-degree block at the level of the AV node. It is uncommon for any of these conduction disturbances to persist after resolution of the acute phase of the infarction. These patients may require temporary pacing if hemodynamically unstable, but they rarely require permanent pacing. All the other answers are class I indications for pacing. Additional class I indications for pacing include: sinus node dysfunction with life-threatening, bradycardiac-dependent arrhythmias, recurrent syncope by carotid sinus stimulation with ventricular asystole of >3 sec, second-degree AV block at any level with symptomatic bradycardia, neuromuscular disease with AV block, and congenital complete AV block with a wide QRS, complex ventricular ectopy, or LV dysfunction.

112. Answer c.

The chest X-ray shows a moderate pneumothorax on the right (*arrows*). A chest tube was inserted and the pneumothorax resolved.

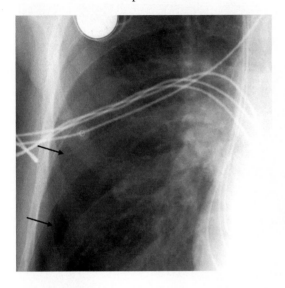

113. Answer b.

Pacemaker syndrome results from inappropriate ventricular pacing or when the ventricular pacing is uncoupled from the atrial contraction. Patients may experience a variety of symptoms that include general malaise, a sensation of fullness in the head and neck, syncope, cough, dyspnea, heart failure, or weakness. They may have cannon A waves on exam and a lower BP when paced. The syndrome is most common when the VVI mode is used and the underlying rhythm is sinus.

114. Answer e.

The episode interrogation showed a fast, sensed rhythm from the ventricular lead. Atrial sense is normal and reveals a regular rhythm, which excludes an inappropriate therapy due to an atrial tachyarrhythmia. The electrogram from the ventricular lead (V_{tip} to V_{ring}) shows considerable artifact with a normal rhythm, as evidenced by a regular R–R interval that marches out, despite the morphologic abnormalities of the tracing. In this case there was a lead fracture. A lead fracture can lead to erratic sensing, a high lead impedance, intermittent or complete loss of capture, and, in this case, an inappropriate shock.

115. Answer b.

The atrial lead has failed to sense the intrinsic P wave and has delivered a regular atrial stimulus at the preset minimal interval. This is an example of atrial lead undersensing. Undersensing may result from lead dislodgement, insulation failure, circuit failure, magnet application, battery depletion, electromagnetic failure, poor or incompatible connection at the connector block, and, for a unipolar device or configuration, air in the pocket.

116. Answer c.

Lead dislodgement is typically characterized by a high voltage and current threshold, but normal lead impedance.

117. Answer a.

The chest X-ray shows migration of the atrial lead that was positioned in the right atrial appendage to a position at the tricuspid valve orifice. There was also failure to capture with the lead. The lead was subsequently repositioned successfully as shown on the follow-up chest X-ray.

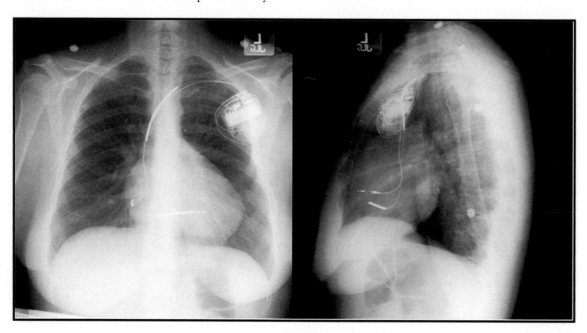

118. Answer e.

AF with rapid ventricular rates does not inhibit the use of CRT. The rapid ventricular rates require careful management to allow the device to consistently pace both ventricles. If this is not medically feasible, then patients can undergo AV node ablation. The COMPANION trial showed a reduction in the primary endpoint of death and hospitalization for any causes with both CRT alone and when combined with an ICD. Multiple trials have demonstrated a benefit in 6-minute walk tests, NYHA functional class, quality of life, oxygen consumption, and functional MR.

SECTION II

Coronary Artery Disease Risk Factors

Charles X. Kim, MD

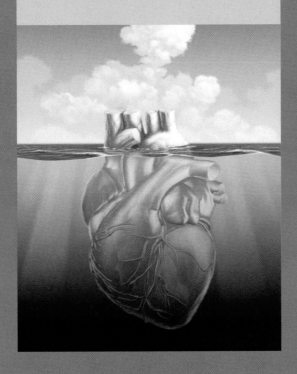

Questions

Pick the best answer(s); some questions have more than one correct answer.

1. In vivo, the subendothelium contains many types of collagen. All the following are types of subendothelial collagen **except:**

   a. Collagen II
   b. Collagen III
   c. Collagen IV
   d. Collagen V
   e. Collagen VIII

2. Endothelium secretes all the following substances in large amounts **except:**

   a. Collagen
   b. Elastin
   c. Glycosaminoglycans
   d. Fibronectin
   e. Mucopolysaccharides

3. Which substance(s) is/are secreted by the endothelium?

   a. Procoagulants
   b. Anticoagulants
   c. Vasoconstrictors
   d. Vasodilators
   e. Pro-proliferative substances

4. Which of the following is/are **not true** about platelets?

   a. Platelet activation can occur through many biochemical pathways and receptors
   b. Platelet aggregation occurs through many different surface receptors
   c. Platelet adhesion occurs principally through subendothelial vWF
   d. Platelet-activating factor also activates monocytes and polymorphonuclear leukocytes
   e. Removal of the endothelium exposes subendothelium and creates intense platelet adhesion

5. Atherosclerosis principally affects which of the following component(s) of the vessel wall?

   a. Intima
   b. Adventitia
   c. Media
   d. Endothelium

Answers to this section start on page 69.

6. The major cell type of the normal coronary artery intima is the:

    a. Macrophage
    b. Smooth muscle cell
    c. Lymphocyte
    d. Endothelial cell
    e. Foam cell

7. The foam cell is a lipid-laden cell derived from:

    a. Macrophage
    b. Smooth muscle cell
    c. Endothelial cell
    d. Lymphocyte
    e. Polymorphonuclear leukocyte

8. Which of the following is/are true about atherosclerotic plaques?

    a. Studies of arteries in patients with atherosclerosis show high rates of proliferation
    b. Intimal cell masses found in normal young patients suggest that proliferation may have an early role in the development of the atherosclerotic lesion
    c. Cells normally accumulate in the coronary arterial intima with aging
    d. Evidence suggests that the fatty streak may not be an early lesion of coronary artherosclerotic plaque
    e. The cells of atherosclerotic plaques are polyclonal in origin; that is, originating from many cells

9. In the "insudation hypothesis" of atherosclerosis, which of the following is/are true?

    a. Lipid accumulation in atherosclerotic plaque comes from circulating lipid
    b. Smooth muscle cell proliferation is induced by lipid accumulation at physiologic lipid concentration
    c. Fatty deposition is required for plaque growth
    d. Lipids in foam cells come from synthesis by local cellular activity

10. Which of the following is/are true of the fatty streak?

    a. It is found frequently in young children and infants
    b. It is found at the same anatomical sites in young persons and adults
    c. T lymphocytes may be found in many fatty streaks
    d. The principal lipid of the fatty streak is unoxidized cholesteryl esters
    e. The fatty streak is found principally in males at older ages

11. Which of the following is/are true of the "vulnerable" plaque?

    a. The vulnerable plaque typically has a fibrous cap covering a lipid-rich layer
    b. These plaques often rupture at the central portion of the fibrous layer, where hydrodynamic forces are increased
    c. Evidence suggests that vulnerable plaque may come from hemorrhage into the coronary artery vessel wall at certain locations
    d. The vulnerable plaque is typically associated with a severe angiographic stenosis
    e. There is evidence suggesting that more than 90% of deaths caused by MIs are associated with plaque rupture or ulceration

12. Which of the following is/are true of calcification of coronary artery plaque?

   a. Coronary calcification may proceed in a biochemical fashion similar to that in bone
   b. The principal component of plaque calcification is calcium carbonate and, thus, is related to vitamin D intake
   c. The degree of calcification is related to the overall volume of atherosclerotic plaque in coronary arteries
   d. Calcific medial sclerosis as a cause of coronary arterial calcification is associated with increased probability of an ACS
   e. The coronary artery develops calcification late in plaque development and nearly always is associated with large plaque burden

13. What is the current accepted practice regarding Lp(a) risk stratification for CAD?

   a. It should be followed serially every 2–4 years to assess for increased risk
   b. It can be targeted by pharmacotherapy to yield reduction in morbidity above and beyond conventional risk factors
   c. An elevated level may prompt moving a patient into a higher risk category and treating to more aggressive LDL and BP goals
   d. The size of Lp(a) isoforms is directly related to its atherogenic potential

14. Which of the following is true about smoking and CV disease?

   a. Smokers have their first CV event approximately 10 years earlier than matched nonsmoking cohorts
   b. Mortality of smokers is 50% greater than nonsmokers and those who quit smoking immediately after a MI
   c. The magnitude of smoking cessation on reducing mortality if EF < 35% is similar to beta blockers and ICDs
   d. There is a dose–response curve between cessation counseling and sustained abstinence up to 8 sessions/300 minutes

For the remainder of the questions in this section, select the **one** best *answer.*

15. Response to which agent can be used to measure endothelial function?

   a. Methergine
   b. Ergonovine
   c. Acetylcholine
   d. Endothelin

16. Functional assessment of an intermediate coronary lesion can be performed by all of the following **except**:

   a. Measurement of coronary flow reserve
   b. Measurement of fractional flow reserve
   c. Quantitative coronary angiography

17. How do ACE inhibitors affect the bradykinin system?

   a. Increase degradation of bradykinin
   b. Decrease degradation of bradykinin
   c. Increase production of bradykinin
   d. Increase kallikrein production

18. NO regulates which of the following processes?

    a. Vasodilation
    b. Platelet aggregation
    c. Matrix synthesis
    d. Smooth muscle cell migration
    e. All of the above

19. The most potent vasoconstrictor is:

    a. Bradykinin
    b. Endothelin
    c. Acetylcholine
    d. PAI-1

20. The endothelium plays a role in which of the following?

    a. Regulation of blood flow
    b. Release of growth factors
    c. Regulation of thrombosis
    d. All of the above

21. Which of the following substances does not directly affect the microcirculation (i.e., arterioles, capillaries, venules)?

    a. Adenosine
    b. Papaverine
    c. NTG
    d. Nitroprusside

22. Atherosclerosis is associated with:

    a. Increase in circulating endothelin concentrations
    b. Increase in oxidative stress
    c. Decrease in NO activity
    d. All of the above

23. Coronary endothelial dysfunction is associated with:

    a. Future cardiac events
    b. Abnormal response to intracoronary adenosine
    c. Abnormal response to intracoronary NTG
    d. Abnormal response to IV Methergine

24. Which of the following substances **is not** an endothelium-dependent dilator?

    a. Acetylcholine
    b. Substance P
    c. Bradykinin
    d. NTG

25. Nitroprusside is an endothelial independent vasodilator. True or false?

    a. True
    b. False

26. All the following are obligate coronary vasodilators **except**:

    a. NTG
    b. NO
    c. Acetylcholine
    d. Hypoxia
    e. Hypercapnia

27. The risk of plaque disruption depends primarily on all of the following factors **except**:

    a. Severity of angiographic stenosis
    b. Plaque morphology
    c. Lipid content of the plaque
    d. Endothelial function

28. Plasma endothelin concentrations are increased in the following states:

    a. Heart failure
    b. Atherosclerosis
    c. Pulmonary HTN
    d. All of the above

29. NO (endothelium-derived relaxant factor) mediates its vasorelaxation effect through:

    a. Specific receptor on the endothelium
    b. Specific receptors on smooth muscle cells
    c. Direct effect on smooth muscle cells
    d. Decrease in intracellular calcium

30. Endothelin exerts its vasoconstriction through:

    a. Activation of cGMP
    b. Direct effect on smooth muscle cells
    c. Injuring the endothelium
    d. Specific endothelin receptors

31. Endothelial dysfunction is characterized by:

    a. Vasoconstriction to endothelial-dependent vasodilator substances
    b. Possible occurrence without significant CAD
    c. Possible causal link to smoking
    d. All of the above

32. Endothelial dysfunction may be reversed by:

    a. Lowering cholesterol
    b. Stent implantation
    c. Thrombolytic therapy
    d. NTG

33. The LDL NCEP goal for treatment of lipids in patients with known CAD or CAD risk equivalent is:

   a. < 190 mg/dL
   b. < 160 mg/dL
   c. < 130 mg/dL
   d. < 100 mg/dL
   e. < 80 mg/dL

34. Which of the following **is not** considered a CAD risk equivalent?

   a. Peripheral arterial disease
   b. Carotid arterial disease
   c. Diabetes
   d. AAA

35. The NCEP ATP-III goal for LDL in the treatment of hyperlipidemia in an asymptomatic patient with no or one risk factor is:

   a. <190 mg/dL
   b. <160 mg/dL
   c. <130 mg/dL
   d. <100 mg/dL
   e. <80 mg/dL

36. If two risk factors are present without CAD or equivalent, a patient can still be treated as a risk equivalent if their 10-year risk is greater than:

   a. >60%
   b. >40%
   c. >20%
   d. >10%
   e. <10%

37. Which of the following drugs would be first-line therapy for a patient without documented heart disease who has the following lipid profile:

   LDL: 138 mg/dL
   HDL: 20 mg/dL
   Triglycerides: 964 mg/dL

   a. Atorvastatin (Lipitor)
   b. Simvastatin (Zocor)
   c. Lovastatin (Mevacor)
   d. Gemfibrozil (Lopid)
   e. Fluvastatin (Lescol)

38. A 55-year-old man presents for risk evaluation. He has a history of HTN (well controlled on medication) and an AAA. He does not smoke, his HDL is 41 mg/dL, and there is no family history of premature CAD.

   His target LDL is:

   a. <160 mg/dL
   b. <130 mg/dL
   c. <100 mg/dL
   d. Unknown, need more information

39. A 50-year-old male lawyer is evaluated because of chest pain for the past 3 mos. His cholesterol level was "high" 1 yr ago. He is trying to follow a low-fat diet and to lose weight but has not had his cholesterol level rechecked. He has no history of DM, HTN, or tobacco use. His family history is unremarkable. He does not report any previous history of chest discomfort or MI. He describes his symptoms as a "central chest burning" that comes on when he is under stress in a courtroom or when he plays doubles tennis. The discomfort has never forced him to stop a courtroom argument or to interrupt his tennis game. In fact, he notes that it frequently resolved while he continued his activity. The discomfort sometimes lasts for an hour or more after he stops playing tennis. He has never taken NTG for this discomfort.

- Physical examination findings are normal
- BP is 130/70 mmHg
- HR is 68 bpm and regular
- ECG is normal

On the basis of this information, what is the probability that the patient has significant CAD?

a. 10%
b. 25%
c. 50%
d. 75%
e. 90%

40. All of the following statements regarding plasma homocysteine are true **except**:

a. Elevated levels increase the risk of atherosclerotic vascular disease
b. Interventions to lower homocysteine levels reduce mortality from CAD
c. Vitamin B12 deficiency tends to raise levels
d. Vitamin B6 and folic acid treatment lowers levels

41. In a 67-year-old man with CCS class II angina, a positive exercise test, normal LV function, and a smooth 70% left main lesion, CABG is indicated for:

a. Prevention of AMI
b. Prevention of CHF
c. Prolongation of life
d. Preservation of hibernating myocardium

42. In a cigarette smoker with a history of intermittent claudication and newly diagnosed HTN, a doubling of the serum creatinine concentration immediately after the addition of an ACE inhibitor suggests:

a. Hemodynamically significant bilateral renal artery stenosis
b. Pheochromocytoma
c. Primary aldosteronism
d. Emboli from arteriosclerosis obliterans of the descending aorta

43. You are asked to see a 53-year-old female dietitian in consultation for HTN. She was found to have an elevated BP on an FAA flight physical 4 yrs ago. She followed her physician's recommendations and uses only sodium substitutes, limits alcohol consumption, and exercises. She adopted a vegetarian lifestyle. Despite these measures, her BP remained above normal and her health care provider prescribed several medication regimens. However, her BP could not be maintained at <160/90 mmHg.

Her medications include:

Metoprolol: 25 mg twice daily
Lisinopril: 20 mg twice daily
Amlodipine: 10 mg daily

Your examination detects the following:

- BP: 188/100 mmHg (seated), 190/100 mmHg (standing); HR: 70 bpm sitting, 80 bpm standing
- Normal funduscopic examination
- Normal peripheral pulses and no abdominal bruits
- Normal cardiopulmonary examination

Of the following statements regarding the clinical presentation, which is correct?

a. The HTN is not "resistant" because the patient is not taking appropriate medications at their maximum doses
b. The absence of an abdominal bruit excludes renovascular HTN as the underlying diagnosis
c. The BP response to postural change suggests a state of low volume–high resistance HTN
d. The next step should be US assessment of renal arterial flow

44. The patient in Question 43 has continued medical therapy and improves somewhat with addition of triamterene/HCTZ (37.5/25 mg) daily. Her BP is now 160 mmHg systolic.

Laboratory results include:

CBC: Normal
Creatinine: 1.9 mg/dL
Sodium: 145 mEq/L
Potassium: 3.5 mEq/L
Uric acid: 3.0 mg/dL
ECG: LVH by voltage criteria
Chest X-ray: Normal

The most likely secondary form of HTN in this setting is:

a. Primary aldosteronism
b. Renovascular stenosis
c. Phenochromocytoma
d. Chronic renal failure

45. In the patient in Question 43, the diagnosis of primary aldosteronism requires each of the following **except:**

a. HTN
b. Hypokalemia (salt replete)
c. Increased 24-hr urinary aldosterone rate
d. Normal renal arteries
e. Suppressed plasma renin activity

46. In the patient in Question 43 the serum aldosterone concentration was 2 ng/dL (Normal: 1–21 ng/dL); which of the following substances might be playing a role in this patient's HTN?

    a. Alcohol
    b. Natural licorice
    c. Diuretic
    d. Premarin

47. Which of the following antihypertensive agents is contraindicated in women who are pregnant?

    a. Triamterene-containing diuretics
    b. Beta blockers
    c. Central alpha agonists
    d. ACE inhibitors

48. All of the following are associated with the syndrome of familial hypercholesterolemia **except**:

    a. Xanthomas
    b. Premature vascular disease
    c. X-linked inheritance
    d. Mutations of the LDL receptor

49. A 55-year-old previously athletic man presents with history of anterior wall MI, poorly controlled HTN, and daytime somnolence. He also has a history of PAF and was found to have elevated CRP. A modifiable risk factor for ischemic heart disease that should be further evaluated in this patient is:

    a. Obstructive sleep apnea
    b. Elevated homocysteine
    c. Elevated Lp(a)
    d. High sensitivity CRP level

50. The diet that has shown to decrease the risk for future CV events or death in patients after MI is:

    a. AHA Step 2 diet
    b. A very low fat diet ($<$10% of the total caloric intake)
    c. Mediterranean diet
    d. Atkins diet
    e. None of the above

51. A 35-year-old female presents for evaluation of chest pain. She describes "central chest pressure" that comes on when she is angry at her students or when she swims. The discomfort is accompanied by shortness of breath and is relieved within a few minutes by leaving the classroom or by rest. She denies any chest pain at rest or at night. She has never used NTG. She has no history of DM or HTN. She smokes one pack per day of cigarettes. She feels that she is overweight and is trying to follow a low-fat diet and to lose weight. Her cholesterol has never been checked. Her father died of an AMI at age 63.

    On physical exam, her BP is 120/70 mmHg and HR is 72 bpm and regular. Her cardiac exam is normal. Her resting ECG is normal.

51. (continued)

On the basis of this information, what is the probability that the patient has significant CAD?

a. 10%
b. 25%
c. 50%
d. 75%
e. 90%

52. In the above case, what is the preferred initial diagnostic test on this patient according to ACC/AHA practice guidelines?

a. TMET
b. Exercise MPI
c. Adenosine MPI
d. Exercise echocardiography
e. Dobutamine echocardiography

53. A 58-year-old male presents with a 15-min episode of central chest tightness with diaphoresis while watching TV, now resolved in the ED. His past medical history includes "borderline blood sugar," and femoral-popliteal peripheral arterial bypass. His family history is significant for a brother with MI at age 59. He is sedentary and is a former smoker (discontinued tobacco 6 months ago). He gained 15 pounds after quitting.

Medications:	Occasional Viagra, Atorvastatin, HCTZ
Exam:	BP 140/88 mmHg, pulse 86 regular; CV exam otherwise normal
ECG:	Nonspecific T abnormality; no comparison available
CXR:	Poor inspiration
Troponin T:	<0.01

The likelihood that his symptoms are due to CAD is:

a. Low
b. Intermediate
c. High

54. The risk of short-term death/MI for the patient described above is:

a. Low
b. Intermediate
c. High

55. A 49-year-old man who received a living-related donor kidney transplant 2 yrs ago is referred to you after an inferior MI that was successfully treated with thrombolysis. He currently has no limitation of his daily activities. His lipid profile is as follows:

Total cholesterol:	300 mg/dL
HDL:	45 mg/dL
LDL:	216 mg/dL
Triglycerides:	195 mg/dL
Glucose:	120 mg/dL
Lp(a):	8 mg/dL
Homocysteine:	8 μmol/L
Fibrinogen:	245 mg/dL

His renal allograft function is normal and he is maintained on prednisone, cyclosporine, and study drug B, a novel antilymphocyte agent.

Which of the following drugs is the best choice for this patient?

    a. Simvastatin

    b. Atorvastatin

    c. Niacin

    d. Pravastatin

    e. Fluvastatin

56. In the patient in Question 55, what would the target LDL cholesterol level be?

    a. 130 mg/dL

    b. 70 mg/dL

    c. 110 mg/dL

    d. 125 mg/dL

    e. 150 mg/dL

57. The patient in Question 55 undergoes exercise stress testing with contrast MPI. He completes stage 2 of a Bruce protocol limited by typical angina and fatigue. The baseline HR is 64 bpm with sinus rhythm and BP of 110/60 mmHg. The peak HR is 134 bpm with BP of 146/84 mmHg. ECG monitoring demonstrates nonspecific ST-T changes. Perfusion imaging demonstrates a large area of anterior and anterolateral ischemia and an inferior infarct. The next step would be to:

    a. Add a beta blocker

    b. Add nitrate therapy

    c. Initiate intensive glycemic control

    d. Order coronary arteriography

58. Increases of the serum fibrinogen value have been associated with an increased risk for development of CAD in some studies. Which of the commonly available lipid-lowering drugs has been consistently shown to **lower** the serum fibrinogen level?

    a. Atorvastatin (Lipitor)

    b. Simvastatin (Zocor)

    c. Lovastatin (Mevacor)

    d. Fenofibrate (TriCor)

    e. Gemfibrozil (Lopid)

59. Which of the following lipid-lowering agents may worsen glycemic control in patients with borderline fasting hyperglycemia?

    a. Simvastatin

    b. Atorvastatin

    c. Niacin

    d. Gemfibrozil

    e. None of the above

60. A 49-year-old chief executive officer of a Fortune 500 company presents to your CV health clinic as part of an executive physical examination program. He runs 15 miles 3 times per week, and was an Olympic athlete during his college years. He recently invested $50,000 in Heart Check America, and as part of the investment he received a complimentary coronary CT scan. He was told he had moderate calcifications in the proximal RCA, but that nothing further was needed at this time. He has a normal ECG, a normal thyroid profile, and no evidence of fasting hyperglycemia. His father died of heart disease at age 88, and his mother is alive at age 92. His lipid profile is as follows:

Total cholesterol:	260 mg/dL
HDL:	85 mg/dL
Triglycerides:	100 mg/dL
LDL:	155 mg/dL

Which of the following approaches to "preventive cardiology" is recommended by the AHA guidelines for this patient?

a. Reassure him that he is free of any CAD
b. Send him for an exercise thallium stress test
c. Start therapy with simvastatin, 40 mg nightly
d. Start therapy with niacin, 1 g daily

61. A 55-year-old father of 6 children is concerned about his lipid profile. His father and mother both died of MIs at age 51 and 58, respectively. He is healthy, does not smoke, and exercises daily by swimming for 45 min. He comes to you for counseling regarding primary prevention. He follows a low-fat diet but does not take any medications. His blood chemistry profile and BP are as follows:

Total cholesterol:	220 mg/dL
HDL:	65 mg/dL
Triglycerides:	125 mg/dL
LDL:	95 mg/dL
Glucose:	95 mg/dL
BP:	110/75 mmHg

Which of the following is appropriate for this patient and is supported by outcomes data?

a. Send him for exercise echocardiography
b. Send him for exercise thallium scanning
c. Prescribe Metoprolol, 25 mg twice daily; aspirin, 162 mg daily
d. Prescribe vitamin E, 400 IU daily; vitamin C, 500 mg daily; aspirin, 81 mg daily
e. Prescribe aspirin, 81 mg daily

62. A 44-year-old police officer was brought to the hospital with an out-of-hospital cardiac arrest due to an acute anterolateral MI. He had quit smoking the day before the acute infarction. He received tPA and "rescue" PTCA and stenting to the proximal LAD. His EF was 45% on the 5th day of hospitalization. One of your associates started therapy with atorvastatin, 10 mg nightly. He comes today for a 6-week examination after completion of cardiac rehabilitation.

He has lost 25 pounds and feels "great." His blood chemistry values and BP are as follows:

Total cholesterol:	165 mg/dL
Triglycerides:	85 mg/dL
HDL:	35 mg/dL
LDL:	113 mg/dL
Fibrinogen:	370 mg/dL
Glucose:	120 mg/dL
BP:	128/82 mmHg
Aspartate aminotransferase:	21 U/L

Which of the following recommendations do you implement in this patient's management?

a. Increase atorvastatin to 40 mg nightly
b. Switch to fluvastatin, 40 mg nightly
c. Add niacin, 500 mg twice a day
d. Arrange to recheck lipid and aspartate aminotransferase values in 3 months
e. Add fenofibrate, 145 mg daily

Answers

1. **Answer a.**
Collagen II is found largely in hyaline cartilage.

2. **Answer e.**
Mucopolysaccharide is secreted from glandular tissue. Endothelium is a layer of thin, specialized epithelium comprised of a single layer of squamous cells in healthy tissue.

3. **Answers a, b, c, d, and e.**

4. **Answers b and c.**
While there is research dedicated to elucidating novel receptors of platelet aggregation, the glycoprotein IIb/IIIa receptor is responsible for a large component of aggregation (as opposed to activation with thromboxane A2). In experiments of a porcine model lacking vWF, initial contact adhesion was not affected. However, activation of platelets was dependent on soluble vWF. It is thought that it is the soluble vWF that attaches to damaged and exposed subendothelium, slowing the platelets enough to allow attachment principally via the glycoprotein IIb/IIIa receptor.

5. **Answers a and c.**

6. **Answer b.**

7. **Answer a and b.**
Smooth muscle cells have a heterogeneity of origin including neurectoderm (neural crest) and mesoderm.

8. **Answers b, c, and d.**

9. **Answer a.**
Seminal work by Anitschkow in the 1920s and 1930s arrived at the hypothesis that circulating lipid accumulated and contributed to atherosclerotic "lipoids" in the plaque. This shaped the way for future investigation and research in targeting lipids in the prevention and treatment of coronary atherosclerosis.

10. **Answers a, b, and c.**

11. **Answers a, b, c, and e.**
Vulnerable plaques are often hemodynamically insignificant (<50%) until rupture and thrombosis causes abrupt flow limitation. It should be noted that vulnerable plaques also often fissure and rupture at the sides as the shear forces are elevated there as well.

11. (*continued*)

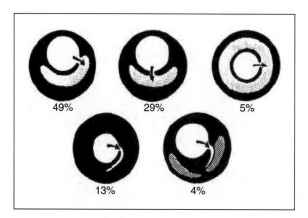

Frequency of sites of tearing in plaques experiencing plaque rupture. *Key: Stippling,* lipid pool; *solid,* fibrous tissue; *cross-hatching,* calcification.

12. Answers a and c.

Of note, in selected young patients presenting with acute atherothrombotic MI, there is little calcification around their vulnerable plaque. Hence, lack of calcification does not completely rule out vulnerable plaque, and presence or absence of calcium is therefore only a tool for risk stratification and should not supplant clinical decision making.

13. Answer c.

The third of the population with the highest Lp(a) levels have increased risk of future CV events. However, there are no specific therapies and it varies little over time. It may be useful to identify higher risk individuals who may benefit from more aggressive conventional risk factor modification.

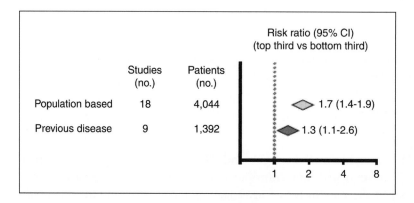

Risk ratios comparing top and bottom thirds of baseline Lp(a) measurements in perspective studies. Diamond symbols indicate the combined risk ratio and its 95% CI for each grouping.

14. Answers a, b, c, and d.

AHA guidelines recommend addressing smoking cessation at every follow up visit. The impact of smoking on CV disease is profound. Epidemiologic studies have found continued smoking after the first MI has a hazard ratio of 1.53 compared to nonsmokers and those who quit smoking during the index hospitalization (J Clin Epidem 2002; 55:654–664). A study of patients with LV EF < 35% by Suskin et al. (JACC 2001) found a 30% mortality reduction in ex-smokers compared to ongoing smokers. This was the same mortality benefit as metoprolol or spironolactone in these patients. It is similar to the benefit seen with ICD implantation in MADIT-II. There is also a known dose–response relationship between amount of counseling and rate of persistent cessation. [Patients can receive free telephone counseling and medications if they are uninsured through the North American Quitline Consortium (www. Naquitline.org).]

15. Answer c.
Acetycholine-mediated vasodilation depends on an intact and functional endothelium to produce NO for relaxation. Methergine is used as a provocative test for coronary spasm and is not used to measure the endothelial function.

16. Answer c.
Angiography only gives a visual estimate of stenosis and does not yield direct functional significance of an intermediate lesion.

17. Answer b.
Degradation of bradykinin relies on ACE. Inhibition with ACE inhibitor allows build-up of bradykinin, which likely mediates the "cough" found in some patients intolerant of ACE inhibitor.

18. Answer e.
All of the above

19. Answer b.
Endothelin is correct. Bradykinin is not a potent vasoconstrictor; acetylcholine mediates constriction if endothelium is denuded or dysfunctional (but not as potently as endothelin); PAI-1 is the main inhibitor of the serine proteases tPA and urokinase and prevents fibrinolysis.

20. Answer d.

21. Answer c.

22. Answer d.

23. Answer a.
Schachinger et al. (Circ 2000; 101:1899) found a significant relationship between endothelial dysfunction as tested by vasoconstriction upon acetylcholine administration and CV events.

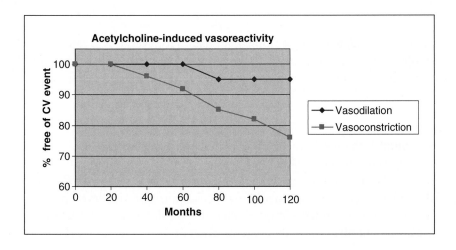

24. Answer d.

NO is released by administration of NTG and works directly on smooth muscle as it diffuses via the bloodstream.

25. Answer a.

True. Nitroprusside is a NO donor and works similar to NTG as an endothelial independent vasodilator.

26. Answer c.

All are known to cause vasodilatation. Only acetylcholine can be a vasoconstrictor if the endothelium is dysfunctional or absent and NO cannot be produced. In this case, it is not an obligate vasodilator.

27. Answer a.

28. Answer d.

29. Answer c.

30. Answer d.

The endothelin receptors are G-protein coupled receptors located on smooth muscle cells. Their role in proliferation and contraction of PA smooth muscle cells is the rationale behind their targeted antagonism with bosentan in pulmonary HTN.

31. Answer d.

32. Answer a.

33. Answer d.

NCEP/ATP III goal <70 mg/dL for "very high risk" individuals (ACS, early/aggressive CAD).

34. Answer b.

Carotid arterial disease must be **symptomatic** to be considered a CAD equivalent by ATP III guidelines. The other items are considered CAD equivalents.

35. Answer b.

The LDL goal is <160 mg/dL and the non-HDL goal is <190 mg/dL.

36. Answer c.

The 10-year risk is calculated using Framingham data. However, this is not a comprehensive model of risk. If, for example, the patient has significant risk of rapid progression due to XRT, it would be reasonable to treat to more aggressive therapeutic goals.

37. Answer d.

Gemfibrozil (Lopid) is the most potent triglyceride-lowering agent among the possible answers. Gemfibrozil reduces plasma triglycerides by 40% to 55%, usually within 1 mo of onset of therapy. Lovastatin and fluvastatin do not appreciably alter the plasma triglyceride values. Atorvastatin will lower plasma triglyceride levels by 25% to 35%, and simvastatin will usually lower plasma triglyceride values by 19% to 25% when used at dosages of 40 mg and 80 mg, respectively.

38. Answer c.

ATP-III guidelines categorize patients with AAA as "CAD risk equivalent" so target LDL is <100 mg/dL. If the patient did not have an abdominal aneurysm, he would have two risk factors: age >45 yr and treated HTN. His goal lipid in that case would depend on his 10-yr CV event risk.

39. Answer c.

The physician should estimate the probability of significant CAD in all patients presenting with chest pain. This patient's chest pain is substernal and provoked by exercise, but it is not consistently relieved by rest. Therefore, it meets the definition of atypical angina. A 50-year-old man with atypical angina has approximately a 50/50 chance of marked CAD. The presence of multiple risk factors may increase the likelihood. In this case, with a single risk factor, the best estimate of CAD is approximately 50%.

40. Answer b.

No trial has demonstrated a definite mortality benefit to lowering homocysteine levels.

41. Answer c.

42. Answer a.

Blockade of angiotensin II mediates afferent arteriolar tone; in the presence of hemodynamically significant bilateral renal artery stenosis it results in a decrease in glomerular filtration because the efferent arterial blood supply cannot increase.

43. Answer a.

JNC (VII) classifies HTN as resistant when it is inadequately controlled despite full doses of three appropriate drugs, ***including a diuretic***. The absence of a bruit does not exclude renal artery stenosis. This patient does not have a decrease in upright BP or reflex tachycardia to suggest volume depletion, although the beta blockade may be blunting this effect.

44. Answer a.

The serum potassium concentration of 3.5 mEq/L in the setting of ACE inhibition, triamterene therapy, and a diet with potassium supplementation (salt substitute) is inappropriately low and suggests a primary mineralocorticoid state like primary aldosteronism.

45. Answer d.

The presence or absence of normal renal arteries is irrelevant if the other four criteria are met.

46. Answer b.

Glycyrrhizic acid present in licorice inhibits the 11-beta-hydroxydehydrogenase enzyme that converts cortisol to its inactive metabolite, cortisone, creating a local "Cushing syndrome" at the level of the renal tubule.

47. Answer d.

ACE inhibitors have been associated with birth defects when used in treating pregnant women.

48. Answer c.

Familial hypercholesterolemia is inherited in an autosomal dominant fashion.

49. Answer a.

A patient need not be obese to have sleep-disordered breathing. It significantly impacts HTN control and mortality especially if patient has systolic dysfunction. The other risk factors are not easily modifiable for clinical effect.

50. Answer c.

The Lyon Diet Heart Study randomized 302 experimental- and 303 control-group subjects into the study. All were patients who had survived a first MI. Follow-up was approximately 46 months. The treatment group consumed a "Mediterranean diet" with the following characteristics:

- High in fruits, vegetables, bread and other cereals, potatoes, beans, nuts and seeds
- Includes olive oil as an important source of monounsaturated fat
- Dairy products, fish, and poultry consumed in low to moderate amounts, little red meat
- Eggs consumed 0 to 4 times weekly
- Wine consumed in low to moderate amounts
- Patients following the Mediterranean-style diet had a 50–70% lower risk of recurrent CAD. The risk was measured by three combinations of outcome measures:

    i.   Cardiac death and non-fatal MI
    ii. The above two plus major events (unstable angina, stroke, heart failure, and pulmonary or peripheral embolism)
    iii. All of these measures plus minor events that required hospitalization

51. Answer b.

52. Answer a.

53. Answer c.

Patient has CAD equivalent with his peripheral artery disease.

54. Answer b.

There are no TIMI high risk features like myocardial necrosis, dynamic T-wave abnormalities, or prior aspirin use.

55. Answer d.

Simvastatin, atorvastatin, and lovastatin are metabolized by the CYP3A4 enzyme. When given with cyclosporine the statin concentration can rise 20-fold and lead to rhabdomyolysis. Pravastatin is not significantly affected by CYP interactions. Fluvastatin is metabolized partly by CYP2C9 and can interact with warfarin and fluconazole.

56. Answer b.

The patient is young and already suffered an AMI. He should at least be treated to LDL goal <100 mg/dL with treatment to <70 mg/dL as a reasonable goal. Due to relative weak potency of pravastatin and his initially very elevated LDL, he may need additional pharmacotherapy such as ezetimibe for further reduction. While limited evidence exists, early reports suggest an approximately 15% increase in cyclosporine levels with co-administration of ezetimibe, so cyclosporine levels should be monitored during addition of these medications.

57. Answer d.

The recent COURAGE trial randomized patients to an initial strategy of intensive medical therapy alone vs. therapy utilizing PCI up front for angiographically defined lesions. It is important to note that all patients in that study had their anatomy defined by angiography first and up to 1/3 of patients eventually crossed over into the PCI arm. Analysis was performed with intention-to-treat.

Also, this patient should have his LV EF assessed, as patients with EF < 30% were excluded from that study.

Beta blocker therapy is indicated; however, the next most important step in management should be coronary arteriography to define the coronary anatomy and evaluate the potential for revascularization, especially in a patient with diabetes who may have decreased LV function.

58. Answer d.

Fenofibrate is a lipid-lowering agent that lowers the serum fibrinogen level approximately 15–25%. Some early reports suggested that atorvastatin may increase the serum fibrinogen level, but these reports were contradicted by later studies. Simvastatin, pravastatin, and fluvastatin have not been reported to increase the serum fibrinogen value. Gemfibrozil does not have potent fibrinogen lowering effects.

59. Answer c.

Niacin worsens fasting hyperglycemia in some patients. Gemfibrozil and simvastatin reduced coronary event rates (including death) in patients with non-insulin-dependent DM in the Helsinki Heart Study and Simvastatin Scandinavian Survival Study, respectively.

60. Answer c.

This patient has a high probability of having at least nonobstructive CAD, as documented by coronary calcification on his coronary CT scan. He is asymptomatic, and the degree of stenosis in the RCA is not quantified. He should be treated for secondary prevention of atherosclerotic heart disease and primary prevention of ischemic heart disease.

61. Answer e.

This patient does not have any evidence of ischemic heart disease or atherosclerotic heart disease. His LDL cholesterol value meets the guidelines of the AHA. Aspirin is the only other agent with proven outcomes data for this patient.

62. Answer a.

This patient has CAD, and the LDL cholesterol value does not meet target guidelines. This should be the primary treatment goal, with secondary goals taking reduced roles until the primary goal is achieved. Increasing the atorvastatin would most likely reduce the LDL cholesterol further and may have mild benefit to the HDL profile. Switching to fluvastatin would most likely provide less effective control of the LDL cholesterol than the current dose of atorvastatin. Adding niacin might worsen the glucose intolerance that is present in this patient. Rechecking the lipid and aspartate aminotransferase values in 3 mos is a good idea after the atorvastatin dosage is doubled. A recent (2006) update to secondary prevention recommends LDL < 100 mg/dL and for "very high risk" patients an optional goal of <70 mg/dL is "reasonable." With this patient's early presentation of ischemic heart disease, aggressive risk factor modification is warranted. Fenofibrate may reduce the fibrinogen level, but once again, it is not a well-defined treatment goal and should be secondary to LDL lowering at this time.

SECTION III

Cardiac Catheterization and Intervention

Charles X. Kim, MD

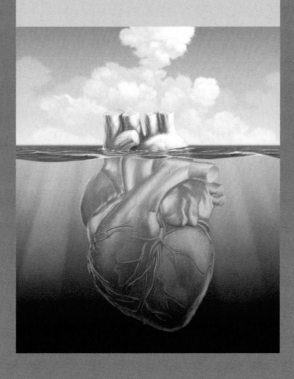

Questions

1. A patient is brought to the catheterization laboratory for evaluation of the severity of MR. A left ventriculogram shows an end-diastolic volume of 150 mL and end-systolic volume of 50 mL. At a rate of 80 bpm, the CO by the Fick method is 6.4 L/min. The calculated regurgitant fraction is:

   a. 20%
   b. 40%
   c. 60%
   d. 80%
   e. 100%

2. A patient is brought to the catheterization laboratory for evaluation of the severity of MS. Calculated using simultaneous measurements of PCWP and LV pressure, the mean diastolic transmitral gradient is 9 mmHg at a HR of 60 bpm and a diastolic filling period of 0.450 sec. The CO by the Fick method is 3.0 L/min. The calculated MVA is approximately:

   a. $0.5\,cm^2$
   b. $1.0\,cm^2$
   c. $1.5\,cm^2$
   d. $2.0\,cm^2$
   e. Insufficient data to calculate the MVA

3. At the time of cardiac catheterization, a patient has a mean aortic valve gradient of 64 mmHg and a CO by the Fick method of 4 L/min. Severe AR is also present. Which of the following is true?

   a. A TCO would give a more accurate AVA
   b. The calculated AVA is lower than the actual AVA
   c. Doppler AVA by continuity equation is less accurate than catheterization
   d. The AR should not affect the calculated AVA
   e. The calculated AVA is $2.0\,cm^2$

4. For assessing the cause of arterial desaturation, which of the following is **not** useful?

   a. Double-sampling dye curves
   b. Repeat determination of the saturation after administration of 100% O_2
   c. Pulmonary vein saturation
   d. Single-sampling dye curve: RA to FA
   e. Saline contrast injection under two-dimensional echocardiography

Answers to this section start on page 97.

5. A patient has a dip-and-plateau pattern in the RV and LV pressure curves with elevation and end-diastolic equalization of the pressures in the LV and RV. Which of the following may be present?

    a. Constrictive pericarditis
    b. Amyloid heart disease
    c. RV infarction
    d. Severe TR
    e. All of the above

6. For the following tracing, what intervention was instituted at time point #2?

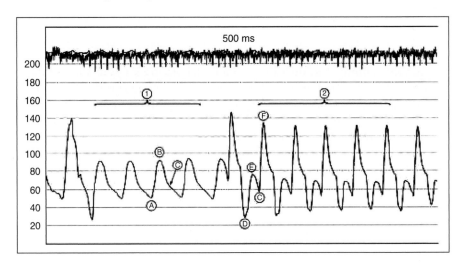

    a. Dobutamine infusion
    b. LVAD activation
    c. RV apical electronic pacemaker
    d. Intra-aortic balloon counterpulsation
    e. Pericardiocentesis

7. What is the diagnosis from the pressure tracing below?

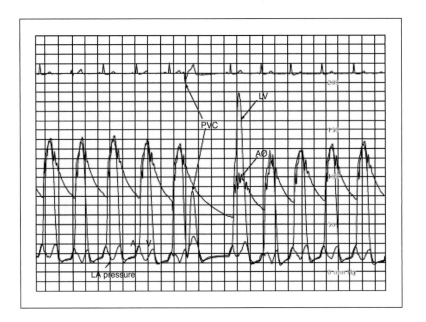

   a. Severe aortic valve stenosis
   b. Severe aortic valve regurgitation
   c. Subaortic stenosis
   d. HCM

8. These are baseline and exercise tracings of a patient with a valvulopathy. Which valve is involved and what is the mechanism?

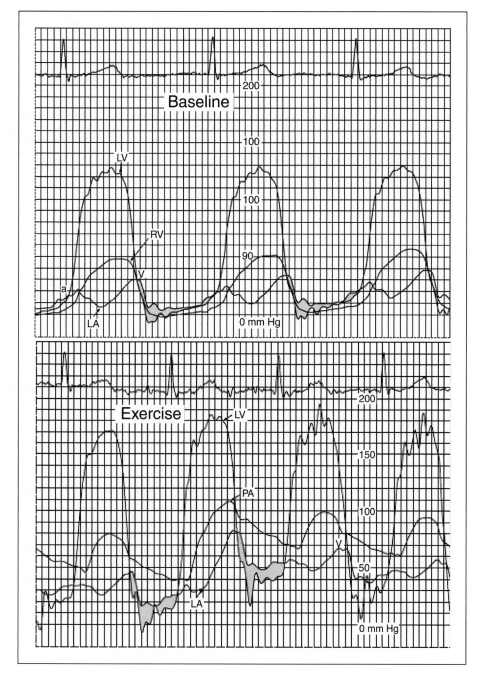

   a. AS
   b. AR
   c. MS
   d. MR
   e. Pulmonic stenosis

9. What is the diagnosis from the pressure tracing below?

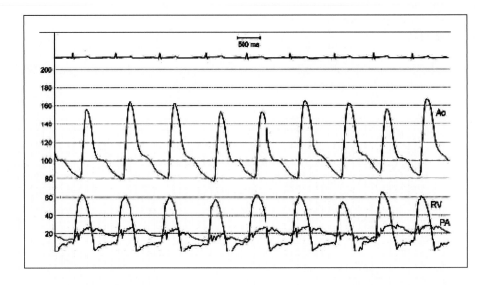

a. TR
b. Tricuspid stenosis
c. Pulmonic regurgitation
d. Pulmonic stenosis

10. What is the diagnosis from the pressure tracing below?

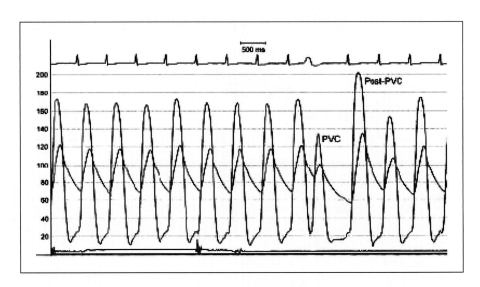

a. HCM
b. AS
c. Coarctation of the aorta
d. AR
e. AS plus AR

11. What is the diagnosis from the ECG and pressure tracing below?

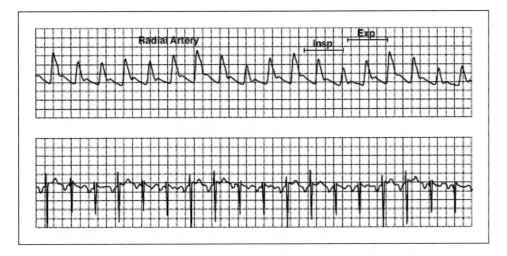

    a. Constrictive pericarditis
    b. Restrictive cardiomyopathy
    c. Ischemic cardiomyopathy
    d. Pericardial tamponade

12. What is the diagnosis from the pressure tracing below?

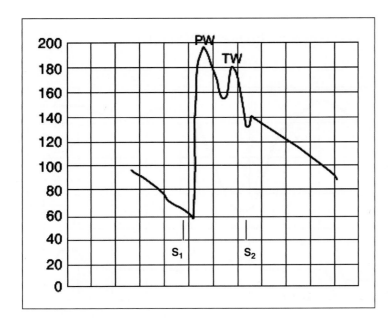

    a. Severe AR
    b. Severe AS
    c. HCM
    d. Severe LV systolic dysfunction

13. What is the diagnosis from the pressure tracing below?

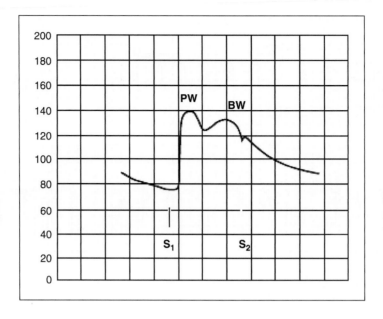

    a. Severe AR
    b. Severe AS
    c. HCM
    d. Severe LV systolic dysfunction

14. What is the diagnosis from the RA pressure tracing below?

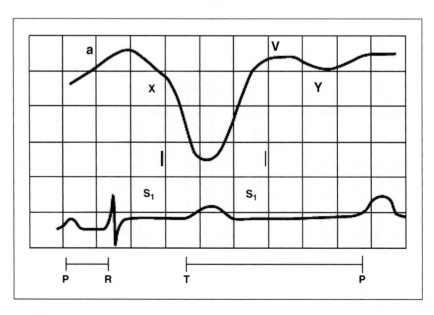

    a. TR
    b. Pericardial tamponade
    c. Constrictive pericarditis
    d. Restrictive cardiomyopathy

15. What is the predominant valvulopathy from the PCWP tracing below?

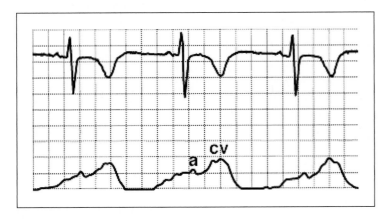

a. Pulmonary HTN
b. TR
c. MR
d. MS

16. LV pressure-volume curves are used to define LV passive diastolic properties. A shift of the pressure-volume curve to the left indicates:

a. A decrease in LV operating chamber compliance
b. An increase in LV operating chamber compliance
c. No changes in operating chamber compliance
d. Curves do not shift in most cardiac disease states

17. A 45-year-old woman presents with DOE and paroxysmal AF. She has a fixed split S2 on exam with a 2/6 SEM at the LSB. Echocardiogram shows:

■ Dilated RV and RA, normal LV
■ Secundum ASD
■ PA systolic, 70 mmHg

The following are found at catheterization:

■ Saturations (%): IVC, 70; SVC, 67; RA, 82; RV, 87; PA, 88; LV, 98; aorta, 98; FA, 98
■ Pressures (mmHg): PA, 70/50; FA, 120/70; PCWP, 10
■ TCO, 6.0 L/min

What is the Qp/Qs?

a. 1.5:1.0
b. 2.0:1.0
c. 2.5:1.0
d. 3.0:1.0
e. Need more information

18. A 77-year-old man presents with increasing symptoms of dyspnea and chest discomfort on exertion over the past 6 mos. He had two episodes of near syncope while climbing stairs. No prior cardiac history.

    ■ BP 130/50 mmHg and pulse 70 bpm
    ■ JVP normal and 2+ carotid delay
    ■ LV sustained and displaced; S4 present
    ■ 2/6 SEM at the base with mid peak
    ■ 2/6 diastolic decrescendo murmur

    Echocardiography

    ■ Moderately dilated LV cavity size
    ■ Mild LVH
    ■ Mild LA enlargement
    ■ Aortic valve calcified
    ■ Mean aortic valve gradient 25 mmHg
    ■ AR probably mild

    What would you do now?

    a. TEE
    b. Coronaries then AVR
    c. TMET
    d. Cardiac catheterization with arterial-venous gradient, CO, root, and coronary angiography
    e. Medical observation

19. The above patient goes to catheterization and the following values are obtained:

    ■ LV 170/10–15 mmHg, aorta 120/50 mmHg, HR 70 bpm
    ■ Mean aortic valve gradient 51 mmHg, SEP 250 msec
    ■ TCO 3.5 L/min, PA saturation 65%
    ■ Normal coronary arteries
    ■ Aortic root—LV fills to same density as root in 4 beats

    What is the calculated AVA?

    a. 0.2 cm^2
    b. 0.5 cm^2
    c. 0.9 cm^2
    d. 1.3 cm^2

20. What can be said about the calculated AVA in the patient in Question 19?

    a. It accurately represents the true AVA
    b. It is smaller than the true AVA
    c. It is larger than the true AVA

21. The LV fills to the same density of the root at 3 to 4 beats.

    What is the severity of AR in the patient in Question 19?

    a. 1+
    b. 2+
    c. 3+
    d. 4+

22. A 45-year-old man with a diagnosis of a severe restrictive cardiomyopathy comes to you for consideration of cardiac transplantation.

   ■ ECG shows low voltage and AF
   ■ Echo shows normal LV size and function and severe biatrial enlargement with moderate MR and TR
   ■ Cardiac catheterization reveals the following:

   PA 60/40 mmHg, mean PAP 50 mmHg, PCWP 20 mmHg (sat 90%)
   TCO = 7.2 L/min
   Saturations (%): SVC 52, IVC 54, RA 53, PA 53, LV and aorta 98
   Hb 14.0 g/dL
   HR 95 bpm, BP 105/70 mmHg, BSA 2.0 m^2

What is the pulmonary arteriolar resistance?

   a. 5.0 Wood units m^2
   b. 7.5 Wood units m^2
   c. 10.0 Wood units m^2
   d. 15.0 Wood units m^2
   e. Need more information

23. In the patient in question 22, you obtain an O$_2$ consumption of 260 mL/min.

   CO by simplified Fick equation:

   $$VO_2/[1.34 \times Hgb \times (FA - PA)] = CO$$

   $$260 \text{ mL/min} / \{10 \text{ dL/L} [1.34 \text{ mL/g} \times 14 \text{ g/dL} \times (0.98 - 0.53)]\} = 3.1 \text{ L/min}$$

What is the pulmonary arteriolar resistance?

   a. 2.5 Wood units $\times$ m^2
   b. 5.0 Wood units $\times$ m^2
   c. 10 Wood units $\times$ m^2
   d. 20 Wood units $\times$ m^2

24. In patients with known stable CAD, which of the following statements is **not** true?
   a. Death and MI can be prevented by percutaneous revascularization
   b. MI can be prevented and LV function preserved with CABG surgery
   c. In nondiabetic patients, CABG surgery and percutaneous revascularization have similar rates of subsequent death, MI, and subsequent revascularization
   d. Improved survival is observed after CABG (compared to medical therapy) for patients with three-vessel disease and either LV dysfunction or class III to IV symptoms

25. The physiological significance of the coronary artery lesion can be assessed in the cardiac catheterization laboratory by:
   a. Quantitative coronary angiography
   b. Intravascular US
   c. Coronary flow reserve to intracoronary adenosine
   d. Response to IV Methergine

26. Well-accepted indications for coronary angiography in patients with recent MI include all of the following **except:**

    a. Angina while walking in the hospital hallway on day 4 post-STEMI
    b. Angina on a submaximal TMET on day 5
    c. Before mitral valve surgery for severe MR
    d. NSTEMI
    e. All of the above are acceptable indications for angiography

27. Among patients with class II angina and one- or two-vessel disease, PCI is indicated for which of the following?

    a. To prevent progression of CAD
    b. Prevention of MI
    c. To alleviate asymptomatic ischemia
    d. To improve symptoms
    e. Prevention of death

28. Rotational atherectomy is contraindicated in which settings:

    a. Bifurcation lesions
    b. Saphenous vein grafts
    c. Heavily calcified lesions
    d. Insulin-dependent diabetes

29. A 58-year-old man presents with atypical chest pain. Coronary angiography reveals a 60% diameter stenosis in the mid-LAD coronary artery. Which of the following intracoronary US or Doppler measurements is the most sensitive for determining if this intermediate stenosis is hemodynamically significant?

    a. Luminal area
    b. Proximal-to-distal velocity ratio
    c. Coronary flow reserve
    d. Percent plaque area in the stenosis
    e. Absolute coronary flow

30. A 78-year-old diabetic male is referred to your clinic for preoperative evaluation prior to left knee replacement. He currently can only walk 1 to 2 blocks before stopping, but he is limited by knee pain and denies angina or shortness of breath. He has an adenosine sestamibi stress test that demonstrates a small area of ischemia at the apex. He did not note any discomfort during the test. He is currently on 81 mg aspirin daily and has adequate beta blockade with metoprolol.

    His vitals are:

HR:	62 bpm
BP:	118/70 mmHg
Lipids:	LDL 68 mg/dL, HDL 45 mg/dL, TG 98 mg/dL

    Your next step is:

    a. Advise patient to postpone surgery for further diagnostic testing
    b. Proceed to coronary angiogram to define the anatomy
    c. Proceed to coronary angiogram to perform PCI on the LAD
    d. Increase aspirin to 325 mg daily and continue beta blocker
    e. Tell patient that nothing further is needed at this time and he should continue his current medical regimen

31. A 62-year-old executive presents for physical examination. He is completely asymptomatic and leads a relatively sedentary life style, playing golf twice per week. His past medical history is significant for chronic mild HTN and hyper-lipidemia, and he is overweight. He does have a positive family history for early CAD in his father. His current medications include hydroclorothiazide.

On physical examination he is found to have a BP of 150/90 mmHg and a HR of 82 bpm. JVP is normal. Carotid upstrokes are normal without bruits. The lungs are clear to auscultation. The heart has a regular rate and rhythm. S1 and S2 are normal. An S4 is present. No murmurs are appreciated. The apical impulse is in normal location and of normal quality. The abdomen is soft with no masses or bruits. The extremities have no clubbing, cyanosis, or edema, and the periph-eral pulses are normal.

Chest X-ray is unremarkable. The resting ECG is normal. His total cholesterol is 252 mg/dL, LDL cholesterol 142 mg/dL, HDL 38 mg/dL, TG 160 mg/dL.

The next best step is:

a. Coronary angiography
b. TMET to diagnose the presence of CAD
c. Begin therapy with antihypertensive, cholesterol-lowering medications, and aspirin therapy
d. Imaging stress test to define the presence of CAD
e. Resting echocardiography to define LV systolic function

32. Over the next 12 months the patient in Question 31 notes classic anginal symp-toms with exertion. These are noted when he climbs the 3 flights of stairs to his office daily. The symptoms are relieved with 1 min of rest at the top of the stairs. He is currently taking atenolol, 50 mg daily; aspirin, 325 mg daily; and pravas-tatin, 20 mg daily. His physical examination is unchanged.

Which of the following does **not** lower risk for subsequent death or MI?

a. Percutaneous revascularization
b. Lipid lowering to an LDL of <100 mg/dL if the current value is >130 mg/dL
c. Lowering LDL to <100 mg/dL if the current value is between 100 and 129 mg/dL
d. Exercise training program

33. A 67-year-old farmer presents with 3 days of intermittent chest pressure and dys-pnea with minimal exertion. He had one episode of nocturnal dyspnea 3 days prior. He is currently asymptomatic. His past medical history includes HTN and hyperlipidemia. He is currently medicated with metoprolol 25 mg twice daily and aspirin 325 mg daily.

On physical examination his BP is 140/85 mmHg and his HR is 76 bpm and regular. His JVP is normal. His carotid upstrokes are normal and without bruits. His lungs are clear to auscultation. His heart has a regular rate and rhythm. The apical impulse is in the normal location and of normal quality. The first and sec-ond heart sounds are normal. There are no murmurs or gallops appreciated. The abdomen is soft with no masses or bruits. The extremities have no clubbing, cyanosis, or edema, and the peripheral pulses are normal.

The ECG shows nonspecific ST-T wave changes without frank elevation or depression. The chest X-ray is interpreted as normal. CBC, electrolytes, and cardiac biomarkers are all negative.

33. (*continued*)

The next best step is:

a. Increase beta blockade and add nitrates, followed by noninvasive stress testing
b. Diagnostic coronary angiography with possible percutaneous revascularization
c. Pharmacologic stress testing
d. Start therapy with tirofiban 0.1 mcg/kg/min
e. Either a or b

34. After appropriate diagnostic workup and medical therapy are commenced, the patient in Question 33 is found to have a 95% stenosis in the middle LAD coronary artery. This was successfully treated with an intracoronary bare metal stent.

With regard to this patient:

a. There is a 4% to 6% risk of in-stent restenosis over the next 6 mos
b. Aspirin 81 mg plus warfarin adjusted to an INR of 2.0 to 2.5 should be commenced
c. Aspirin 325 mg and clopidogrel 75 mg daily should be commenced
d. Noninvasive stress testing is required at 3 to 6 mos following the percutaneous procedure regardless of the patient's symptom status

35. One year later the patient in Question 33 is in need of cholecystectomy. He remains asymptomatic. The surgeon arranged for a TMET before you visited with the patient. The patient exercised to an equivalent of 9.0 METS with a normal HR and BP response. The ECG was interpreted as nondiagnostic (<1 mm of upsloping ST depression) at peak exercise and resolved by 3 min into recovery.

At this point, which of the following is true?

a. Repeat coronary angiography and possible coronary revascularization will improve the patient's operative outcome
b. Repeat stress testing was not necessary at this point in time as the patient was active and asymptomatic
c. The operation should be postponed until an imaging stress test can be obtained
d. You should recommend IV beta blockers and IV NTG with PA catheter monitoring and to proceed with the cholecystectomy

36. A 53-year-old man with limited CAD risk factors presents with a 6-month history of DOE and exertional chest fullness. He has had orthopnea and an episode of paroxysmal nocturnal dyspnea. He has a very significant alcoholic history.

- ECG: Nonspecific ST abnormalities
- Echocardiography: Moderately dilated LV; EF 25%; global hypokinesis

The next step in diagnostic evaluation should be:

a. Exercise MUGA scanning
b. Stress test with measurement of maximal O_2 consumption
c. Coronary angiography
d. Transplant consultation

37. A 58-year-old man with multiple CAD risk factors presents with a 1-year history of DOE and exertional chest pressure. He has had orthopnea and an episode of paroxysmal nocturnal dyspnea.

   ■ Laboratory findings: serum potassium 4.5; creatinine 3.2
   ■ ECG shows nonspecific ST abnormalities
   ■ Echocardiography shows a mildly dilated LV; EF 25% to 30%; global hypokinesis
   ■ Coronary angiography shows an 80% stenosis of proximal LAD, 85% proximal LFX, 90% mid-RCA; distal vessels are good caliber

   The appropriate next step includes:

   a. Surgical consultation for CABG
   b. Rest thallium test with delayed imaging
   c. Initiation of spironolactone therapy
   d. All of the above

38. Which of the following is **incorrect** regarding a patient who has had an anaphylactoid reaction to a contrast agent in the past?

   a. The patient is at increased risk for a second anaphylactoid reaction if exposed again to a contrast agent
   b. The likelihood of a second anaphylactoid reaction can be reduced by the use of a low osmolar contrast agent
   c. The likelihood of a second anaphylactoid reaction can be reduced by the administration of corticosteroids before the second procedure
   d. May have been exposed to NPH insulin in the past, because NPH insulin increases the likelihood of an anaphylactoid contrast reaction

39. Most coronary artery anomalies:

   a. Are clinically significant
   b. Are abnormal fistula connections between the coronary arteries and other cardiac structures
   c. Are identified in children
   d. Must be visualized by the angiographer

40. Ventriculography:

   a. Must be performed in the LAO view in addition to the RAO view to visualize the posterior portion of the LV
   b. Can be used to quantify MR and AR
   c. Is associated with a significantly higher risk of complications than coronary angiography
   d. Permits the accurate and reproducible assessment of both MR and LV wall motion

41. A 74-year-old man with diabetic nephropathy is seeing you in clinic on Friday in preparation for his scheduled coronary angiogram on Monday. He currently takes NPH insulin, metformin, lisinopril, furosimide, and aspirin. On physical exam he is euvolemic. Which of these medications should he stop prior to his angiogram?

    a. NPH insulin
    b. Metformin
    c. Lisinopril
    d. Furosimide
    e. Aspirin

42. In comparison to balloon angioplasty the major benefit of elective coronary artery stenting is:

    a. Prevention of death
    b. Prevention of death/MI
    c. Reducing the need for further procedures
    d. Reducing length of stay and hospital costs

43. Reduction of restenosis by bare metal stents when compared to balloon angioplasty results from all of the following mechanisms **except:**

    a. Reduced neointimal proliferation
    b. Reduced residual stenosis
    c. Reduced elastic recoil
    d. "Tacking up" of the dissection flaps and improved blood rheology

44. Abrupt closure following coronary angioplasty:

    a. Is more common in men than women
    b. Is reduced in high risk patients pretreated with abciximab (Reopro)
    c. Occurs most frequently in LAD lesions
    d. Occurs less frequently with directional atherectomy in comparison to balloon angioplasty

45. Which of the following is characteristic of a type C lesion?

    a. Angulated segments > 60 degrees
    b. Discrete
    c. Proximal lesion with large amount of myocardium at risk
    d. Vein grafts

46. A 71-year-old male was admitted to the hospital with unstable angina. The ECG demonstrated anterolateral ST depression, and cardiac enzymes revealed a mild increase in total CK and the CK-MB fraction. Because of continued angina, the patient was taken to the catheterization lab and coronary angioplasty was performed.

    Which of the following agents would be **least** beneficial to the patient in terms of short-term clinical outcome?

    a. tPA
    b. Aspirin
    c. Abciximab (Reopro)
    d. Heparin

47. In the (SIRIUS) Sirolimus-coated stent in treatment of de novo coronary artery lesions trial, what was the target vessel revascularization rate for the sirolimus-eluting stent at 9 months?

a. 0%

b. 4%

c. 8%

d. 16%

48. Which of the following factors is the most important in terms of reducing the incidence of late stent thrombosis with DESs?

a. Pretreatment with abciximab

b. Optimal stent deployment (complete apposition of stent with vessel wall)

c. The introduction of more potent antiplatelet agents (eg, ticlopidine, clopidogrel)

d. Aggressive anticoagulation with warfarin and aspirin

49. A 63-year-old male presents with symptoms of progressive angina pectoris. Coronary angiography is performed and reveals a high grade, heavily calcified, eccentric lesion in the mid LAD. Which of the following interventional approaches would be associated with the best initial outcome?

a. Balloon angioplasty

b. Directional atherectomy

c. Excimer laser angioplasty

d. Rotational atherectomy

50. A 45-year-old male who received bare metal stent to LAD 1 yr ago is found to have exertional angina and a markedly positive exercise stress test. He undergoes angiography and has this LAO caudal view:

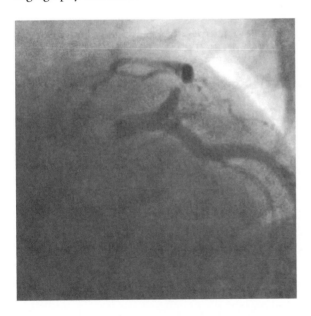

Initial attempt at dilation with PTCA is only partially successful, with 40% residual in-stent stenosis. What is the next step in management?

a. Aggressive medical therapy with high dose statin and lifelong dual antiplatelet therapy

b. LIMA to LAD coronary bypass surgery

c. Brachytherapy to lesion

d. Directional atherectomy

e. DES placement

*The following questions pertain to **chronic CAD only**.*

Note: The following questions may have more than one correct answer.

51. In patients with stable CAD, CABG has been shown to improve survival in which of the following anatomical subgroups?

    a. Left main artery disease
    b. Three-vessel disease
    c. Two-vessel disease with normal LV EF
    d. One-vessel disease, except for the main LCA or proximal LAD

52. In the CABG pooling project, the odds ratio for death over long-term follow-up (CABG versus medical treatment) was almost identical for patients who had normal and abnormal LV EF; however, CABG is thought to have greater benefit in patients with LV dysfunction. Possible reasons for this include:

    a. The higher absolute risk of death while receiving medical treatment
    b. Because of small sample sizes, improvement in mortality with CABG could not be detected among patients with normal LV EF in individual trials
    c. In the Coronary Artery Surgery Study, CABG was initially shown to have a survival advantage for patients with three-vessel disease and LV dysfunction
    d. All survival curves converge with time

53. Of the three major CABG versus medical therapy trials, which of the following showed an *overall* survival benefit for CABG?

    a. CASS
    b. ECSS
    c. VA multicenter study

54. At the time of the CABG versus medical therapy randomized trials, which of the following medical therapies were widely used for CAD?

    a. Aspirin
    b. Beta blockers
    c. HMG CoA reductase inhibitor
    d. Calcium channel blockers
    e. Nitrates
    f. Clopidogrel

55. In the historic CABG versus medical therapy trials, which of the following subgroups were well represented?

    a. Females
    b. Patients older than 65 years
    c. Patients with an EF $< 35\%$
    d. Asymptomatic patients
    e. Patients with a previous infarction
    f. Smokers
    g. Patients with HTN

56. Because numerous technological advances in CABG have occurred since these randomized trials, which of the following statements can be expected to be true?

   a. CABG would be even more efficacious if trials were repeated today
   b. CABG in fact would be less efficacious because medical therapy has improved as well
   c. Because medical therapy has improved markedly, a much larger number of patients would be necessary to show a survival benefit, if any, for CABG

57. Which of the following statements are true for PTCA versus CABG trials for multivessel disease?

   a. In comparison with the older CABG versus medical therapy trials, patients of equivalent risk were enrolled in more recent trials
   b. They showed that overall survival was better after CABG
   c. They showed survival was better after CABG only in the diabetic subgroup
   d. Repeat procedures were necessary more often after PTCA
   e. Although relief of angina was initially superior after CABG, the differences diminish with time
   f. Because of the risk of perioperative infarction, PTCA was superior to CABG in preventing MI

58. In patients with stable CAD, CABG has been shown to improve survival in which of the following anatomical subgroups?

   a. Left main or three-vessel disease
   b. "Left main equivalent"; ie, stenosis of at least 50% of both the LAD and circumflex coronary arteries proximal to their major branches
   c. RCA + LCX disease with normal LV function
   d. One-vessel disease (excluding left main or proximal LAD)

59. You are counseling a 56-year-old euglycemic man with class III angina, two-vessel CAD, and normal LV function.

   Which of the following statements are true for PTCA versus CABG for multivessel disease?

   a. Angina relief is equivalent
   b. Mortality rates were lower after CABG
   c. Repeat procedures were necessary more often after PTCA
   d. Because of the risk of perioperative infarction, PTCA was superior to CABG in preventing MI

Answers

1. Answer a.

For MR, the RF is the percentage of the total amount of blood ejected by the LV which goes back into the LA. The RF is the regurgitant volume divided by the total amount of blood the ventricle ejects in one beat (TV). TV is derived from the left ventriculogram by subtracting the end systolic volume from the end diastolic volume. The FFV is the amount of blood the ventricle ejects out the aortic valve and is equal to the systemic flow. Thus, this FFV is obtained from the Fick equation. The regurgitant volume is the TV minus the FFV.

TV = End-diastolic volume − End-systolic volume (from left ventriculography)
FFV = CO/HR
Regurgitant Volume = TV − FFV
RF = Regurgitant volume/Total ventricular volume

TV = 150 mL − 50 mL = 100 mL
FFV = 6400 mL/min / 80 bpm = 80 mL
Regurgitant Volume = 100 mL − 80 mL = 20 mL
RF = 20/100 = 0.2 = 20%

2. Answer b.

Using the Gorlin equation:

"Discharge coefficient" for mitral valves = $37.7 \, cm/(sec \times \sqrt{mmHg})$
This is $0.85 \times$ the discharge coefficient of aortic valves (44.3) = 37.7

Area = Flow/$[37.7 \times \sqrt{(\Delta P)}]$
ΔP = Mean diastolic pressure gradient between the LA and LV
Mitral flow = $1000 \times CO/(HR \times diastolic \, filling \, period)$
Mitral flow = $1000 \, mL/L \times 3 \, L/min/(60 \, bpm \times 0.450 \, sec/beat)$ =
            $111 \, mL/sec = 111 \, cm^3/sec$
Area = $111 \, cm^3/sec \, / \, \{[37.7 cm/(sec \times \sqrt{mmHg})] \times \sqrt{(9 \, mmHg)}\} = 0.98 \, cm^2$

3. Answer b.

In severe concomitant AR, both the Fick and thermodilution methods underestimate aortic flow, yielding an underestimate of the AVA.

4. Answer a.

The double-sampling dye curve is used in assessing L-to-R shunts and involves injecting dye into the pulmonary trunk and simultaneously sampling in the ascending aorta and RV. If L-to-R shunt, RV dye will appear early. The other answer choices may be used to determine R-to-L shunts.

5. Answer a.

The dip-and-plateau pattern and equalization of end-diastolic pressures are not specific for constrictive pericarditis and should be interpreted in the appropriate clinical context.

5. (*continued*)

Specifically, discriminating between constrictive pericarditis and restrictive cardiomyopathy is subtle, but can be determined by discordance of the RV systolic pressure and LV systolic pressure with respiration, and variation in gradient between early LV diastolic pressure and PCWP during inspiration when compared with expiration >5 mmHg.

6. Answer d.

This aortic pressure tracing (*see page 80*) shows the aortic contours before (*1*) and after (*2*) application of 1:1 intra-aortic balloon counterpulsation. Before balloon counterpulsation (*1*), the unassisted aortic end-diastolic pressure (*A*), unassisted systolic pressure (*B*), and dicrotic notch (*C*) can be seen. After initiation of balloon counterpulsation (*2*), the aortic end-diastolic pressure (*D*) and systolic pressure (*E*) are reduced as a result of decreased afterload; this results in decreased myocardial oxygen demand. Simultaneously the aortic diastolic pressure (*F*) is augmented resulting in increased myocardial perfusion, since most of coronary arterial flow occurs during diastole.

7. Answer d.

This is the *Brockenbrough sign* in HCM (*see page 80*). The post-extrasystolic behavior of a gradient across the aortic outflow tract can differentiate between a fixed and a dynamic obstruction. In a patient with HCM, the post-extrasystolic beat develops more severe obstruction, with a marked increase in gradient and decrease in aortic pressure (Ao). This feature is characteristic of dynamic LVOT obstruction. In fixed obstructions such as AS (in the presence of normal LV function), the gradient increases with the increase in stroke volume but not to the extent that occurs in HCM. Also, the aortic pulse pressure should increase. This patient demonstrates an increased gradient for several beats after a PVC before it returns to baseline. Also, the dynamic nature of the gradient with beat-to-beat variation should be noted. Note the decrease in the aortic pulse pressure in the post-extrasystolic beat along with the increase in the LV systolic pressure.

8. Answer c.

The shaded area (*see page 81*) is the pressure gradient across the mitral valve. It is mild at rest, but increases significantly with exercise and is associated with increased right heart pressures.

9. Answer d.

Note the gradient of ~40 mmHg from RV systolic and PA pressures (*see page 82*).

10. Answer b.

By the difference in systolic and diastolic pressures, the tracings (*see page 82*) are identified as aortic and LV pressures. Note that the post-PVC aortic pressure is increased as contrasted to the reduced systemic pressure post-PVC in HCM.

11. Answer d.

The marked respiratory variation could be consistent with constriction, restriction, or tamponade (*see page 83*). With restrictive cardiomyopathy from infiltrative disease, there is often reduced QRS voltage and conduction disturbance. The electrical alternans more likely suggests effusion, thus supporting a diagnosis of tamponade.

12. Answer a.

This bifid pulse can also be seen in combined AS with regurgitation (*see page 83*). Note the wide pulse pressure indicating AR. PW is the percussion wave and TW is the tidal wave.

13. Answer c.

This is the "spike-and-dome" or "bisferiens" pulse of HCM (*see page 84*). PW is the initial percussion wave and SW is the late systolic secondary wave.

14. Answer b.

Pericardial tamponade. Note the sharp X descent, but minimal or absent Y descent, consistent with minimal passive atrial emptying (*see page 84*). In constrictive pericarditis, there would be a sharp X and Y descent.

15. Answer c.

MR leading to a large CV wave (*see page 85*).

16. Answer a.

With pressure plotted on the Y axis (vertical) and volume on the X axis (horizontal), the slope of this curve is the *compliance*. A shift of a curve to the left means that for any given volume on the initial curve, the shifted curve has a higher pressure (ie, less compliant).

17. Answer d.

Qp/Qs = Total shunt flow / Total systemic flow

Total shunt flow = O_2 consumption / (PV O_2 content − PA O_2 content)

Total systemic flow = O_2 consumption / (FA O_2 content − MV O_2 content)

Qp/Qs = 1/(PV O_2 content − PA O_2 content)/[1/(FA O_2 content − MV O_2 content)]

Qp/Qs = (FA O_2 content − MV O_2 content)/(PV O_2 content − PA O_2 content)

O_2 content = 10 dL/L(1.34 mL/g × Hgb g/dL × O_2 saturation)

Cancelling out the Hgb and correction factor:

Qp/Qs = (FA O_2 sat − MV O_2 sat)/ (PV O_2 sat − PA O_2 sat)

Mixed venous sat = (3SVC + IVC)/4 = (3 × 67% + 70%)/4 = 68% FA O_2 sat − MV O_2 sat = 98% − 68% = 30%

There is no pulmonary vein saturation listed, however since the LV saturation is 98%, it is a left-to-right shunt through the ASD so the PV saturation is the same as the LA and LV.

PV O_2 sat − PA O_2 sat = LV O_2 sat − PA O_2 sat = 98%−88% = 10%
Qp/Qs = 30% / 10% = 3.0:1.0

18. Answer d.

This gentleman has increasing symptoms. Based on the physical examination he has at least moderate AS and moderate to severe AR. The echocardiogram is discrepant with the clinical information, showing only mild AS and mild AR. Therefore, further evaluation is warranted to determine the true severity of the aortic valve lesion.

19. Answer b.

The Haake equation can be used. This is the CO/$\sqrt{\text{mean gradient}}$ (3.5/7 = the AVA). The calculated AVA is 0.5 cm^2.

20. Answer b.

In this instance, the AVA is calculated by the systemic flow. However, the true flow of the LVOT is higher due to the concomitant AR. Therefore, the calculated AVA is smaller than the true AVA. The patient has severe AS and moderate to severe AR. He is markedly symptomatic. He should have the valve replacement.

21. Answer c.

22. Answer e.

To calculate the pulmonary arteriolar resistance, one needs to have the oxygen consumption. Although a thermal dilution CO has been performed, this is erroneous due to the patient's AF. One would know that thermal dilution and CO are not giving proper numbers as the PA saturation is only 53%, indicating that the CO should be low, not high. It is important to correlate measured numbers with the patient's physiology for consistency. (For institutions that do not use Wood units: 1 Wood unit = 80 dynes/s/cm^{-5})

23. Answer c.

The pulmonary arteriolar resistance is the mean PAP − LAP/CO. Thus, it is (50 mmHg − 20 mmHg)/3 L/min ≈ 10 Wood units × m^2.

24. Answer d.

Percutaneous revascularization has been shown to relieve symptoms. In patients with stable CAD (as opposed to ACS), percutaneous revascularization has not been shown to improve mortality or prevent infarction. Diabetic patients appear to have improved survival with CABG as compared to PCI. The other groups that have shown improved survival with CABG (as compared to medical therapy) include those with left main disease and those with three-vessel disease plus LV dysfunction or severe symptoms.

25. Answer c.

26. Answer e.

The 2002 update of the ACC/AHA guidelines upgraded the recommendation of angiography for patients after NSTEMI from a class IIB indication to class I in the setting of an early invasive strategy.

Recommendations for Coronary Angiography during the Hospital-Management Phase (Patients with Q-Wave and Non-Q-Wave Infarction):

Class I:

1. Spontaneous myocardial ischemia or myocardial ischemia provoked by minimal exertion, during recovery from MI. (*Level of evidence: C*)
2. Before definitive therapy of a mechanical complication of MI such as acute MR, VSD, pseudoaneurysm, or LV aneurysm. (*Level of evidence: C*)
3. Persistent hemodynamic instability. (*Level of evidence: B*)

Class IIa:

1. When MI is suspected to have occurred by a mechanism other than thrombotic occlusion at an atherosclerotic plaque (eg, coronary embolism, arteritis, trauma, certain metabolic or hematologic diseases, or coronary spasm). (*Level of evidence: C*)
2. Survivors of AMI with LV EF < 0.40, CHF, prior revascularization, or malignant ventricular arrhythmias. (*Level of evidence: C*)
3. Clinical heart failure during the acute episode, but subsequent demonstration of preserved LV function (LV EF > 0.40). (*Level of evidence: C*)

Class IIb:

1. Coronary angiography to find a persistently occluded infarct-related artery in an attempt to revascularize that artery (open artery hypothesis). (*Level of evidence: C*)
2. Coronary angiography performed without other risk stratification to identify the presence of left main or three-vessel disease. (*Level of evidence: C*)
3. Recurrent VT and/or VF, despite antiarrhythmic therapy, without evidence of ongoing myocardial ischemia. (*Level of evidence: C*)

Class III:

1. Patients who are not candidates for or who refuse coronary revascularization. (*Level of evidence: C*)

27. Answer d.
Of note, all patients should also have intensive medical regimen and an *initial strategy* of medical therapy alone in appropriately selected patients does not have adverse effects on morbidity or mortality (COURAGE trial).

28. Answer b.
Because of the higher likelihood of a saphenous vein graft to contain thrombus and subsequent microembolization with no reflow, this is considered to be a contraindication to rotational atherectomy. The location of a vein graft can make perforation particularly catastrophic as well. Debulking heavily calcified lesions prior to stent deployment is a useful application of rotational atherectomy.

29. Answer c.
Coronary flow reserve is the most sensitive measurement for determining the hemodynamic significance of an intermediate stenosis. The anatomical measurements made with intracoronary US are useful for assessing the quantitative and qualitative aspects of atherosclerosis but are less accurate for determining physiology. Proximal-to-distal velocity ratio is one measurement of lesion severity, but it has been shown to be less accurate than coronary flow reserve.

30. Answer e.
The patient is moderate risk for a moderate risk surgery. Medical management including aggressive beta blockade is indicated to reduce perioperative MI risk. There are no data proving that full-dose aspirin is more effective in preventing future MI.

By the 2005 AHA/ACC guidelines on PCI:

Class III:

PCI is not recommended in patients with asymptomatic ischemia or CCS class I or II angina who do not meet the criteria as listed under the class II recommendations or who have one or more of the following:

  a. Only a small area of viable myocardium at risk (*Level of evidence: C*)
  b. No objective evidence of ischemia. (*Level of evidence: C*)
  c. Lesions that have a low likelihood of successful dilatation. (*Level of evidence: C*)
  d. Mild symptoms that are unlikely to be due to myocardial ischemia. (*Level of evidence: C*)
  e. Factors associated with increased risk of morbidity or mortality. (*Level of evidence: C*)
  f. Left main disease and eligibility for CABG. (*Level of evidence: C*)
  g. Insignificant disease (<50% coronary stenosis). (*Level of evidence: C*)

31. Answer c.

This case is an asymptomatic 62-year-old male with multiple risk factors for CAD. The most important step to take in managing his subsequent CV risk is to treat his modifiable risk factors. These are principally his HTN and hyperlipidemia. Coronary angiography would not be indicated as an initial step for this asymptomatic individual. Exercise testing to diagnose coronary disease is not particularly useful for someone in this age group who already has pretest probability of harboring CAD. The more appropriate use of functional testing for this type of individual would be for prognostic information.

32. Answer a.

Once he had developed chronic stable angina, all of the modalities listed decrease subsequent death and nonfatal MI rates except for percutaneous revascularization. This modality has been proven to relieve symptoms but not to improve survival in patients with stable CAD.

33. Answer e.

By definition this patient has an unstable angina syndrome. Generally, noninvasive stress testing without intensification of anti-ischemic therapy is contraindicated in unstable syndromes. He does not have markers of increased risk (positive biomarkers, evidence of CHF, ongoing or prolonged chest pain, ECG changes, etc.); therefore, the administration of glycoprotein IIb/IIIa inhibitors is not strictly indicated. Multiple studies have suggested that both conservative strategies and early invasive strategies can be used with similar outcomes for patients like this one.

34. Answer c.

Bare metal intracoronary stents have a 15% to 20% restenosis rate in the first 6 mos. Subsequent death, MI, and ischemic stroke are dramatically reduced using the combination of aspirin and clopidogrel (or aspirin and ticlopidine). Warfarin is not part of standard care following intracoronary stenting and should be used only if there is another indication. Follow-up testing is not mandated after percutaneous revascularization and generally is performed only when indicated based on clinical symptoms.

35. Answer b.

Patients who have undergone coronary revascularization within the last 5 yrs and *remain active and asymptomatic* do not need preoperative cardiac testing. In this case, the patient did undergo TMET that demonstrated good exercise capacity (9 METS), confirming his relatively good prognosis. Preoperative PA catheterization is not supported by trial data. He should continue on aspirin as long as possible before and restart as soon as possible after surgery, as well as maintain aggressive beta blockade and statin therapy throughout the surgery.

36. Answer c.

Even though this could be alcoholic cardiomyopathy, coronary angiography is indicated to rule out an ischemic cause and assess potential for revascularization that may improve LV function.

37. Answer b.

This similar patient has severe three-vessel coronary disease and cardiomyopathy with depressed LV systolic function. Revascularization (likely with CABG) is indicated if there is salvageable myocardium. The degree of renal failure limits initiation of aldosterone-blocking agent at this time.

38. Answer d.

The risk of an anaphylactoid reaction to contrast media is increased if a previous reaction has occurred but is not related to use of NPH insulin. Previous NPH use increases the risk of anaphylaxis to protamine (used to reverse heparin effect).

39. Answer d.

Coronary artery anomalies are frequently incidental findings but should always be visualized. The most common coronary anomaly is a "pants leg" or separate coronary ostia of the LAD and LCX. If not looking specifically for a separate ostia, an occlusion or entire territory can be missed angiographically, especially in an emergency setting.

40. Answer a.

Biplane ventriculography is needed for complete visualization of the LV.

41. Answer b.

Especially in light of his nephropathy and upcoming contrast administration, he should stop his metformin and remain off the medication 24 to 48 hr post procedure to limit the potential for developing lactic acidosis. Metformin-associated lactic acidosis is thought to be type B (overproduction rather than tissue hypoxia) because it inhibits the gluconeogenesis from alanine, pyruvate, and lactate. The other medications may be continued with special attention: with the NPH, the patient should not have protamine reversal of heparin post procedure. In addition, it would be reasonable to either have the patient increase oral intake or hold lasix to support his volume status and decrease chance of contrast nephropathy. The patient should receive aggressive IV hydration 1 hr prior to angiogram and for 6 hr after with a sodium bicarbonate or saline solution to further limit contrast nephropathy. Other considerations to limit further nephropathy are limiting volume of contrast and avoiding high osmolar ionic contrast dye.

42. Answer c.

Stent reduces need for target vessel revascularization. It also reduces significance of coronary artery dissection caused by angioplasty.

43. Answer a.

Reduced neointimal proliferation is the mechanism that DESs use to reduce restenosis. The reduction of restenosis of bare metal stents compared to angioplasty (22% vs. 32%) was documented in the BENESTENT trial (1994).

44. Answer b.

With balloon angioplasty, the rate of abrupt vessel closure is 3% to 8% and attributed to thrombus or dissection. Abciximab reduces platelet aggregation and can facilitate dissolution of thrombus. In the current stent era, abciximab (ADMIRAL), when given early in STEMI, decreases the need for urgent target vessel revascularization by 30 days. This benefit does not necessarily apply to neointimal hypertrophy and in-stent restenosis: the ERASER trial had 4-mos follow-up IVUS that did not show any significant difference with or without abciximab at the time of implant.

45. Answer d.

By ACC definition:

Descriptions of a High-Risk Lesion (Type C Lesion):

- Diffuse (length >2 cm)
- Excessive tortuosity of proximal segment
- Extremely angulated segments (>90°)
- Total occlusions more than 3 mos old and/or bridging collaterals*
- Inability to protect major side branches
- Degenerated vein grafts with friable lesions*

*The high risk with these criteria is for technical failure and increased restenosis, not for acute complications.

46. Answer a.

Direct comparison of thrombolysis versus PCI shows better outcomes for PCI if door-to-balloon times and door-to-needle times are equivalent. In addition, this patient is **not** having an STEMI. Thrombolysis is not appropriate for NSTEMI.

47. Answer b.

In the SIRIUS trial, target vessel restenosis was reduced in DESs versus bare metal stent (4.1% vs. 16.6%) at 9 mos. Major adverse CV events were reduced as well (7.1% vs. 18.9%). The mechanism of reduced events was attributed to decreased neointimal hyperplasia. TAXUS-IV was the similar paclitaxel-eluting stent trial that had decreased angiographic restenosis at 9 mos (7.9% vs. 26.6%) when compared to bare metal stent.

48. Answer b.

With the recent widespread implementation of DESs, late thrombosis data started appearing 1 yr after placement. In May, 2007, Cook et al. (Circulation 115:2426−2434) published an IVUS study on 13 patients with late stent thrombosis with a mean of 630 days ± 166 after DES implantation. They found incomplete stent apposition in 77% of these patients versus 12% of controls (IVUS done at 8 mos and no stent thrombosis > 2 yrs post implant). Whether the incomplete apposition was due to technical limitation or the positive remodeling by local inflammation is unknown. They also found that patients with thrombosis had longer lesions, longer stents, more stents-per-lesion, and more stent overlap.

49. Answer d.

Rotational atherectomy utilizes a miniature burr that is able to debulk calcified lesions by grinding them into microscopic fragments that theoretically pass through the capillaries and microcirculation of the myocardium. Balloon angioplasty is unlikely to have much success dilating a heavily calcified lesion. Directional atherectomy was previously used to debulk plaque, but when compared to balloon angioplasty had no clear benefit. With the advent of bare metal stents, directional atherectomy was reduced to a more limited role. The calcification would also make use of this technology difficult in this setting. Directional atherectomy has enjoyed renewed use in treatment of peripheral vascular disease. Excimer is short for "excited dimer" and typically uses a combination of an inert gas and a reactive gas to create UV laser light that can be absorbed by biological tissue causing vaporization of the organic compound. This is the technology behind LASIK surgery. It is currently used for in-stent restenosis and is less effective in calcified lesions and also carries a higher risk of complication such as perforation. With the advent of DESs, the frequency of in-stent restenosis has dropped dramatically and, therefore, one of the primary roles of this technology has fallen out of favor. There is novel research investigating its role in vaporizing thrombus and plaque in the setting of AMI.

50. Answer e.

The TAXUS V ISR (in-stent restenosis) trial and SISR trials were both published in JAMA (2006) and compared paclitaxel and sirolimus-eluting stents (DES) versus vascular brachytherapy for bare metal stent restenosis. DES was superior to brachytherapy with reduction in target vessel restenosis. In the TAXUS V study, the rates were 10.5% versus 17.5% target vessel restenosis at 9 mos. In the SISR study, there was also less target vessel restenosis in the sirolimus-eluting stent (12% vs. 22%) at 9 mos. Brachytherapy and DES implantation are the only remaining FDA-approved treatments for restenosis of bare metal stents at this time.

51. Answers a and b.

52. Answers a, b, c, and d.

53. Answer b.

The ECSS trial was published in 1980 and studied 768 patients. The surgical arm, however, actually had better compliance with beta blocker therapy than the medical therapy arm. It could be considered a "surgery versus no surgery" trial. The 5-yr survival was 93% for CABG and 84% without. The VA multicenter study was published in 1977 and did not show an overall survival benefit. There was improved survival (87% vs. 74%) in patients with left main disease.

54. Answers b and e.

The CASS trial was conducted from 1975 to 1979. They used nitrates and beta blockers, but only had 64% compliance with beta blockers at 5 yrs. The ECSS and VA multicenter studies are discussed above. However, the MASS-II trial recently finished 5-yr follow-up in 2007. This was the most modern application of medical therapy including ASA, nitrates, beta blockers, calcium channel blockers, ACE inhibitors, and statins. Patients in all three arms received aggressive medical therapy. Medications were provided free of charge to patients. This trial did not show any mortality difference between the three randomized arms. Nonfatal MI was more common in the medical therapy and PCI arms than the CABG arm, as was the need for revascularization procedures.

55. Answers e, f, and g.

Understanding which patients were **not** well represented is important to critically assess applicability of trial data to specific patients.

56. Answer c.

The 10-yr results from the BARI trial were recently published. There was no significant long-term advantage of an initial strategy of PTCA compared with CABG. However, the trial was started prior to stent implantation and glycoprotein IIb/IIIa inhibition, rendering some question on modern applicability of the trial. However, the only survival advantage by 10 yrs was in the diabetic population. Ongoing trials such as BARI 2D and FREEDOM will help clarify the role of multivessel intervention in the modern PCI era.

57. Answers c, d, and e.

58. Answer a.
Left main equivalent is more properly considered a variant of multivessel CAD with major differences in operative mortality compared to true left main disease (0.8% vs. 4%) and natural history (5-yr survival 98% vs. 76%) (Tyras et al., Circulation 1981).

59. Answer b.
The sicker the patient, the more likely it is that CABG will prolong life. Thus, patients are likely to live longer after CABG if they have left main disease; three-vessel disease with LV dysfunction (EF < 50%), class III or IV angina, provocable ischemia, or disease in the proximal LAD; two-vessel disease with proximal LAD involvement; and two-vessel disease with class III or IV angina as well as either severe LV dysfunction alone, or moderate LV dysfunction together with at least one proximal lesion.

SECTION IV

Myocardial Infarction

Charles X. Kim, MD

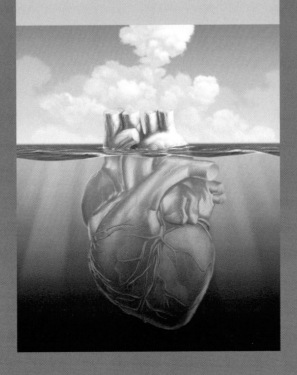

Questions

1. A 67-year-old man is admitted with an acute inferior wall MI. He is taken directly to the catheterization laboratory and at coronary angiography is found to have an occluded RCA. He has minor disease in the LAD. The most likely pre-existing culprit lesion that precipitated the acute coronary occlusion is which of the following coronary lesions?

   a. The highest grade stenosis
   b. The most proximal stenosis
   c. A non-flow limiting (<50%) stenosis
   d. A coronary aneurysm

2. You are asked to see a 41-year-old woman who presents in her 32nd week of pregnancy with sudden onset severe chest discomfort. She has a history of systemic HTN prior to pregnancy controlled on two oral hypotensive agents. Control of HTN has been excellent during pregnancy. She has a past history of smoking but has not used tobacco during the pregnancy. The patient presented to the ED for evaluation. She is markedly diaphoretic. When you see her, she has received 2 SL NTG and has persistent chest pain. She denies cocaine usage.

   An ECG is obtained and shows 2 mm ST segment elevation in the anterior precordial leads V2, V3, V4. You would recommend which of the following?

   a. Perform an emergency coronary angiography and PCI if indicated by the coronary anatomy
   b. Administer thrombolytic therapy with tPA in order to minimize radiation exposure to the baby
   c. Start a glycoprotein IIB/IIIA inhibitor and wait 1 hr to assess the clinical response and then, if needed, proceed to cardiac catheterization only if there is no improvement in symptoms or ECG findings
   d. Perform a CT scan of the chest to rule out aortic dissection or pulmonary embolism
   e. Start aspirin therapy, administer IV NTG, and admit to the CCU for observation

3. A 50-year-old man went to the ED because he had substernal chest pressure for 2 hrs. He has been healthy and has no history of heart disease, HTN, hyperlipidemia or DM. He smokes one pack of cigarettes daily. His initial HR was 124 bpm, sinus rhythm and BP was 150/100 mmHg. Cardiac examination was otherwise normal. ECG showed 3 mm ST segment elevation in leads II, III, and aVF and was otherwise normal.

   He was given a thrombolytic agent and the chest pain and ECG changes resolved within 1 hr. Treatment with a beta blocker and aspirin was initiated and the patient was admitted to the coronary care unit. Four hours later he had an asymptomatic 7-beat run of VT. Occasional single ventricular premature contractions were observed over the next 24 hrs. He was transferred to a step-down bed. His hospital course was uncomplicated. The patient was ready for dismissal on day 3.

Answers to this section start on page 123.

3. (*continued*)

   Which of the following clinical variables is associated with increased 30-day mortality risk?

   a. Age 50 years
   b. Male sex
   c. History of cigarette smoking
   d. Initial HR of 120 bpm
   e. Initial BP of 150/100 mmHg

4. Which of the following is correct concerning invasive and non-invasive assessment of arrhythmia potential after MI?

   a. Complex ventricular ectopy predicts risk of recurrent MI but not cardiac death
   b. Late potentials on signal-averaged ECG are of little predictive value
   c. Decreased HR variability fails to identify high-risk patients
   d. The therapeutic implications of positive noninvasive test results are uncertain
   e. Invasive EP testing early after MI is predictive of long-term ventricular arrhythmias

5. Which of the following statements is true about post-MI stress testing in patients treated with thrombolytic therapy versus patients not treated with this therapy?

   a. The positive predictive value of stress testing is lower in the thrombolytic patients
   b. Mid-LV cavity obliteration during dobutamine echocardiography is a more powerful prognostic variable in the thrombolytic patients
   c. Increased lung uptake on a adenosine technetium-99 m sestamibi scan has similar prognostic value in both thrombolytic and non-thrombolytic patients
   d. ST-segment elevation during exercise is of prognostic value only in thrombolytic patients
   e. Positive test results are associated with a higher risk of three-vessel disease in thrombolytic versus non-thrombolytic patients

6. Which of the following clinical and stress testing variables is associated with the worst prognosis in patients after AMI?

   a. Inability to perform an exercise test
   b. ST-segment depression in the lateral precordial leads
   c. ST-segment elevation at the site of Q waves
   d. An increase in systolic BP > 60 mmHg above baseline
   e. Ventricular bigeminy during the first 2 mins of recovery

7. A 65-year-old man presents with unstable angina and an elevated troponin level. Comorbidities include adult-onset DM treated with metformin and essential HTN treated with metoprolol. Angiography shows three-vessel CAD with three discrete proximal flow limiting lesions and normal LV function. Treatment of choice is:

   a. Medical therapy and functional testing to assess the extent of myocardial ischemia
   b. Multivessel PTCA starting with the tightest stenosis
   c. Multivessel stenting starting with the proximal LAD stenosis
   d. CABG including a LIMA graft

8. The percentage of patients presenting post-MI without any major modifiable conventional CV risk factor is:

    a. <10%
    b. 20% to 40%
    c. 60% to 70%
    d. >90%

9. For patients with significant CAD, which of the following has **not** been shown to improve survival and decreased coronary events?

    a. Statin drugs
    b. Beta blockers
    c. ACE inhibitors
    d. Aspirin
    e. Vitamin E

10. A 74-year-old man was admitted to the ED because of chest pain that started 1 hr ago. He is now pain free, following morphine that was administered in the ambulance. He had a right-sided cardioembolic stroke 3 yrs ago and has minimal residual left arm weakness. ECG was performed.

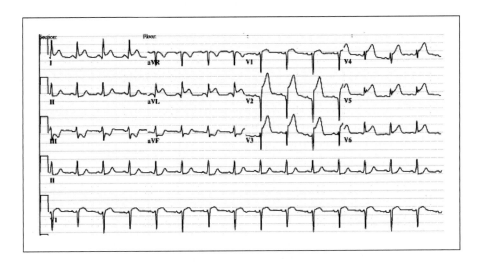

    The next best step for management would be:

    a. Thrombolytic therapy
    b. Emergency cardiac catheterization
    c. Echocardiography
    d. Indomethacin
    e. Pericardiocentesis
    f. Urgent cardiac catheterization only if pain returns

11. In AMI survivors, mortality between hospital discharge and 1 yr is:

    a. 18% to 20%
    b. 7% to 8%
    c. 3% to 4%
    d. 2% or less

12. Which variable is associated with increased 30-day mortality in a patient treated with thrombolytic therapy?

    a. Systolic: BP > 160 mmHg
    b. HR < 65 bpm
    c. ST segment elevation in anterior leads V1–V4 on the ECG
    d. Weight > 100 kg

13. Measurement of LV EF in the AMI setting:

    a. Is a class I indication in patients treated with thrombolytic therapy
    b. Can be performed by either echocardiography or equilibrium radionuclide angiography (MUGA), but in patients with AF is preferably performed using radionuclide angiography
    c. Should be delayed for 72 to 96 hrs to allow the effects of "myocardial stunning" to resolve
    d. Could accurately predict long-term mortality in the pre-thrombolytic era but not in patients treated with reperfusion therapy

14. Which statement concerning exercise testing post-MI is true?

    a. A maximal test at 4 to 6 wks is preferable to a submaximal test at 4 to 5 days
    b. ST segment depression is the strongest prognostic variable
    c. Due to the effect of beta blockers on HR, all patients taking a beta blocker should undergo pharmacologic imaging rather than exercise testing
    d. Patients not referred for cardiac stress testing have a higher mortality than patients referred for stress testing

15. You are the back-up cardiologist on-call for the weekend at your local hospital. You receive a phone call at 11:30 pm Saturday night from the ED physician. He is calling you because he has been unable to reach the primary cardiologist on-call for the past 2 hrs. A 50-year-old man presented to the ED 2 hrs ago with 3 hrs of substernal chest pressure with radiation into his jaws. The patient has no prior history of heart disease. He takes no medications. CAD risk factors include MI in his father at age 56, cigarette smoking 2 packs/day for 33 yrs, borderline HTN, no diabetes, and unknown lipid status.

    Physical exam upon presentation revealed BMI 32.4; BP 145/92 mmHg; HR 112 bpm; lungs clear; heart apical impulse not palpable, normal S1 and S2, soft apical S4, no S3 or murmur or rub; extremities no edema; peripheral pulses normal.

    The ECG showed Q waves and 3 mm ST segment elevation in the inferior leads. The patient was treated with SL NTG, aspirin and tPA followed by a heparin drip. His chest pain resolved and he has been pain-free for the past hour. The ST elevation resolved but the Q waves in the inferior leads persist. The initial Troponin T was 0.03 ng/ml (normal <0.10 ng/ml). His ECG monitor shows 8 to 10 single ventricular premature contractions per min. You visit and examine the patient and confirm the findings of the ED physician.

The next step in this patient's management should be:

a. CT chest scan with contrast to rule out aortic dissection
b. Coronary angiography
c. Echocardiogram
d. Lidocaine 100 mg IV bolus followed by lidocaine 2 mg/min IV drip
e. Metoprolol 50 mg PO followed by metoprolol 50 mg PO BID.

16. Which of the following features is associated with increased 30-day mortality risk in the patient in Question 15 according to the TIMI STEMI risk score?

a. Age 50 yrs
b. Cigarette smoking history
c. BP 146/92 mmHg
d. HR 112 bpm
e. 3 mm ST elevation in the inferior leads

17. A 72-year-old male underwent coronary angiography for a history of chest pain with positive serum biomarkers. He was found to have a 75% middle RCA stenosis, a 40% mid-LAD stenosis, and three 30% lesions in the left CFX. The coronary flow reserve in the RCA was 0.82. Medical treatment was recommended.

Statistically this patient's risk for future MI is:

a. Highest in the left CFX
b. Highest in the LAD
c. Highest in the RCA
d. Improved by stenting of the 75% RCA stenosis

18. A major reason for performing post-MI risk stratification is:

a. To identify patients most likely to benefit from statins
b. To identify patients most likely to benefit from aspirin and beta blockers
c. To identify patients at highest risk for future events
d. To identify patients requiring referral to a cardiac rehabilitation program

19. Which of the following statements concerning post-MI exercise stress ECG testing is true?

a. If a patient has had coronary angiography, exercise stress testing adds little to future risk stratification
b. The most useful prognostic variable is ST-segment depression
c. In uncomplicated patients treated with thrombolytic therapy, stress testing an safely be performed at 24 to 48 hrs
d. Patients selected for angiography should first undergo stress imaging to aid in the functional assessment of any borderline coronary stenoses seen at angiography

20. A class I indication for coronary angiography following a medically managed AMI includes:

    a. An elevated EBCT calcium score in the non-infarct zone vessels
    b. A high-sensitivity CRP level three times normal
    c. Delayed resolution of ST-segment elevation by filtered ECG monitoring
    d. 1.5 mm ST-segment depression at 4 METS during a submaximal exercise test

21. A 61-year-old male with long standing essential HTN on drug treatment had two episodes of chest "heaviness" in the last 24 hours.

    Risk factors include an LDL-cholesterol of 148 mg/dL; his initial troponin 0.1 ng/mL. He develops transient recurrent chest pain. The ECG monitor now shows new 2-mm ST depression with T-wave inversions in V5–V6. The patient is seen in the ED before admission.

    The best initial treatment now is:

    a. ASA, unfractionated heparin, beta blocker
    b. ASA, unfractionated heparin, IIb/IIIa inhibitor, beta blocker
    c. ASA, clopidogrel, nifedipine
    d. ASA, clopidogrel, IIb/IIIa inhibitor, immediate angiography

22. The patient described in Question 21 stabilizes on medical therapy. Elective catheterization shows:

    ■ An EF 68%, no areas of ventricular hypokinesis
    ■ 70% stenosis of the second OM with TIMI III flow
    ■ 40% to 50% lesions in remaining vessels
    ■ The OM lesion is suitable for PCI with stent

    You elect to:

    a. Perform PCI with stent, dismiss on ASA, clopidogrel, dietary modification
    b. Perform PCI with stent, dismiss on ASA, clopidogrel, Lovenox 7 days
    c. Perform PCI with stent, IIb/IIIa inhibitor, dismiss on ASA, clopidogrel, beta blocker and statin
    d. Intensive medical therapy with ASA, beta blocker, diet, increased dose of statin, and follow-up exercise test in 7 to 10 days

23. Which of the following is true about the patient in Question 21?

    a. ASA reduces mortality
    b. Clopidogrel reduces mortality
    c. IIb/IIIa agents reduce mortality
    d. Dalteparin reduces morality
    e. None of the above

24. Identify the true statement:

    a. Randomized trials demonstrated that an urgent (6–12 hr) invasive strategy is superior to initial medical management of unstable angina in respect to preservation of hibernating myocardium
    b. An early invasive strategy is generally indicated in patients with recent PCI (within 6 mos) or prior bypass graft
    c. PCI is contraindicated in diabetic patients with ACS
    d. IIb/IIIa agents are equally beneficial in high and low risk ACS
    e. Ticlopidine should be administered to all ACS patients in the ED before planned PCI

25. All of the following are considered absolute contraindications to the administration of a thrombolytic agent to a patient with an AMI **except:**

    a. Embolic CVA 6 mos earlier
    b. Remote history of incidentally discovered unruptured cerebral aneurysm on CT brain scan
    c. Gastrointestinal bleed secondary to duodenal ulcer 4 wks earlier
    d. Severe dementia

26. A 55-year-old retired financial services company chief executive officer arrives in the ED where you are moonlighting as a cardiology fellow. He has a history of mild CAD and PAF. He is on a daily aspirin and beta blocker. His chief complaint is new onset of a dense left-sided hemiplegia that was spontaneous in onset ~1 hr prior to admission. With the stress of the new neurological deficit, he is markedly anxious and notes some chest heaviness and shortness of breath. Vital signs are: HR 90 bpm, BP 160/80 mmHg, RR 20/min. His initial ECG does not show evidence of ischemia. Head CT suggests MCA stroke without hemorrhage. The local neurologist is available within ~30 mins.

    Your next clinical step is:

    a. Administer clopidrogel 300 mg immediately
    b. 4ASA, heparin 5000 units as a bolus and 1000 units per hour, metoprolol
    c. 4 × 81 mg ASA, heparin, metoprolol, IIb/IIIa inhibitor
    d. Metoprolol only and call for an emergency neurological opinion

27. All of the following ECG signs are associated with high-risk inferior MIs and identify patients most likely to gain benefit from reperfusion therapy **except:**

    a. ST elevation in V3R and V4R
    b. ST segment depression in V1 and V2
    c. Complete AV block
    d. Sum of the ST segment elevation >0.8 mV
    e. Onset of AF

28. According to the ACC/AHA guidelines which of the following is a class I indication for coronary angiography?

    a. A patient with new onset chest pain, no ST segment deviation but an elevated troponin T
    b. A patient with a new finding of an LV EF of 45% by echocardiography
    c. A patient with apical ischemia on exercise perfusion study at 11 METS
    d. A patient with CRP in the upper quintile not associated with cardiac symptoms

29. According to the ACC 2005 update for PCI, which of the following is a **contraindication** (class III indication) for PCI in the setting of unstable angina/NSTEMI?

    a. Three-vessel disease and diabetes
    b. Significant proximal LAD disease and no contraindication for CABG
    c. Significant left main CAD and no contraindication for CABG
    d. Cardiogenic shock secondary to proximal LAD occlusion

30. Which of the following statements is true concerning the comparison of primary PCI and thrombolysis in the treatment of AMI?

    a. Survival with PCI in an 74-year-old diabetic female who presented 2 hrs after the onset of MI with cardiogenic shock is likely to be better than with aggressive medical treatment including thrombolysis

    b. Survival benefit with primary PCI compared to thrombolysis is confined to anterior MI

    c. Successful PCI and survival benefit with primary PCI is not associated with operator volume

    d. Survival is higher among elderly patients if treated with thrombolytic agents rather than primary PCI

    e. Success rates of rescue PCI after failed thrombolysis are similar to those of primary PCI

31. The administration of aspirin in AMI:

    a. Has been shown to reduce 30-day mortality only among patients with ST elevation on the initial ECG

    b. Is less beneficial in patients treated with thrombolytic therapy than other patients

    c. Is statistically as effective as streptokinase at reducing 30-day mortality but is added in benefit when used in conjunction with streptokinase or another thrombolytic agent.

    d. Is optional in the setting of AMI if the patient is therapeutic on warfarin (INR 2–3)

32. Among patients suffering an MI with true contraindications to aspirin, which of the following should be administered in its place?

    a. Coumadin

    b. Dipyridamole

    c. Ticlopidine

    d. Clopidogrel

33. All the following are true concerning the use of beta blockers in AMI **except**:

    a. More than 50% of patients have contraindications to their use when first seen in the ED

    b. There are data indicating that their use reduces the frequency of myocardial rupture

    c. Their beneficial effect is partly due to an increase in myocardial blood flow

    d. They should generally be administered acutely even to patients known to have a chronically low EF of 35%

34. IV NTG:

    a. Has been shown in randomized trials to reduce mortality in patients with anterior wall MI receiving thrombolytic therapy

    b. May reduce infarct size even in patients with hypotension

    c. Reduces preload and may dilate collaterals

    d. Reduces the frequency of reinfarction when administered with thrombolytic therapy

35. In the setting of thrombolytic therapy, which adjunctive therapy is **least** useful?

    a. Aspirin
    b. Plavix
    c. Gp IIb/IIIa inhibitor
    d. Heparin

36. For a patient with NSTEMI and high risk features proceeding to PCI, which of the following therapies is **least** likely to improve outcomes?

    a. Aspirin + heparin
    b. Aspirin + IIb/IIIa inhibitor
    c. Plavix + heparin
    d. Half-strength tenecteplase
    e. Aspirin + bivalirudin

37. Which of the following glycoprotein IIb/IIIa inhibitors can be reversed by platelet transfusion?

    a. Abciximab
    b. Tirofiban
    c. Eptifibatide

38. A 45-year-old male is hospitalized at the local outreach hospital with 3-mm ST-segment elevation in leads II, III, aVF. There is no ST-elevation in right-sided chest leads. He is given tPA and is transported by helicopter to your institution. He arrives in the CCU 40 mins after administration of aspirin, tPA, and heparin infusion. He is also receiving a low dose NTG drip. His vital signs are: HR 75 bpm, BP 110/50 mmHg, RR 16/min. He is still complaining of "3/10" chest heaviness and is mildly agitated. A repeat ECG showed residual inferior wall ST elevation of 1 to 1.5 mm. What is your next step?

    a. Add IIb/IIIa inhibitor to his medical regimen
    b. Increase NTG dose and add oral metoprolol
    c. Activate the cardiac catheterization laboratory for emergent mechanical revascularization and "rescue" PCI
    d. Consult cardiac surgery for emergency CABG
    e. Inset an aortic balloon pump to improve diastolic perfusion pressure

39. A 62-year-old diabetic smoker arrives at the local community hospital after 6 hrs of continuous crushing substernal chest pain. There is 2-mm ST elevation in leads V2–V4. Vital signs are: HR 80 bpm, BP 126/78 mmHg, respiratory rate 18/min. Physical exam demonstrates mild JVD, but clear lungs and no S3. The nearest catheterization laboratory is 60 mins away by ambulance. A helicopter is unavailable because of adverse weather conditions.

    The most appropriate treatment option is:

    a. Aspirin, heparin, IIb/IIIa inhibitor, clopidogrel, metoprolol
    b. Aspirin, heparin, IIb/IIIa inhibitor, metoprolol, tPA
    c. Aspirin, heparin, metoprolol, tPA
    d. Aspirin, heparin, IIb/IIIa inhibitor, metoprolol, transfer to awaiting catheterization laboratory
    e. Half strength streptokinase, aspirin, heparin, metoprolol

40. A 38-year-old who had an anterior STEMI followed by prompt revascularization of a proximal LAD lesion with a sirolimus-coated DES is recovering uneventfully in the coronary care unit. On hospital day 4, the nurse alerts you to a new rash that he has developed. It is on his knees, elbows, and scalp and is well-demarcated with red-raised skin and silvery scale. Which of his new medications is likely the cause?

   a. Sirolimus in the stent
   b. Clopidogrel
   c. Ramipril
   d. Metoprolol

41. In patients with unstable angina who undergo coronary angiography, what percentage have angiographically normal coronary arteries or minimal CAD?

   a. <10%
   b. 10% to 20%
   c. 40% to 50%
   d. 60% to 70%
   e. >80%

42. Which of the following is **not** a contraindication to intra-aortic balloon pump use in patients with unstable angina?

   a. Severe peripheral vascular disease
   b. Severe AS
   c. Severe aortic insufficiency
   d. Severe aortoiliac disease
   e. Helium allergy

43. Which of the following is **least** likely to be a cause of unstable angina?

   a. Anemia
   b. Fever
   c. Hypothyroidism
   d. Severe AS
   e. Severe HTN

44. Which of the following drugs has been shown to decrease CV events in patients with unstable angina who are allergic to aspirin?

   a. Ticlopidine
   b. Sulfinpyrazone
   c. Dipyridamole
   d. All of the above
   e. None of the above

45. Which patients with unstable angina who have the following ECG subsets have been shown to benefit from acute IV thrombolytic therapy?

   a. ST-segment depression >1 mm in leads V5–V6
   b. T-wave inversion >2 mm in leads V1–V4
   c. Peaked T waves >2 mm in leads V1–V4
   d. All of the above
   e. None of the above

46. Which of the following diagnoses should be considered in the differential diagnosis of unstable angina?

    a. Aortic dissection
    b. Pericarditis
    c. Pneumothorax
    d. Pulmonary embolus
    e. None of the above
    f. All the above

47. Which of the following historic features indicates the **lowest** risk of death or non-fatal MI in patients with unstable angina?

    a. Rest pain >20 mins
    b. Pulmonary edema associated with ischemia
    c. Angina associated with ST-segment depression ≥1 mm
    d. Angina with new MR murmur
    e. Angina provoked at a workload lower than normal

48. Which of the following is an indication for the use of calcium channel blockers in patients with unstable angina?

    a. Vasospastic angina
    b. Ischemic symptoms associated with subacute stent thrombosis
    c. Unstable angina occurring in association with AS
    d. Unstable angina in the setting of hyperparathyroidism
    e. Unstable angina in the periopertive period

49. IV lidocaine:

    a. Reduces ventricular ectopy in AMI and should be administered to all patients prophylactically
    b. Reduces mortality in AMI
    c. Should be routinely administered before primary angioplasty for AMI
    d. May increase mortality in AMI

50. Calcium channel blockers:

    a. Should be routinely used in patients with NSTEMI for secondary prevention of coronary vasospasm
    b. Are indicated after MI for the treatment of angina or HTN, when the patient has a normal EF
    c. May increase mortality after AMI, especially in patients with reduced ventricular function
    d. Are recommended in patients with combined cerebrovascular disease and MI

51. Lipid-lowering agents:

    a. Are effective for reducing long-term mortality, even in patients with advanced CAD
    b. Should not be used early in the post-infarction period
    c. May paradoxically increase mortality in patients with low levels of HDL cholesterol
    d. Were frequently stopped because of congestive hepatitis in trials among patients with a history of heart failure

52. Which of the following is true?

    a. Warfarin prevents reocclusion more effectively than aspirin after thrombolytic therapy
    b. Clopidogrel is less effective than aspirin for reducing adverse CV events in patients with vascular disease
    c. Aspirin is roughly as effective both early and late after MI for reducing adverse CV events
    d. Beta blockers should not be administered after MI until after an exercise test has been performed; this avoids false negatives and higher sensitivity on the test

53. The administration of beta blockers after MI:

    a. Should be avoided in patients with reduced ventricular function
    b. Is less likely to benefit patients with reduced ventricular function than patients with normal ventricular function
    c. May paradoxically reduce symptoms of CHF in certain patients with a low EF
    d. Should never be considered in patients with a history of CHF

54. Angiography after MI:

    a. Predicts patients who will have reinfarction
    b. Predicts mortality
    c. Often leads to revascularization
    d. Is a cost-effective risk-stratification strategy
    e. Is necessary in all patients after MI

55. TMET after MI in patients who have had thrombolysis:

    a. Predicts reinfarction
    b. Predicts mortality
    c. Is vastly inferior to nuclear or exercise echocardiography
    d. Is useful for exercise prescription and reassurance of the patient
    e. Is mandatory in all patients after MI

56. Clinical risk factors for a poor outcome after MI include all **except:**

    a. Shock
    b. Pulmonary congestion
    c. Age 70 years or older
    d. Cigarette smoking on admission
    e. Recurrent rest angina

57. The average 1-yr post-dismissal mortality rate for patients receiving thrombolytic therapy in a clinical trial is:

    a. 1%
    b. 2% to 4%
    c. 8%
    d. >15%
    e. >40%

58. The average 1-yr post-dismissal mortality rate in a large observational registry of patients after reperfusion (primary percutaneous transluminal coronary angioplasty or thrombolysis) was:

    a. 1%
    b. 3%
    c. 5% to 6%
    d. 10% to 15%
    e. >20%

59. In GISSI II:

    a. There was a high (>50%) rate of angiography after MI
    b. There was considerable (>40%) revascularization after MI
    c. TMET gave incremental prognostic information over clinical assessment
    d. A resting EF < 40% was associated with a 6 mo mortality rate of more than 8%
    e. Female patients had a higher mortality rate than male patients

60. All of the following are true about the GUSTO I trial **except:**

    a. 20% of patients had an uncomplicated MI
    b. The 30-day mortality rate was 1%, and the 1-yr additional mortality rate was 3.5%
    c. Patients with uncomplicated infarction by day 4 had 1% 30-day and 2.6% additional 1-yr mortality rates
    d. Age, hypotension, Killip class II or higher, increased HR, and location of infarct were the five most important clinical predictors of morality at 30 days

61. For patients **not** receiving thrombolysis or primary percutaneous transluminal coronary angioplasty:

    a. Mortality is lower than in candidates for thrombolysis
    b. Angiography and stress testing are useful to select patients for revascularization versus medical therapy
    c. Ancillary therapy (aspirin, beta blockers, ACE inhibitors) is unimportant
    d. Revascularization prolongs survival in asymptomatic patients with well-preserved EF and single-vessel (not left main) disease

62. Which patient is at the highest risk after MI?

    a. Received thrombolysis as part of a clinical trial
    b. Received primary percutaneous transluminal coronary angioplasty as part of a clinical trial
    c. Received thrombolysis or angioplasty in a nontrial setting within 1 hr of presentation
    d. Received thrombolysis, is in Killip class II with a LV EF of 36%
    e. Received thrombolysis, uncomplicated hospital course, asymptomatic 1-mm ST depression on rehabilitation TMET at 6 METS

Answers

1. Answer c.

In an ACS, in contrast to chronic stable angina or demand ischemia secondary to cardiac arrhythmia or hypotension, the pre-existing "vulnerable plaque" is often NOT hemodynamically significant until the time of rupture. Currently research is attempting to find improved methods of identifying coronary plaques with a higher likelihood of future rupture. This finding highlights the importance of aggressive long-term coronary risk factor management for all patients in addition to emergency revascularization by PCI.

2. Answer a.

Due in part to the availability of assisted reproductive techniques, there has been an increase in pregnancy rates among middle-aged women. CAD including ACS may be infrequently encountered during pregnancy. This patient has features of an acute anterior wall MI by clinical and ECG parameters. Emergency coronary angiography is indicated. If coronary intervention is required, additional therapy with other medications could be considered. The diagnosis of acute coronary disease should be confirmed before therapy is instituted. The differential diagnosis should include spontaneous coronary artery dissection, aortic dissection with ostial coronary involvement (bilateral upper extremity pulses and BP should be evaluated as well as a careful cardiac auscultation for the diastolic murmur of AR) and pulmonary embolism. Note ascending aortic dissection usually involves the RCA rather than the left main coronary artery or its branches.

3. Answer d.

Tachycardia on presentation is associated with increased 30-day mortality. The other variables are not associated with an increased short-term risk.

4. Answer d.

Complex ventricular ectopy following MI predicts a higher risk of future cardiac death. Both late potentials on signal-averaged ECG and decreased HR variability identify patients at increased risk of sudden death; the therapeutic implications of these findings are uncertain.

5. Answer a.

Although a positive stress test following thrombolytic therapy may identify patients at higher risk, the positive predictive value for future CV events is lower than patients with stable chronic angina.

6. Answer a.

In studies from the pre-thrombolytic era and studies of patients treated with thrombolysis, the highest risk patient subset has consistently been those unable to perform an exercise test for any reason.

7. **Answer d.**

CABG is still the preferred option in diabetic patients with significant three-vessel CAD and high-risk features (positive biomarkers in this presentation of unstable angina). However, PCI in low-risk unstable angina carries a class IIb recommendation, even with multivessel disease (2005 ACC update to PCI). However, "formal surgical consultation is recommended" in these scenarios.

Class IIa:

1. It is reasonable that PCI be performed in patients with UA/NSTEMI and single-vessel or multivessel CAD who are undergoing medical therapy with focal saphenous vein graft lesions or multiple stenoses who are poor candidates for reoperative surgery. *(Level of evidence: C)*

2. In the absence of high-risk features associated with UA/NSTEMI, it is reasonable to perform PCI in patients with amenable lesions and no contraindication for PCI with either an early invasive or early conservative strategy. *(Level of evidence: B)*

3. Use of PCI is reasonable in patients with UA/NSTEMI with significant left main CAD (>50% diameter stenosis) who are candidates for revascularization but are not eligible for CABG. *(Level of evidence: B)*

Class IIb:

1. In the absence of high-risk features associated with UA/NSTEMI, PCI may be considered in patients with single-vessel or multivessel CAD who are undergoing medical therapy and who have 1 or more lesions to be dilated with reduced likelihood of success. *(Level of evidence: B)*

2. PCI may be considered in patients with UA/NSTEMI who are undergoing medical therapy who have two- or three-vessel disease, significant proximal LAD CAD, and treated diabetes or abnormal LV function. *(Level of evidence: B)*

Short-Term Risk of Death or Nonfatal MI in Patients with Unstable Angina:

Feature	High risk (At least 1 of the following features must be present)	Intermediate risk (No high-risk feature but must have 1 of the following features)	Low risk (No high- or intermediate-risk feature but may have any of the following features)
History	Accelerating tempo of ischemic symptoms in preceding 48 hrs	Prior MI, peripheral or cerebrovascular disease, or CABG; prior aspirin use	
Character of pain	Prolonged ongoing (>20 min) rest pain	Prolonged (>20 min) rest angina, now resolved, with moderate or high likelihood of CAD Rest angina (<20 min or relieved with rest or sublingual NTG)	New-onset or progressive CCS Class III or IV angina in the past 2 wk without prolonged (>20 min) rest pain but with moderate or high likelihood of CAD

Clinical findings	Pulmonary edema, most likely related to ischemia New or worsening MR murmur S3 or new/worsening rales Hypotension, brady-cardia, tachycardia Age >75 yr	Age >70 yr	
ECG findings	Angina at rest with transient ST-segment changes >0.05 mV Bundle-branch block, new or presumed new Sustained VT	T-wave inversions >0.2 mV pathological Q waves	Normal or unchanged ECG during an episode of chest discomfort
Cardiac markers	Elevated (eg, TnT or TnI > 0.1 ng/mL)	Slightly elevated (eg, TnT > 0.01 but <0.1 ng/mL)	Normal

8. Answer a.

Over 90% of patients with AMI have a modifiable CV risk factor.

9. Answer e.

Statins, beta blockers, ACE inhibitors and aspirin have all be shown to improve survival in patients with CAD while Vitamin E does not improve survival.

10. Answer b.

The ECG shows features typical of acute anterior MI. While he is pain free, there is continuing evidence of myocardial injury on the ECG. Cardiac catheterization can be performed promptly with consideration of acute reperfusion, using balloon angioplasty and stenting. If a cardiac catheterization laboratory is not available, the benefits and risk of thrombolytic therapy must be carefully weighed while considering the past history of a cardioembolic stroke 3 yrs ago. In this case, since there was no catheterization laboratory available, the patient received thrombolytic therapy and the ST segments normalized. Note that a history of hemorrhagic stroke is an absolute contraindication to thrombolytics, while a history of embolic stroke is a relative contraindication if greater than 1 year prior. These ECG changes should be distinguished from those of acute pericarditis. Thrombolytic therapy in acute pericarditis can result in hemorrhagic pericarditis.

11. Answer b.

In the current era overall mortality between hospital discharge and 1 yr is 7% to 8%. Before 1980 mortality was approximately 20%. In patients selected for randomized trials and treated with reperfusion therapy, 1-yr post discharge mortality is between 2% and 4%, highlighting the selected subset of patients enrolled in clinical trials.

12. Answer c.

Mortality risk is higher in anterior wall MI as in this case. Hypotension (< 100 mmHg systolic) and high HR (> 100 bpm) are also associated with higher mortality. Low body weight (in the TIMI STEMI risk score < 67 kg) is associated with increased mortality.

13. Answer a.

Measurement of LV EF is considered a class I indication in AMI patients. LV EF has been one of the strongest prognostic variables in both the pre-thrombolytic and the current eras. LV EF measurements performed by equilibrium radionuclide angiography are not reliable in patients in AF due to the irregular HR. The effects of stunning may take weeks to resolve.

14. Answer d.

The most consistent finding of studies on exercise testing post AMI in both the pre-thrombolytic and current eras is that patients not referred for exercise testing have considerably higher mortality than patients referred for testing. ST segment depression has been considered the hallmark of an abnormal test but is a weaker prognostic variable than exercise duration. Beta blockers may lower the sensitivity of the exercise ECG, but most MI patients are commonly tested on beta blockers. 2002 ACC/AHA Exercise Testing Guidelines state that an early submaximal test or a later maximal test are both class I indications. Some studies have suggested that the early submaximal test has better prognostic value.

Exercise Testing after MI

Class I:

1. Before discharge for prognostic assessment, activity prescription, evaluation of medical therapy (submaximal at about 4 to 76 days).

2. Early after discharge for prognostic assessment, activity prescription, evaluation of medical therapy, and cardiac rehabilitation if the predischarge exercise test was not done (symptom limited; about 14 to 21 days).

3. Late after discharge for prognostic assessment, activity prescription, evaluation of medical therapy, and cardiac rehabilitation if the early exercise test was submaximal (symptom limited; about 3 to 6 weeks).

Class IIa:

1. After discharge for activity counseling and/or exercise training as part of cardiac rehabilitation in patients who have undergone coronary revascularization.

Class IIb:

1. Patients with the following ECG abnormalities:
   - Complete LBBB
   - Pre-excitation syndrome
   - LVH
   - Digoxin therapy
   - >1 mm of resting ST-segment
   - Depression
   - Electronically-paced ventricular rhythm

2. Periodic monitoring in patients who continue to participate in exercise training or cardiac rehabilitation.

Class III:

1. Severe comorbidity likely to limit life expectancy and/or candidacy for revascularization.

2. At any time to evaluate patients with AMI who have uncompensated CHF, cardiac arrhythmia, or noncardiac conditions that severely limit their ability to exercise. (Level of evidence: C)

3. Before discharge to evaluate patients who have already been selected for, or have undergone, cardiac catheterization. Although a stress test may be useful before or after catheterization to evaluate or identify ischemia in the distribution of a coronary lesion of borderline severity, stress imaging tests are recommended. *(Level of evidence: C)*

15. Answer e.

The patient underwent successful pharmacologic reperfusion with thrombolysis. While coronary angiography is useful to define the anatomy, it becomes an elective procedure in the setting of successful thrombolysis. Aggressive medical management should always accompany pharmacologic or percutaneous revascularization strategies.

16. Answer d.

The TIMI STEMI Risk Score assigns points for the following:

TIMI Risk Score for STEMI

Historical	
Age 65–74	2 points
≥75	3 points
DM/HTN or Angina	1 point
Exam	
SBP < 100 mmHg	3 points
HR > 100 bpm	2 points
Killip II–IV	2 points
Weight <67 kg	1 point
Presentation	
Anterior ST elevation or LBBB	1 point
Time to rx >4 hrs	1 point
Risk score = Total	*(0–14)*

The odds ratio of death by 30 days (referenced to average mortality) is 0.1 for a score of 0 points, 1.2 for score of 4 points and 8.8 for a score >8.

17. Answer a.

More MIs occur from the rupture of stenoses with <50% luminal diameter obstruction than in those >50%. The best answer is the vessel with the greatest extent of coronary disease. This is reflective of the fact that there are generally far more "mild-moderate" stenoses in the coronary arterial tree in patients with CAD. It could reasonably be argued that all three coronary vessels likely have multiple non-flow limiting stenoses, not all of which will be evident on angiography. It is the stability of the plaque, rather than the size or luminal encroachment of the plaque, that is crucial. There are currently no methods available to absolutely determine the stability of a plaque, although virtual histology with IVUS may be an important future imaging modality.

18. Answer c.

In the absence of contraindications all MI patients should receive a statin, beta blocker, and aspirin and be referred for cardiac rehabilitation.

19. Answer a.

Due to lack of sensitivity and specificity, current guidelines do not have a risk-stratification role for TMET in the setting of coronary angiography.

Exercise Testing after AMI: 2002 ACC/AHA Guideline Update for Exercise Testing

Class III:

1. Severe comorbidity likely to limit life expectancy and/or candidacy for revascularization.
2. At any time to evaluate patients with AMI who have uncompensated CHF, cardiac arrhythmia, or noncardiac conditions that severely limit their ability to exercise. *(Level of evidence: C)*
3. Before discharge to evaluate patients who have already been selected for, or have undergone, cardiac catheterization. Although a stress test may be useful before or after catheterization to evaluate or identify ischemia in the distribution of a coronary lesion of borderline severity, stress imaging tests are not routinely recommended. *(Level of evidence: C)*

20. Answer d.

Marked ST-segment depression at 4 METS during a submaximal TMET is marker of significant myocardial ischemia.

21. Answer b.

This patient has high risk features of ACS and will likely need coronary angiography with PCI in an "early invasive strategy." In addition to traditional medical management with aspirin, heparin, and a beta blocker, an IV glycoprotein IIb/IIIa inhibitor has evidence of benefit in this setting. The CURE trial studied patients with NSTEMI or unstable angina with ECG changes and demonstrated clopidogrel loading with 300 mg >6 hrs prior to coronary angiography has benefit. An alternative strategy is to wait until the coronary anatomy has been defined before administering clopidrogel, in case the patients has "surgical-type" CAD and needs urgent CABG. It would also be a reasonable choice to select clopidrogel for the initial management of this patient. However, answer **d** is not appropriate as heparin administration, an important component of unstable angina management, is omitted.

22. Answer c.

PCI and coronary stenting are indicated in the presence of a flow-limiting stenosis associated with unstable coronary symptoms.

23. Answer a.

The only drug that has been conclusively proven to reduce mortality in unstable angina is aspirin.

24. Answer b.

While initial studies such as VANQWISH did not demonstrate benefit from early aggressive angiography and PCI, further studies and ACC guidelines in 2002 determined that, compared with conservative management, early invasive treatment of patients with unstable angina or NSTEMI using coronary angiography (<48 hrs) with or without revascularization reduces re-hospitalization and refractory angina within the first year and significantly reduces mortality and MI at 2 to 5 yrs. However, patients undergoing early invasive treatment are more likely to have short-term complications such as bleeding and procedure-related MI. Clopidogrel given as a loading dose (300 mg) >6 hrs prior to PCI has significant benefit (CREDO, CURE trials); however, this should be balanced by the potential delay or increased bleeding if a surgical revascularization is needed. Ticlopidine has been replaced by clopidrogel because of the occurence of blood dyscrasias with ticlopidine. Consideration should be given to the potential need for emergent CABG in patients with suspected severe three-vessel or left-main CAD.

25. Answer a.

From ACC/AHA STEMI Guidelines:

Contraindications and Cautions for Fibrinolysis in STEMI MI:

Absolute contraindications:

- Any prior ICH
- Known structural cerebral vascular lesion (eg, arteriovenous malformation)
- Known malignant intracranial neoplasm (primary or metastatic)
- Ischemic stroke within 3 mos EXCEPT acute ischemic stroke within 3 hrs
- Suspected aortic dissection
- Active bleeding or bleeding diathesis (excluding menses)
- Significant closed-head or facial trauma within 3 mos

Relative contraindications:

- History of chronic, severe, poorly controlled HTN
- Severe uncontrolled HTN on presentation (SBP > 180 mmHg or DBP > 110 mmHg)
- History of prior ischemic stroke >3 mos, dementia, or known intracranial pathology not covered in contraindications
- Traumatic or prolonged (>10 mins) CPR or major surgery (<3 wks)
- Recent (within 2 to 4 wks) internal bleeding
- Noncompressible vascular punctures
- For streptokinase/anistreplase: prior exposure (more than 5 days ago) or prior allergic reaction to these agents
- Pregnancy
- Active peptic ulcer
- Current use of anticoagulants: the higher the INR, the higher the risk of bleeding

26. Answer d.

This patient may be a candidate for IV thrombolysis. This question highlights the differences in current guidelines for thrombolytic administration for CVA versus STEMI. If thrombolytics are to be given, other anticoagulation (heparin) and antiplatelet agents (ASA, clopidogrel, IIb/IIIa inhibitor) are relatively contraindicated within 24 hrs. This is due to the increased risk of intracranial hemorrhage. However, this is in contrast to aspirin and heparin co-administration for thrombolysis in STEMI. If the patient had **clear** evidence of MI, clinical decision-making would dictate pharmacotherapy.

27. Answer e.

AF is not directly an ischemic rhythm. In select cases, a large MI can increase LVEDP and left atrial pressures. This increased stretch and pressure on the atrium can trigger AF. However, in a patient predisposed to AF, the rhythm can be triggered merely by the increased catecholamines of the event and is not a high-risk feature.

28. Answer a.

The updated (2002) ACC/AHA guideline for ACS considers coronary angiography a class I indication for a patient with unstable angina/NSTEMI and high risk features like elevated troponin T or I. Angiography is a class I indication in patients with more severely reduced LV EF (<0.40). In the first edition of the ACC/ AHA AMI guidelines, non-Q wave MI was considered a class I indication for coronary angiography but now is a class IIb indication. An elevated CRP has been shown to predict higher mortality but its role in patient management has yet to be determined.

Class I:

1. An early invasive strategy in patients with unstable angina/NSTEMI without serious comorbidity and who have any of the following high-risk indicators: *(Level of evidence: A)*

    a. Recurrent ischemia despite intensive anti-ischemic therapy. *(Level of evidence: A)*
    b. Elevated troponin level. *(Level of evidence: A)*
    c. New ST-segment depression. *(Level of evidence: A)*
    d. CHF symptoms or new or worsening MR. *(Level of evidence: A)*
    e. Depressed LV systolic function. *(Level of evidence: A)*
    f. Hemodynamic instability. *(Level of evidence: A)*
    g. Sustained VT. *(Level of evidence: A)*
    h. PCI within 6 mos. *(Level of evidence: A)*
    i. Prior CABG. *(Level of evidence: A)*

2. In the absence of any of these findings, either an early conservative or an early invasive strategy may be offered in hospitalized patients without contraindications for revascularization. *(Level of evidence: B)*

29. Answer c.

Unstable angina/NSTEMI with left main disease should be referred for CABG unless contraindications exist. PCI is indicated for the other options barring contraindications.

Class IIa:

1. It is reasonable that PCI be performed in patients with unstable angina/NSTEMI and single-vessel or multivessel CAD who are undergoing medical therapy with focal saphenous vein graft lesions or multiple stenoses who are poor candidates for reoperative surgery. *(Level of evidence: C)*
2. In the absence of high-risk features associated with unstable angina/NSTEMI, it is reasonable to perform PCI in patients with amenable lesions and no contraindication for PCI with either an early invasive or early conservative strategy. *(Level of evidence: B)*
3. Use of PCI is reasonable in patients with unstable angina/NSTEMI with significant left main CAD (>50% diameter stenosis) who are candidates for revascularization but are not eligible for CABG. *(Level of evidence: B)*

Class IIb:

1. In the absence of high-risk features associated with unstable angina/NSTEMI, PCI may be considered in patients with single-vessel or multivessel CAD who are undergoing medical therapy and who have 1 or more lesions to be dilated with reduced likelihood of success. *(Level of evidence: B)*
2. PCI may be considered in patients with unstable angina/NSTEMI who are undergoing medical therapy who have two- or three-vessel disease, significant proximal LAD CAD, and treated diabetes or abnormal LV function. *(Level of evidence: B)*

Class III:

In the absence of high-risk features associated with unstable angina/NSTEMI, PCI is not recommended for patients with unstable angina/NSTEMI who have single-vessel or multivessel CAD and no trial of medical therapy, or who have 1 or more of the following:

- Only a small area of myocardium at risk. *(Level of evidence: C)*
- All lesions or the culprit lesion to be dilated with morphology that conveys a low likelihood of success. *(Level of evidence: C)*
- A high risk of procedure-related morbidity or mortality. *(Level of evidence: C)*
- Insignificant disease (<50% coronary stenosis). *(Level of evidence: C)*
- Significant left main CAD and candidacy for CABG. *(Level of evidence: B)*

30. Answer a.

The SHOCK Trial Registry showed that mechanical revascularization was superior to medical therapy in the setting of cardiogenic shock and AMI. The magnitude of benefit to early revascularization was 132 lives saved at 1 yr per 1000 patients.

Largely based on this study, the 2004 ACC/AHA STEMI update recommends the following:

Pre-hospital Destination Protocols

Class I:

1. Patients with STEMI who have cardiogenic shock and are <75 yrs of age should be brought immediately or secondarily transferred to facilities capable of cardiac catheterization and rapid revascularization (PCI or CABG) if it can be performed within 18 hrs of onset of shock. *(Level of evidence: A)*
2. Patients with STEMI who have contraindications to fibrinolytic therapy should be brought immediately or secondarily transferred promptly (ie, primary-receiving hospital door-to-departure time <30 mins) to facilities capable of cardiac catheterization and rapid revascularization (PCI or CABG). *(Level of evidence: B)*
3. Every community should have a written protocol that guides EMS system personnel in determining where to take patients with suspected or confirmed STEMI. *(Level of evidence: C)*

Class IIa:

1. It is reasonable that patients with STEMI who have cardiogenic shock and are 75 yrs of age or older be considered for immediate or prompt secondary transfer to facilities capable of cardiac catheterization and rapid revascularization (PCI or CABG) if it can be performed within 18 hrs of onset of shock. *(Level of evidence: B)*
2. It is reasonable that patients with STEMI who are at especially high risk of dying, including those with severe CHF, be considered for immediate or prompt secondary transfer (ie, primary-receiving hospital door-to-departure time <30 mins) to facilities capable of cardiac catheterization and rapid revascularization (PCI or CABG). *(Level of evidence: B)*

31. Answer c.

In ISIS-2, streptokinase reduced mortality by 25%, aspirin by 23%, and the combination of aspirin with streptokinase reduced mortality by 42%.

32. Answer d.

A IIb/IIIa inhibitor can also be added if clinically indicated. Ticlopidine has been associated with TTP and agranulocytosis, and has largely been supplanted by the use of clopidogrel.

33. Answer a.

While contraindicated in cardiogenic shock and overt systolic heart failure, beta blockers can be safely given to patients with compensated systolic heart failure and AMI. Clinical assessment should dictate administration and caution with IV administration in those settings.

34. Answer c.

There are no data supporting increased survival or decreased morbidity with nitroglycerin use in AMI.

35. Answer c.

Thrombolytics create highly thrombogenic split products that require the use of heparin anticoagulation. Aspirin should always be co-administered. Full and half-dose glycoprotein IIb/IIIa inhibitors have been studied in combination with thrombolytics; there is increased bleeding and no significant net benefit.

36. Answer d.

Thrombolytics do not improve outcome in unstable angina. The ACUITY trial studied 14,000 patients with moderate to high risk ACS (including both UA and NSTEMI), compared bivalirudin (IV direct thrombin inhibitor) to heparin + IIb/IIIa inhibitor, and found that bivalirudin alone was **non-inferior** to heparin + IIb/IIIa and had less major bleeding. When IIb/IIIa inhibitor was added to bivalirudin for "bailout," bleeding rates were not significantly different than heparin + IIb/IIIa.

37. Answer a.

Abciximab is a monoclonal antibody directed against the platelet glycoprotein IIb/IIIa molecule and prevents fibrinogen binding to activated platelets. It has a short plasma half-life and binds strongly to the platelet receptors. This can cause an abrupt and profound thrombocytopenia within 2 to 4 hrs. The platelets affected by abciximab administration are permanently inhibited and recovery depends on either production or transfusion of new platelets. The small molecule IIb/IIIa inhibitors (tirofiban and eptifibatide) reversibly bind platelet receptors. They are able to inactivate any new platelets transfused and metabolic clearance of the drug is needed for eventual reversal of action.

38. Answer b.

This patient received thrombolysis 40 mins prior to arriving at your institution. In the absence of evidence of cardiogenic shock requiring emergent mechanical revascularization, it is too early to determine if pharmacologic reperfusion therapy has failed. However, depending on the time required to mobilize the catheterization laboratory, it may be prudent to forewarn them of impending pharmacologic failure. The REACT trial (NEJM 2005) was a randomized trial comparing medical therapy, rescue PCI, or repeat thrombolysis in the setting of acute STEMI initially treated with thrombolysis. They used non-resolution of ST-segments by 50% by 90 mins as criteria for failure. They found that "rescue" PCI was associated with event-free survival of 85% at 6 mos compared to ~70% with conservative management or repeat thrombolysis.

By ACC/AHA 2004 STEMI update:

Assessment of Reperfusion
Class IIa:
It is reasonable to monitor the pattern of STE, cardiac rhythm, and clinical symptoms over the 60 to 180 mins after initiation of fibrinolytic therapy. Noninvasive findings

suggestive of reperfusion include relief of symptoms, maintenance or restoration of hemodynamic and or electrical stability, and a reduction of at least 50% of the initial ST-segment elevation injury pattern on a follow-up ECG 60 to 90 mins after initiation of therapy. *(Level of evidence: B)*

39. Answer d.

The patient is presenting >6 hrs of symptoms, making thrombolysis markedly less effective. In addition, the patient is within 1 hr of transport time making a "medical contact-to-balloon time" within ~90 mins.

From 2004 ACC/AHA STEMI guidelines

Primary PCI

Class I:

1. General considerations: If immediately available, primary PCI should be performed in patients with STEMI (including true posterior MI) or MI with new or presumably new LBBB who can undergo PCI of the infarct artery within 12 hrs of symptom onset, if performed in a timely fashion (balloon inflation within 90 mins of presentation) by persons skilled in the procedure (individuals who perform more than 75 PCI procedures per year).

2. The procedure should be supported by experienced personnel in an appropriate laboratory environment (a laboratory that performs more than 200 PCI procedures per year, of which at least 36 are primary PCI for STEMI, and has cardiac surgery capability). *(Level of evidence: A)*

3. Specific considerations:

    ■ Primary PCI should be performed as quickly as possible with a goal of a medical contact-to-balloon or door-to-balloon interval of within 90 mins. *(Level of evidence: B)*

    ■ If the symptom duration is within 3 hrs and the expected door-to-balloon time minus the expected door-to-needle time is:
        i.   Within 1 hr, primary PCI is generally preferred. *(Level of evidence: B)*
        ii. Greater than 1 hr, fibrinolytic therapy (fibrinspecific agents) is generally preferred. *(Level of evidence: B)*

    ■ If symptom duration is >3 hrs, primary PCI is generally preferred and should be performed with a medical contact-to-balloon or door-to-balloon interval as short as possible and a goal of within 90 mins. *(Level of evidence: B)*

    ■ Primary PCI should be performed for patients <75 yrs old with ST elevation or LBBB who develop shock within 36 hrs of MI and are suitable for revascularization that can be performed within 18 hours of shock unless further support is futile because of the patient's wishes or contraindications/unsuitability for further invasive care. *(Level of evidence: A)*

    ■ Primary PCI should be performed in patients with severe CHF and/or pulmonary edema (Killip class 3) and onset of symptoms within 12 hrs. The medical contact-to-balloon or door-to-balloon time should be as short as possible (ie, goal within 90 mins). *(Level of evidence: B)*

Class IIa:

1. Primary PCI is reasonable for selected patients 75 yrs or older with ST elevation or LBBB or who develop shock within 36 hrs of MI and are suitable for revascularization that can be performed within 18 hrs of shock. Patients with good prior functional status who are suitable for revascularization and agree to invasive care may be selected for such an invasive strategy. *(Level of evidence: B)*

39. (*continued*)

2. It is reasonable to perform primary PCI for patients with onset of symptoms within the prior 12 to 24 hrs and 1 or more of the following:

- Severe CHF (*Level of evidence C*)
- Hemodynamic or electrical instability (*Level of evidence: C*)
- Persistent ischemic symptoms. (*Level of evidence: C*)

Class IIb:

The benefit of primary PCI for STEMI patients eligible for fibrinolysis is not well established when performed by an operator who performs fewer than 75 PCI procedures per year. (*Level of evidence: C*)

Class III:

1. PCI should not be performed in a non-infarct artery at the time of primary PCI in patients without hemodynamic compromise. (*Level of evidence: C*)
2. Primary PCI should not be performed in asymptomatic patients more than 12 hrs after onset of STEMI if they are hemodynamically and electrically stable. (*Level of evidence: C*)

40. Answer d.

This patient has new onset psoriasis precipitated by addition of a beta blocker. This is a known association and often resolves completely with discontinuation of the medication. It is important to recognize drug reactions from allergies to prevent unnecessary discontinuation of necessary pharmacotherapy.

41. Answer b.

Normal or minimally diseased epicardial coronary arteries are found in 10% to 20% of patients with unstable angina.

42. Answer b.

AR—but not AS—is a contraindication to intra-aortic balloon pump implantation.

43. Answer c.

Hyperthyroidism—but not hypothyroidism—may precipitate unstable angina.

44. Answer a.

Ticlopidine—but not sulfinpyrazone or dipyridamole—decreases cardiac events in patients with unstable angina.

45. Answer e.

Thrombolytic agents have no documented benefit in the *absence* of acute STEMI, with the exception of patients with LBBB in whom a new MI is masked or in patients with a posterior infarct and ST-segment depression in leads V1–V3.

46. Answer f.

The differential diagnosis of unstable angina includes all the above.

47. Answer e.

Unstable angina associated with any of the following is associated with a worse prognosis: rest pain, ST-segment depression ≥1 mm, a new MR murmur, or pulmonary edema.

48. Answer a.
Aspirin, heparin, beta blockers, and nitrates have been shown to be beneficial in unstable angina. Calcium channel blockers are indicated in subsets of patients with vasospastic angina or increased systolic BP or in those refractory to conventional treatment.

49. Answer d.
Lidocaine reduced ventricular ectopy in AMI but may increase the incidence of conduction disturbances and should not be administered to patients prophylactically. There is no substantial evidence that lidocaine reduces mortality in AMI.

50. Answer c.
Dihydropyridine calcium channel blockers can be useful in treating HTN and angina, especially if there is a vasospastic component. However, pharmacotherapy should utilize mortality-reducing medications (beta blockers and ACE inhibitors) preferentially in the setting of AMI. Calcium channel blockers *may* increase mortality after AMI, especially in patients with reduced ventricular function. Recent studies have suggested that there is no increased risk.

51. Answer a.
Statins should be started in the hospital on all patients with MI with a few exceptions such as patients with liver disease or a history of rhabdomyolysis.

52. Answer c.

53. Answer c.
Patients, especially with depressed LV EF benefit from titration of beta blockers. Mortality is decreased by ~30% with therapeutic doses of beta blockers, especially after MI.

54. Answer c.
Angiography after MI frequently leads to revascularization, including angioplasty, stent placement, or CABG. It is not a good predictor of mortality and does not predict reinfarction with any degree of accuracy. Angiography is not necessary in low-risk patients and is not a cost-effective risk-stratification method if applied to all patients. Angiography is best applied to high-risk patients, including those with ongoing ischemia, CHF, significant ventricular arrhythmias beyond the immediate post-infarction period and evidence of ischemia on stress testing.

55. Answer d.
TMET after MI in patients who have received thrombolysis differs significantly from that in patients treated in the pre-thrombolytic area or in those who have not received thrombolytic therapy. TMET does not accurately predict either mortality or reinfarction. It is, however, useful for exercise prescription and reassurance of the patient. Although stress testing in combination with either nuclear or exercise imaging has improved diagnostic accuracy, in general, compared with TMET alone, the incremental prognostic value of stress imaging after thrombolysis is not large.

56. Answer d.
Risk factors associated with poor outcome after MI include shock or advanced Killip class on presentation; the presence of CHF, including pulmonary congestion; advanced age, especially older than 70 yrs; or recurrent ischemia or rest angina. Patients who quit smoking during the hospitalization for AMI have similar rates of death compared to nonsmokers. Patients who continue to smoke have a hazard ratio of ~1.7 with regard to mortality.

57. Answer b.

The average 1-yr post-dismissal mortality rate for a patient receiving thrombolytic therapy in a clinical trial is 2% to 4%. Clinical trials often exclude high-risk patients and must be critically interpreted to assess applicability to individual patients.

58. Answer c.

The average 1-yr post-dismissal mortality rate in a large observational registry after reperfusion with either thrombolysis or PTCA was 5% to 6%, which is significantly higher than that for patients in clinical trials referred to in Question 57, which was 2% to 4%. Selection bias for patients included in clinical trials is thought to explain the difference.

59. Answer d.

In the GISSI II trial, an EF < 40% was associated with a mortality rate of more than 8% 6 mos after MI. Female patients did not have a higher mortality rate than male patients. Exercise testing did not provide any incremental prognostic information over good clinical assessment. The GISSI II trial was notable in that there was a relatively low rate of angiography after MI in comparison to present-day practice in the United States.

60. Answer a.

In the GUSTO I trial, the 30-day mortality was approximately 1% and the additional 1-yr mortality rate was 3.5%. Patients with uncomplicated infarction by day 4 had a 1% 30-day mortality rate and 2.6% additional 1-yr mortality rate. Older age, hypotension, Killip class II or higher, increased HR, and location of infarct were the strongest clinical predictors of mortality at 30 days. In comparison, the uncomplicated infarction rate was 57% higher in the GISSI study.

61. Answer b.

For patients not receiving thrombolysis or primary PTCA, the mortality is generally higher than in those receiving thrombolysis or considered candidates for thrombolysis. Angiography and stress testing are useful to select patients for revascularization therapy or those who may be safely managed with medical therapy. In patients who do not receive thrombolysis, the importance of ancillary therapy (including aspirin, beta blockers, and ACE inhibitors) is comparable to that in patients receiving thrombolysis. There is no evidence that revascularization prolongs survival in patients who are asymptomatic with good ventricular function and have single-vessel CAD, excluding flow-limiting left main CAD or proximal LAD disease.

62. Answer d.

The highest risk of death after MI occurs in patients presenting in Killip class II or higher with significantly decreased LV function. Patients considered to be at relatively low risk are those who received thrombolysis or primary PTCA as part of a trial, because trials generally seem to select patients at lower risk than those excluded from participation. Patients who are not part of a clinical trial but who present early are also in a favorable prognostic category. Patients with uncomplicated MI after thrombolysis also have a favorable prognosis, even with the presence of 1 mm of asymptomatic depression on rehabilitation treadmill at 6 METS.

SECTION V

Congestive Heart Failure and Cardiac Transplantation

Brian P. Shapiro, MD

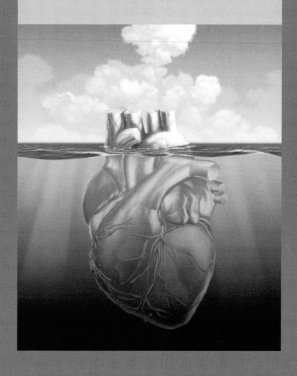

Questions

1. An 83-year-old man presents to the ED with worsening dyspnea, paroxysmal nocturnal dyspnea, and edema over the last week. He has a history of CAD with a prior MI and CABG at the age of 74. He developed heart failure 3 years ago but has done well since then with stable NYHA class II symptoms. He has been free of angina, palpitations, or syncope. He follows a low salt diet and is compliant with medications. He denies fever, chills, sweats, or productive cough. His weight has increased by 8 pounds in the past week and has been unresponsive to taking an extra dose of furosemide (60 mg) per day. The patient has had increasing pain in his left great toe for one week and has been using ibuprofen 400 mg TID for the past 7 days. His past medical history is significant for hyperlipidemia, chronic obstructive lung disease, and mild renal insufficiency.

   - Medications
Enalapril:	10 mg BID
Carvedilol:	3.125 mg BID
Digoxin	0.125 mg QD
Furosemide:	60 mg BID (increased to 60 mg TID 6 days ago)
Ibuprofen:	400 mg TID (started 7 days ago)

   - Vital signs
BP:	147/86 mmHg
HR:	90 bpm, regular

   - Physical examination
Lungs:	Bilateral lower lung crackles
Cardiac:	JVP 12 cm, point of maximal impulse enlarged and displaced inferolaterally, +S3, 2/6 holosystolic murmur at apex
Extremities:	Lower extremity edema to the knee bilaterally

   - Laboratory
Sodium:	131 mEq/L
Creatinine:	3.8 mg/dL (previously 1.7 mg/dL)
Troponin T:	0.10 ng/mL (no change)
BNP:	1250 pg/mL

   - ECG: Regular sinus rhythm rate 75 bpm; old LBBB
   - TTE:
     EF 25%
     Mild-moderate mitral valve regurgitation

Answers to this section start on page 173.

1. (*continued*)

   ■ Portable chest radiograph:

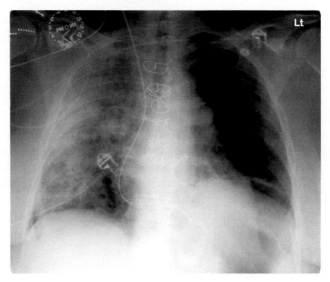

   Which factor(s) was most likely responsible for the patient's clinical decompensation?

   a. Reduction in renal blood flow
   b. Myocardial ischemia
   c. Inhibition of renal production of prostaglandins
   d. Mitral valve regurgitation
   e. All of the above
   f. a, b, c
   g. a and c

2. Myocardial contraction occurs due to release of large stores of Ca^{2+} from the SR, which activates the Ca^{2+}/troponin/actin/myosin cascade.

   Which of the following best characterizes the events that occur in LV relaxation?

   a. LV relaxation is an active, energy-dependent process
   b. Ca^{2+} reuptake into the SR is dependent on the SERCA pump
   c. In diastolic dysfunction, Ca^{2+} reuptake into the SR is slowed/abnormal
   d. All of the above

3. A 78-year-old man with DM and HTN presents to your office with progressive dyspnea (NYHA functional class III) and lower extremity swelling. In addition to ordering an echocardiogram for assessment of LV systolic function, what is currently the most appropriate next test to assess his diastolic function?

   a. Cardiac MRI
   b. Echocardiography-Doppler imaging techniques
   c. Echocardiography-Strain imaging techniques
   d. Left heart catheterization
   e. BNP

4. A 35-year-old woman who is 37 weeks pregnant presents to the ED with progressive dyspnea, lower extremity edema, weight gain, and fatigue. The patient was previously asymptomatic and has no history of CV disease.

■   Physical examination
Lungs: Crackles are noted in both lungs
Cardiac: JVP of 13 cm, diffuse apical impulse, apical holosystolic
                 murmur, +S3

Based on the clinical presentation, what is the mostly likely diagnosis?

a. Severe AS
b. Severe TR
c. ASD
d. Peripartum cardiomyopathy

5. A leftward shift in the LVEDP volume curve (see figure below) suggests which
    one of the following?

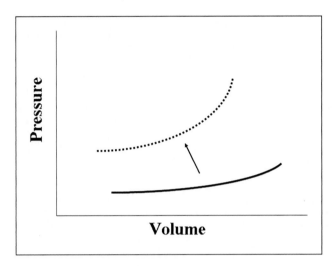

a. Increased LV compliance
b. Decreased LV compliance
c. Pericardial constraint
d. Decreased LV systolic function

6. Agents that promote NO synthesis or activity have recently gained interest in the
    treatment of heart failure. Which one of the following best describes the action
    of NO?

a. Promotes vasodilatation
b. Promotes ventricular hypertrophy and fibrosis
c. Contributes to essential HTN
d. Contributes to atherosclerosis
e. Activates the renin–angiotensin–aldosterone system

7. Patients with isolated chronic mitral or aortic valve regurgitation often have nor-
    mal filling pressures despite significant LV enlargement. The mechanism by
    which this may occur is known to include which one of the following?

a. A rightward shift in the LV pressure–volume relationship
b. A leftward shift in the LV pressure–volume relationship
c. An increase in the speed of LV relaxation
d. None of the above

8. A 91-year-old woman presents to the ED with severe shortness of breath at rest. She has a history of HTN for 35 years. A recent echocardiogram revealed an EF of 65%, LVH, and a pseudonormal pattern of ventricular diastolic filling.

- Vital Signs

BP:	192/45 mmHg
HR:	108 bpm, irregularly irregular
Respiration:	34 per min, labored
Oxygen saturation:	86%, room air

- Laboratory

Creatinine:	1.4 mg/dL
Troponin T:	< 0.01 ng/mL

- ECG:

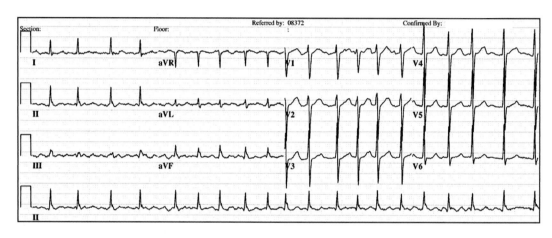

- Portable chest radiograph:

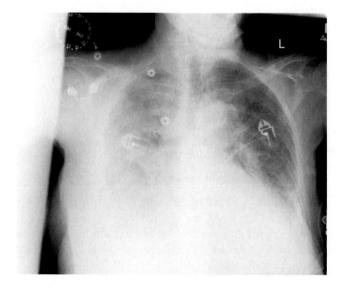

What would be the next most appropriate step in management?

a. Reduce BP
b. Control HR
c. Diuresis
d. TEE with electrical cardioversion
e. All of the above

9. A 42-year-old man with significant dyspnea, fatigue, peripheral edema, and orthostatic hypotension presents to the ED for evaluation.

■ Vital signs
   BP: 96/60 mmHg supine and 74/45 mmHg standing
   HR: 88 bpm

■ Physical examination
   Lungs: Bibasilar crackles and decreased breath sounds at base
   Cardiac: Regular rate and rhythm, JVP 15 cm, S3 present
   Extremities: 2+ lower extremity pedal edema bilaterally

■ ECG:

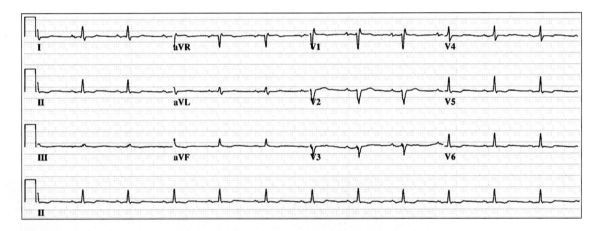

What is the most likely diagnosis given these findings?

a. Amyloid heart disease
b. HCM
c. Hypertensive heart disease
d. Severe mitral valve regurgitation

10. You are asked to evaluate a 35-year-old man in the ICU who was in a motor vehicle accident as a potential donor for cardiac transplantation. CT of the brain revealed brainstem herniation and the neurologist informs you that he is officially and irreversibly brain dead.

   To assess suitability as a cardiac donor, which of the following tests would **not** be part of the routine evaluation?

a. Endomyocardial biopsy
b. Echocardiography
c. ECG
d. Measurement of pulmonary vascular resistance
e. Coronary angiography

11. The abnormal LV filling pattern that demonstrates a reduced proportion of filling in early diastole and an increased proportion at atrial contraction is termed:

    a. Pseudonormal
    b. Impaired relaxation
    c. Restrictive
    d. None of the above

12. A 62-year-old man with ischemic cardiomyopathy (EF 25%) and NYHA class III symptoms presents to the ED with worsening dyspnea. Despite increased ventricular filling pressures, cardiopulmonary baroreceptor reflexes are attenuated in this patient, resulting in which of the following?

    a. Decreased adrenergic activity
    b. Increased adrenergic activity
    c. Systemic vasodilatation
    d. Suppression of the renin–angiotensin–aldosterone system

13. An 85-year-old woman with a history of DM and HTN presents to your office with mild DOE. She has no previous history of heart failure requiring hospitalizations. She denies orthopnea, palpitations, leg swelling, paroxysmal nocturnal dyspnea, or chest pain.

    ■ Vital signs
        BP: 165/50 mmHg
        HR: 80 bpm, regular

The ECG and chest radiogram are normal. A TTE revealed a normal EF and the following Doppler mitral inflow and tissue Doppler pattern:

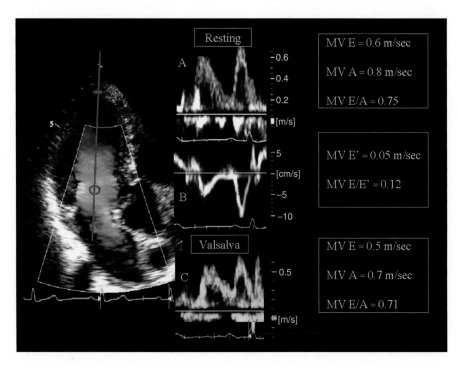

Based on this presentation, the most likely reason for her dyspnea would include:

a. Diastolic dysfunction
b. Pulmonary HTN
c. Heart failure with normal EF
d. Ischemic heart disease

14. You discuss medical management with a 52-year-old man with idiopathic cardiomyopathy (EF 35%) who describes NYHA function class III symptoms. You inform him that an ACE inhibitor is appropriate since it has been shown to do which one of the following?

a. Increase LV end-systolic volume
b. Improve survival and hospitalization rate
c. Increase LV mass
d. Promote vasoconstriction

15. A 38-year-old man with a 5-year history of heart failure due to idiopathic dilated cardiomyopathy presents with increasing dyspnea (unable to walk > 200 feet). Coronary angiography 4 years ago showed normal coronary arteries with an EF of 20% by ventriculography. EF by echocardiography 2 months ago was essentially unchanged.

- Medications
Lisinopril	10 mg once daily
Digoxin:	0.125 mg once daily
Furosemide:	40 mg twice daily
Warfarin:	5 mg once daily
Metolazone:	2.5 mg once daily

He comes in for routine follow-up. He is slightly more dyspneic and fatigued (has difficulty climbing one flight of stairs) and is requiring more frequent use of furosemide to control peripheral edema.

- ECG:

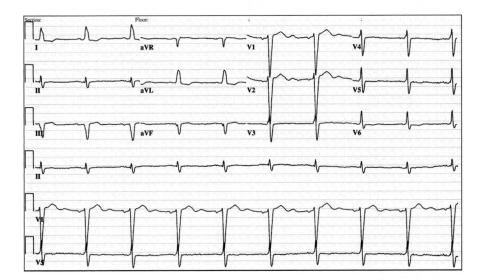

15. (*continued*)

The most appropriate next step in management includes which one of the following?

a. Coronary angiography
b. Echocardiogram
c. Stress testing, with measurement of oxygen consumption
d. Holter monitoring

16. With the exception of heart transplant evaluation, which of the following therapies would **not** be indicated in this above patient (Question 15)?

a. ICD
b. Carvedilol
c. Increase digoxin to 0.25 mg daily
d. Increased diuresis
e. Spironolactone
f. ICD and cardiac resynchronization device
g. All of the above are indicated

17. A 56-year-old woman who is active and completely asymptomatic presents to your office for her routine evaluation and has the following findings:

- ECG: Regular sinus rhythm, rate 68 bpm, no conduction abnormalities

- Chest radiograph: Mildly enlarged LV, no pulmonary congestion

- Echocardiogram:
  EF of 30%
  Moderate LV dilatation

The patient is otherwise normal, but has a family history of a mother who had sudden death at the age of 45 and a sister that was recently told of an enlarged heart. She has 3 children of childbearing age.

Exercise stress testing revealed no evidence of coronary ischemia and her maximal oxygen consumption was 75% predicted.

Further recommendation(s) should include:

a. Digoxin, a diuretic, an ACE inhibitor, a beta blocker, genetic counseling, and ICD
b. An ACE inhibitor, a beta blocker, genetic counseling, and ICD
c. Genetic counseling, close follow-up, and initiation of therapy when symptoms of heart failure develop
d. Transplant evaluation
e. A biventricular pacemaker

18. A 57-year-old woman presents with DOE, pedal edema, fatigue, and orthopnea. She has a long history of HTN and DM with suboptimal control. She does not have angina and is a nonsmoker with normal cholesterol levels.

- Medications
  Metoprolol: 50 mg twice daily
  Hydrochorothiazide: 25 mg once daily

- Vital signs
  BP: 170/90 mmHg
  HR: 64 bpm, regular

- Physical examination
  Lungs: Clear to auscultation
  Cardiac: JVP 12 cm, LV impulse prominent and sustained,
                      +S3, no murmurs
  Extremities: 2+ lower extremity pedal edema bilaterally

- ECG: Regular sinus rhythm, rate 65 bpm.

- Chest radiograph:

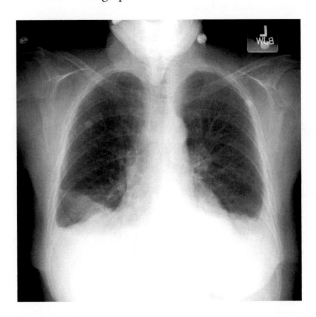

The next step in management should include which of the following?

a. Digoxin
b. Echocardiography
c. ACE inhibitor
d. Coronary angiography

19. A 91-year-old woman with exertional dyspnea and a HR of 88 bpm underwent echocardiography with assessment of ventricular filling pressures. She has a normal EF, mild LVH and moderate biatrial enlargement. The RV function is mildly reduced and the estimated RVSP is 52 mmHg (systolic BP 162/50 mmHg). Which abnormal LV filling pattern is **least** likely to benefit from therapies to reduce the HR?

a. Impaired relaxation
b. Pseudonormal LV filling
c. Restrictive LV filling
d. None of the above

20. Endothelin production is up-regulated in heart failure. An endothelin-receptor antagonist may be expected to do which one of the following?

a. Up-regulate the renin–angiotensin–aldosterone system
b. Improve survival in patients with left-sided heart failure and severe pulmonary HTN
c. Promote vasoconstriction
d. Promote vasodilatation

21. An 80-year-old woman without known heart failure presents to the ED with a one-week history of palpitations, progressive dyspnea, orthopnea, and peripheral edema. She has a history of HTN for 30 years.

- Vital signs
  BP: 190/60 mmHg
  HR: 135 bpm, irregularly irregular

- Physical examination
  Lungs: Diffuse crackles in bases bilaterally
  Cardiac: Irregularly irregular rhythm, no murmurs, JVP 13 cm
  Extremities: 1+ bilateral lower extremity edema

- ECG:

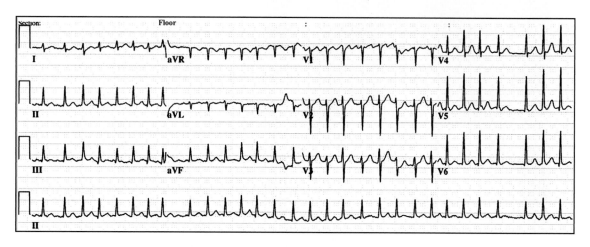

- Portable chest radiograph:

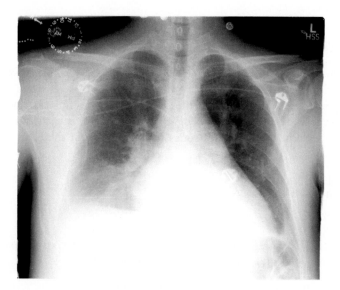

- Echocardiogram:
  EF 30%
  Severe biatrial enlargement
  Borderline LVH

What is the next most appropriate step in managing this patient?

a. Unfractionated heparin
b. IV calcium channel blocker
c. BP control
d. TEE with electrical cardioversion
e. All of the above

22. Which of the following is most accurate regarding current survival following cardiac transplantation?

a. One-year overall survival of 65% to 70%
b. Survival statistics are uniform from center-to-center
c. Highly dependent on recipient age
d. Posttransplant outcome is independent of donor heart ischemic time

23. Administration of recombinant BNP to a patient with heart failure should result in which one of the following changes?

a. Natriuresis
b. Reduced filling pressures
c. Decreased CO
d. a, b, and c
e. a and b

24. Which one of the following patients with heart failure would be expected to derive the greatest benefit from cardiac transplantation?

a. 45-year-old man with an EF of 18%, peak oxygen uptake (VO$_2$max) of 16 mL/kg/min, and BNP level of 1,650 pg/mL
b. 59-year-old woman with an EF of 30%, VO$_2$max of 10 mL/kg/min, and BNP of 650 pg/mL
c. 49-year-old woman with an EF of 20%, VO$_2$max of 14 mL/kg/min, and BNP of 1,200 pg/mL
d. 77-year-old man with an EF of 15%, VO$_2$max of 10 mL/kg/min, and BNP of 1,800 pg/mL

25. An 89-year-old woman with a 30-year history of HTN presents to the ED with worsening shortness of breath and 8-pound weight gain. She was in her usual state of health last week, but resting BP taken by her primary care physician was 175/50 mmHg. The present ED evaluation revealed the following:

■ Vital signs
   BP: 210/55 mmHg
   HR: 90 bpm, irregularly irregular
■ Laboratory
   Creatinine: 2.4 mg/dL (1.3 mg/dL a week ago)

25. (continued)

- ECG:

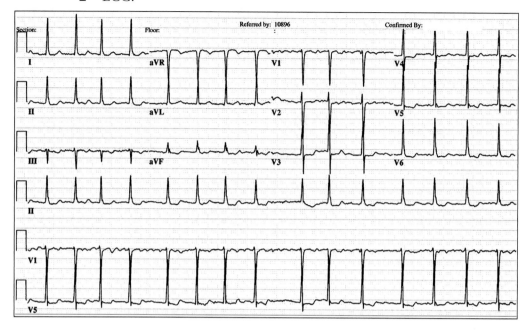

- Chest radiograph: Bilateral pleural effusions.

In the ED, she was administered IV NTG, which lowered her BP to 125/50 mmHg and improved her symptoms. Which answer best describes the arterial baroreflex response to the abrupt drop in BP?

a. Stimulation of efferent parasympathetic activity
b. Inhibition of efferent sympathetic activity
c. Decreased HR
d. Decreased carotid sinus baroreceptor discharge rate

26. A 76-year-old woman complains of mild exertional dyspnea, which she started to notice several weeks ago while walking around her neighborhood. An echocardiogram performed one year ago revealed an EF of 30% and an ICD was implanted at that time. She becomes dyspneic with walking fast or on hills but still walks approximately ¼ mile per day. She denies paroxysmal nocturnal dyspnea, orthopnea, or rest dyspnea. She has had mild edema in the evenings for years. She denies angina, palpitations, or syncope. She is a nonsmoker. She has a history of HTN.

- Medications
  Lisinopril: 20 mg once daily
  Metoprolol: 50 mg twice daily
  Furosemide: 40 mg twice daily
  Potassium: 20 mEq once daily

- Vital signs
  BP: 178/95 mmHg
  HR: 62 bpm, regular

- Physical examination
  Lungs: Clear to auscultation
  Cardiac: JVP normal with normal waveform, S1
                 S2 are paradoxically split, no S3 but there is an S4 present
  Extremities: Trace edema bilaterally

- Laboratory
  Creatinine: 2.5 mg/dL (at baseline)
  Potassium: 4.5 mEq/L

- ECG: Regular sinus rhythm, rate 60 bpm, LBBB

- Chest radiograph: Enlarged LV, mild pulmonary congestion. ICD with good position of the atrial and RV lead.

- Echocardiogram:
  LV end-diastolic dimension 6.5 cm
  EF 25%
  Normal valves

- Coronary angiography:
  Normal coronary arteries

The most appropriate next additional therapy includes:

a. Hydralazine titrated to 75 mg 4 times daily and isosorbide dinitrate titrated to 40 mg TID
b. Digoxin 0.125 mg once daily
c. Metolazone 2.5 mg once daily 30 minutes prior to furosemide
d. CRT

27. A 55-year-old man has a 6-month history of dilated cardiomyopathy (EF 35%, NYHA functional class II). The patient was previously healthy and his only traditional CV risk factor is age. He also has a one-year history of systolic HTN.

- Medications
  Metoprolol: 100 mg twice daily
  HCTZ: 25 mg once daily
  Lisinopril: 20 mg once daily
  Amlodipine: 10 mg once daily

Despite this treatment, the patient's BP remains elevated (165/78 mmHg) with a resting HR of 92 bpm. This clinical presentation is most consistent with which one of the following?

a. Renal artery stenosis
b. Pheochromocytoma
c. Viral myocarditis
d. Amyloid heart disease

28. You are asked to evaluate a 31-year-old woman who has a history of peripartum cardiomyopathy for suitability of cardiac transplantation. She delivered a normal healthy baby 6 weeks ago without complications, but since then has had NYHA functional class III/IV symptoms requiring hospitalization. Her EF is 15%. Which of the following tests would **not** be necessary for her work-up to assess suitability for cardiac transplantion recipients?

a. Psychosocial assessment
b. Right heart catheterization
c. CT of chest, abdomen, and pelvis
d. Echocardiography
e. Exercising testing for VO_2 assessment

29. An 87-year-old woman was referred for a second opinion after 4 hospitalizations for heart failure in the last 6 months. She has a long history of HTN. She denied having angina or CAD. She describes symptoms consistent with NYHA functional class III. An ICD was placed 6 months ago and since then there has been no ventricular arrhythmia noted or shocks delivered.

- Medications

Lisinopril:	5 mg once daily
Digoxin:	0.125 mg once daily
Carvedilol:	6.25 mg twice daily
Spironolactone:	25 mg once daily
Furosemide:	20 mg once daily
Potassium:	10 mEq once daily

- Vital signs

BP:	152/84 mmHg
HR:	70 bpm, regular

- Physical examination

Lungs:	Clear to auscultation
Cardiac:	JVP elevated to 12 cm with a large V wave, S3 present
Extremities:	2+ edema to knee bilaterally

- ECG:

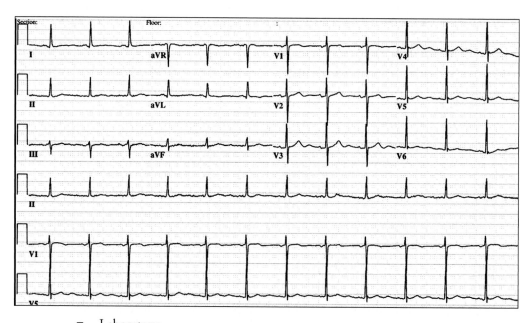

- Laboratory

Creatinine:	1.2 mg/dL
Potassium:	4.7 mEq/L

- Echocardiogram:
  LV end-diastolic dimension 6.0 cm
  EF 30%
  Global hypokinesis
  LV wall thickness 13 mm

The most appropriate therapeutic change at this point includes which one of the following?

a. Add metolazone
b. Add amlodipine
c. Titrate up lisinopril to 20 to 40 mg once daily and increase dose of furosemide
d. CRT

30. A 41-year-old woman who underwent heart transplantation 2 years ago for severe dilated cardiomyopathy returns to clinic following a cardiac biopsy. She is currently on cyclosporine and low-dose prednisone for maintenance immuno-suppressive therapy and has had no prior evidence of transplant rejection. Patient is currently experiencing fatigue, worsening dyspnea, and 10-pound weight gain over the past 3 weeks. She is hemodynamically stable, echocardiography reveals a normal EF with normal RV size and function, and her PA pressures are stable.

Cardiac biopsy reveals the following:

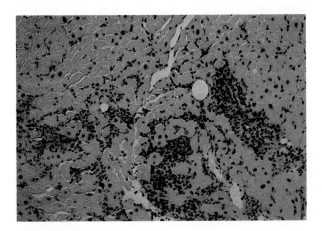

The next most appropriate step would include:

a. Reassuring her that this is a normal finding and that she is not undergoing rejection
b. Initiating ACE inhibitor
c. Admitting her and initiating Nesiritide and/or IV diuresis
d. Admitting her and initiating IV corticosteroids

31. Which one of the following does **not** represent abnormal LV diastolic function?

a. Restrictive filling pattern
b. Impaired LV relaxation filling pattern
c. Pseudonormal LV filling pattern
d. Diastolic predominant filling pattern

32. Which of the following LV diastolic filling patterns would suggest the highest PCWP?

    a. Pseudonormal
    b. Impaired relaxation
    c. Restrictive
    d. None of the above

33. An 88-year-old female with a history of ischemic cardiomyopathy (EF 25%) and moderate RV dysfunction presents to your office with progressive dyspnea (NYHA class III), 20-pound weight gain, and peripheral edema.

    ■ Medications
      Lisinopril: 10 mg once daily
      Carvedilol: 6.25 mg twice daily
      Aspirin: 81 mg once daily
      Atorvastatin: 40 mg once daily
      Furosemide: 60 mg twice daily
      Potassium: 20 mEq once daily

    ■ Vital signs
      BP: 125/55 mmHg
      HR: 65 bpm, regular

    ■ Physical exam
      Lungs: Bilateral crackles halfway up
      Cardiac: +S3, 3/6 holosystolic murmur over apex, JVP elevated to angle of the jaw
      Extremities: 3+ pedal edema to groin

    ■ Laboratory
      Sodium: 133 mEq/L
      Creatinine: 1.8 mg/dL
      Potassium: 3.5 mEq/l
      BNP: 1050 pg/mL
      Troponin T: 0.03 ng/mL

    ■ ECG: Regular sinus rhythm, rate 70 bpm

    ■ Portable chest radiograph:

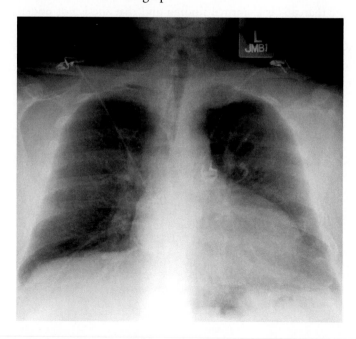

You decide to admit the patient into the hospital and initiate recombinant BNP (Nesiritide) therapy. This would be expected to do which of the following?

a. Improve survival
b. Enhance sodium excretion
c. Have no effect on PCWP
d. Have no effect on systemic BP

34. The above patient (Question 33) is administered IV recombinant BNP (Nesiritide) infusion and, after 6 hours, is breathing more comfortably. Her urine output during this time has exceeded 1.5 L. Her BP has declined to 88/45 mmHg.

The most appropriate next step would include:

a. Stopping the Nesiritide infusion, waiting for BP to improve, then reinitiating Nesiritide at a reduced dose (ie, 30% lower dose) without a bolus
b. Checking a BNP level and, if still markedly elevated, continue Nesiritide
c. Starting dobutamine and continuing Nesiritide
d. Discontinuing the angiotenin-converting enzyme inhibitor

35. A 42-year-old man with known idiopathic dilated cardiomyopathy for 7 years is on a transplant list in another state. An ICD was placed 4 years ago. While on vacation, he had acutely decompensated heart failure with dyspnea at rest, nightly paroxysmal nocturnal dyspnea, orthopnea, edema, and lightheadedness. His EF has been documented at 12% and a recent metabolic stress test showed a peak oxygen consumption of 10 mL/kg/min.

- Medications
  Lisinopril: 20 mg once daily
  Digoxin: 0.25 mg once daily
  Furosemide: 120 mg twice daily
  Warfarin: 2 mg once daily

- Vital signs
  BP: 82/64 mmHg
  HR: 120 bpm, regular
  Respiratory rate: 36 per min, moderately labored
  Oxygen saturation: 86% on room air; increased to 94% on 4 L nasal canula

- Physical examination
  General: Moderate respiratory distress at rest, has difficulty completing sentences due to breathlessness
  Lungs: Crackles halfway up posterior chest wall on auscultation
  Cardiac: JVP located at the angle of jaw with large V waves, dilated point of maximal impulse that is inferolaterally displaced, S1 and S2 split paradoxically, S3 is present, II/VI holosystolic murmur at apex
  Extremities: Cool, grade 3+ edema

- Laboratory
  Potassium: 3.5 mEq/L
  Sodium: 132 mEq/L
  Creatinine: 2.5 mg/dL (previously, 1.8 mg/dL)
  BNP: 1880 pg/ml
  Troponin T: 0.16 ng/ml

35. (*continued*)

■   ECG:

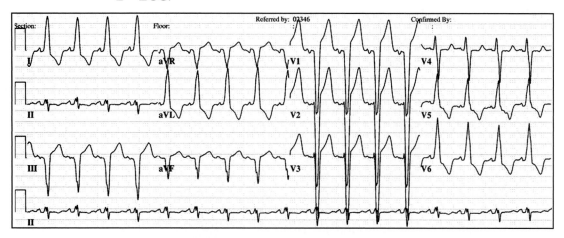

■   Portable chest radiograph:

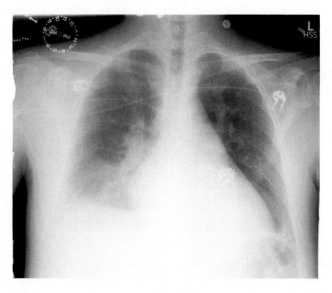

The most appropriate medical therapy at this point includes which one of the following?

a. Carefully reinitiate carvedilol
b. Titrate lisinopril up to 40 mg/day
c. Add spironolactone
d. Initiate IV inotropic and diuretic therapy and transfer to a cardiac transplant center as soon as possible
e. Add metolazone

36. You are asked to evaluate a 60-year-old woman who is hospitalized for treatment of cellulitis and is doing well, but nurses on the general medical floor have been refusing to administer her captopril due to low BP. She has stable NYHA functional class II symptoms. She denies any orthostatic lightheadedness, syncope, or presyncope. She insists that her BP is always "low." A review of her medical record shows BP in the range of 70/50 to 80/55 mmHg. She has not received captopril since admission. Her EF has been stable at 28%.

- Medications
  Captopril: 50 mg TID
  Carvedilol: 12.5 mg twice daily
  Furosemide: 40 mg once daily
  Digoxin: 0.25 mg once daily
  Cephalosporin: intravenously

- Vital signs
  BP: 75/50 mmHg supine, 72/55 mmHg standing
  HR: 66 bpm, regular

- Physical examination
  Lungs: Clear to auscultation
  Cardiac: Within normal limits
  Extremities: Cellulitis in left lower extremity, no edema, warm extremities, normal capillary refill time

- Laboratory
  Creatinine: 1.2 mg/dL
  Potassium: 4.2 mEq/L

Which one of the following represents the most appropriate next step in management?

a. Hold captopril completely
b. Reduce dose of captopril by half and follow-up with her cardiologist as an outpatient
c. Resume captopril at previous dose
d. Discontinue furosemide
e. Discontinue captopril and start hydralazine/isosorbide dinitrate
f. Refer for CRT

37. A 53-year-old man with multiple atherosclerotic risk factors, including HTN, hyperlipidemia, and tobacco use, presents with a 6-month history of DOE and exertional chest tightness. He has orthopnea and paroxysmal nocturnal dyspnea.
    Echocardiography reveals a severely dilated LV with an EF of 20% and global ventricular hypokinesis. The ECG is normal.

    The next step in diagnostic evaluation should be:

    a. Holter monitor
    b. Stress test with measurement of maximal oxygen consumption
    c. Coronary angiography
    d. Heart transplant evaluation

38. In the patient listed above (Question 37), coronary angiography reveals the following stenotic lesions:

    Left main: 20%
    Proximal LAD: 80%
    Proximal circumflex: 85%
    Mid-RCA: 90%

38. (*continued*)

Distal vessels are adequate in size. The most appropriate next step includes:

a. Surgical consultation for CABG

b. Viability study

c. Initiation of therapy with an ACE inhibitor and beta blocker

d. All of the above

39. A 78-year-old man with ischemic cardiomyopathy (cardiac bypass 21 years ago) for 7 years comes for his regular checkup. He has stable NYHA functional class II symptoms and has noted no change in his exercise tolerance or fluid retention. His EF is 20%. He has no palpitations, syncope, or presyncope. He has a past medical history significant for gout (last episode one year ago) and acute femoral arterial occlusion treated with embolectomy 3 years ago.

- Medications

Lisinopril:	30 mg once daily
Metoprolol:	50 mg once daily
Furosemide:	60 mg once daily
Digoxin:	0.25 mg once daily
Potassium:	20 mEq once daily
Warfarin:	5 mg once daily
Allopurinol:	200 mg once daily

- Vital signs

BP:	105/65 mmHg
HR:	80 bpm, regular

- Physical examination

Lungs:	Clear to auscultation
Cardiac:	JVP is normal with positive hepatojugular reflex; apex beat in sixth mid-axillary line, S1, S2 normal, no S3 + S4 present
Extremities:	1+ edema, peripheral pulses strong without bruits

- Laboratory

Creatinine:	1.2 mg/dL
Potassium:	4.3 mEq/L
INR:	2.3

- ECG:

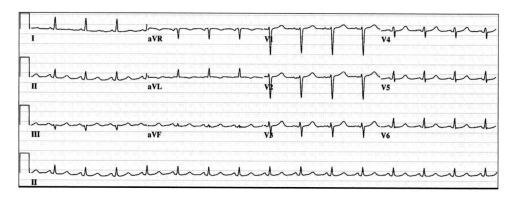

Which of the following is the most appropriate next step in management?

a. Invasive EP testing
b. Amiodarone
c. ICD
d. Discontinue warfarin
e. ICD plus CRT

40. Which of the following best describes the biologic actions of an ACE?

a. Promotes degradation of angiotensin II
b. Directly stimulates the synthesis of aldosterone
c. Stimulates the production of norepinephrine
d. Converts angiotensin I to angiotensin II
e. All of the above

41. A 62-year-old woman has ischemic cardiomyopathy (EF 30%) and is unable to walk > 100 feet on level ground due to DOE. She describes two-pillow orthopnea and lower extremity swelling that is stable, but denies paroxysmal nocturnal dyspnea, palpitations or syncope. Several years ago, a dual-chamber pacemaker was placed for symptomatic high grade AV block.

- Medications
  Enalapril: 10 mg twice daily
  Carvedilol: 12.5 mg twice daily
  Spironolactone: 25 mg twice daily
  Furosemide: 40 mg twice daily
  Aspirin: 81 mg once daily
  Simvastatin: 40 mg once daily

- ECG:

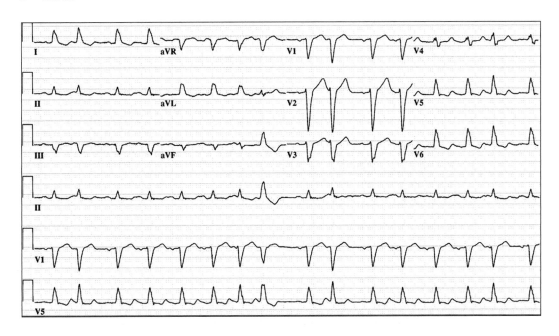

41. (*continued*)

- Portable chest radiograph:

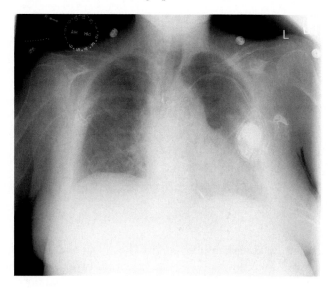

The next most appropriate step in management should include which of the following?

a. Increase furosemide dose
b. Initiate ARB
c. Initiate recombinant BNP (Nesiritide)
d. Upgrade to CRT

42. A 76-year-old man was admitted to the hospital with pulmonary edema. He has a long history of CAD and has had 2 prior MIs, but has not been evaluated by a physician in the last 2 years.

- Medications
Aspirin:	81 mg once daily
Metoprolol:	25 mg twice daily
Furosemide:	40 mg once daily
Isosorbide dinitrate:	30 mg TID

While in the hospital, he was treated with furosemide intravenously and had a 9-kg weight loss in 2 days. He was then switched to oral furosemide 80 mg twice daily on the third hospital day. An echocardiogram reveals an EF of 15%, with a dyskinetic apex. On the fourth hospital day, he was started on digoxin 0.125 mg once daily and lisinopril 10 mg once daily. On that same day, his BP decreased from 100/50 to 70/40 mmHg and he became lightheaded. You are asked to recommend additional medical therapy.

- Vital signs
BP:	90/50 mmHg supine and 80/40 mmHg standing
HR:	100 bpm, regular

- Physical examination
Lungs:	Clear to auscultation
Cardiac:	JVP flat, S1, S2 normal, no S3, no S4
Extremities:	No edema, mucous membranes are dry

■ Laboratory
  Creatinine: 1.3 mg/dL on admission, 2.3 mg/dL 2 days later (prior to first Lisinopril dose)
  Potassium: 3.7 mEq/L

■ ECG: Regular sinus rhythm, rate 90 bpm

■ Chest radiograph:

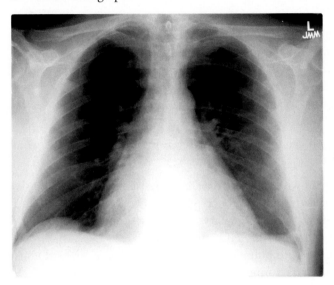

■ Adenosine sestamibi: Fixed anterior, septal, and apical perfusion defects, but no ischemia; EF 18%

Which one of the following would constitute the next most appropriate step to pharmacologic management?

a. Start inotropic therapy
b. Hold diuretics and isosorbide dinitrate, but continue the rest of his cardiac medicines with careful monitoring
c. Stop lisinopril and switch to losartan
d. Hold metoprolol

43. Which of the following medications is **not** associated with a survival benefit in systolic heart failure patients?

a. ACE inhibitor
b. Digoxin
c. Beta blockers
d. Aldosterone antagonists
e. Isosorbide dinitrate/hydralazine
f. All of the above improve survival

44. Which component of the cardiac cycle is most responsible for LV filling?

a. LV end-systolic volume
b. Transmitral pressure gradient
c. Rate of ventricular relaxation
d. Mean left atrial pressure
e. Viscoelastic properties of the LV

45. What percentage of heart failure patients have a normal EF?

    a. 20%
    b. 40% to 50%
    c. 60%
    d. 70%

46. Which of the following answers is **incorrect** regarding central sleep apnea and chronic heart failure?

    a. Characterized by repetitive episodes of apnea and hyperventilation
    b. Occurs predominantly during non-REM sleep
    c. Occurs in 33% to 70% of stable heart failure patients
    d. Is not associated with severity or prognosis of heart failure
    e. Optimization of heart failure therapy is the mainstay in treatment

47. Which one of the following patients with severe systolic heart failure would be the most appropriate for cardiac transplantation?

    a. 72-year-old woman with pulmonary vascular resistance of 2 Wood units
    b. 48-year-old man with transpulmonary gradient of 18 mmHg
    c. 32-year-old woman with pulmonary vascular resistance of 5 Wood units which does not change during NO administration
    d. 41-year-old woman with pulmonary vascular resistance of 8 Wood units that drops to 3 Wood units during NO administration

48. Which of the following is **incorrect** regarding initial, routine diagnostic work-up of heart failure that is supported by the ACC/AHA guidelines (2005)?

    a. Echocardiogram with Doppler
    b. Endomyocardial biopsy
    c. Coronary angiogram if there is evidence of angina or ischemia
    d. Thyroid-stimulating hormone

49. In which of the following scenarios is IV inotropic support most appropriate?

    a. In acute hemodynamically unstable heart failure
    b. In a patient awaiting transplantation who is hemodynamically unstable while receiving maximal oral therapy
    c. As palliative therapy to allow dismissal of the patient with refractory heart failure receiving oral therapy who is not a candidate for transplantation or other surgical therapy
    d. All of the above

50. Cardiac transplant rejection is most reliably detected by assessment of which of the following tests?

    a. Peripheral leukocyte count
    b. Echocardiography
    c. Endomyocardial biopsy
    d. Coronary angiogram

51. A 67-year-old man with severe, diffuse three-vessel CAD presents for outpatient follow-up after a recent heart failure hospitalization. He has been hospitalized for cardiac reasons 6 times this past year. A typical episode starts with chest tightness and quickly progresses to pulmonary edema. The patient has had numerous surgical consultations and has not been offered surgery because of "non-graftable" distal vessels. He also has a history of COPD, but currently not requiring medical or oxygen therapy. Viability testing has shown large areas of ischemia without fixed defects. His EF is 35%.

- CV risk factors:
  Insulin dependent DM for 20 years
  Hyperlipidemia for 10 years
  HTN for 20 years
  Tobacco abuse (50-pack-year history, quit 12 years ago)
  Family history (father had his first MI at the age of 40 years)

- Medications

Lisinopril:	40 mg once daily
Furosemide:	80 mg twice daily
Digoxin:	0.25 mg once daily
Aspirin:	325 mg once daily
Clopidogrel:	75 mg once daily
Isosorbide dinitrate:	60 mg TID
Atorvastatin:	40 mg once daily
Nifedipine:	30 mg once daily

- Vital signs

BP:	125/75 mmHg
HR:	90 bpm, regular

- Physical Examination

Lungs:	Clear to auscultation
Cardiac:	JVP 12 cm, S3 present
Extremities:	No edema

- Laboratory

Creatinine:	1.3 mg/dL
Potassium:	4.7 mEq/L

- ECG:

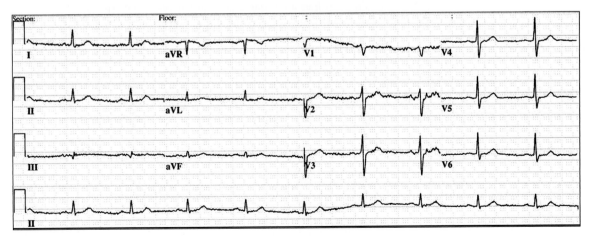

51. (*continued*)

■   Chest radiograph:

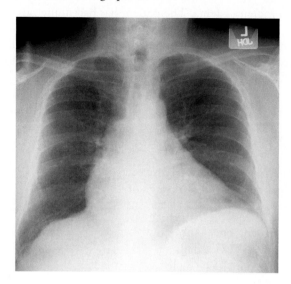

The most appropriate next step in management includes which one of the following?

a. Add a low dose of a cardioselective beta-receptor antagonist and titrate up as tolerated

b. Stop nifedipine and add hydralazine

c. Stop nifedipine and add amlodipine

d. Refer for EECP

52. Biologic actions of ANPs and BNPs include which of the following?

a. Inhibition of natriuresis

b. Activation of the renin–angiotensin–aldosterone system

c. Pro-fibrotic

d. Vasodilatation

e. Inhibition of guanylate cyclase

53. A 25-year-old man had a cardiac transplant 4 years ago due to severe myocarditis. He has done well post-transplant, but has noticed progressive DOE over the past 6 months.

■   ECG (reflects new changes):

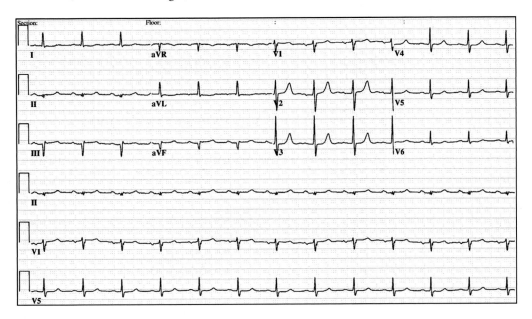

■   Echocardiogram:
EF 50%
Apical and inferior hypokinesis

The most likely cause for clinical deterioration includes which one of the following?

a. Acute T cell rejection
b. Non-Hodgkin's lymphoma
c. Coronary artery vasculopathy
d. None of the above

54. A 53-year-old man is referred by his orthopedist after a routine pre-anesthetic ECG showed the following abnormality:

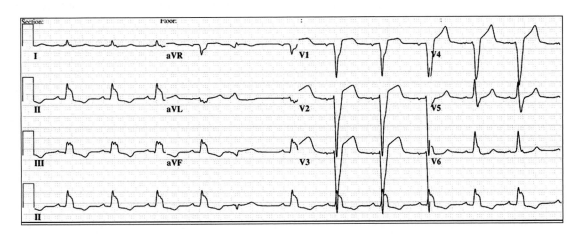

54. (continued)

Otherwise, he is healthy without a history of CV disease. He is a physically active construction worker and denies angina, exertional dyspnea, edema, palpitations or syncope. There is no family history of sudden death or heart disease. He has no specific CV risk factors and does not drink alcohol or take recreational drugs.

- Vital signs
  BP: 115/65 mmHg
  HR: 65 bpm, regular

- Physical examination
  Lungs: Clear to auscultation
  Cardiac: JVP and waveforms are normal, apical beat normal in location and character, S1, S2 paradoxically split, no S3, but + S4 present
  Extremities: No edema

- Laboratory
  Creatinine: 1.0 mg/dL
  Potassium: 4.2 mEq/L

- Chest radiograph:
  No pulmonary congestion

- Echocardiogram:
  LV end-diastolic dimension 7.0 cm
  EF 30%
  Normal cardiac valves

- Exercise stress test:
  No evidence of infarction or ischemia, VO_2 max 110% predicted

The most appropriate therapy for this patient includes which one of the following?

a. Digoxin 0.25 mg once daily, lisinopril titrated to 40 mg once daily, furosemide 20 mg once daily

b. Carvedilol titrated to 25 mg twice daily and lisinopril titrated to 40 mg once daily

c. Hydralazine titrated to 75 mg 4 times daily and isosorbide dinitrate titrated to 30 mg TID

d. Carvedilol titrated to 25 mg twice daily, lisinopril titrated to 40 mg once daily and ICD

e. Enalapril titrated to 40 mg once daily

f. Carvedilol titrated to 25 mg twice daily, lisinopril titrated to 40 mg once daily, spironolactone 25 mg once daily and ICD

g. Since he is asymptomatic, monitor without therapy with close follow-up

55. A 70-year-old man is referred for a second opinion after a recent hospitalization in which he had a perioperative anterior MI following radical prostate surgery. He did not receive thrombolysis or coronary angiography due to concern regarding postoperative bleeding. In the first hospitalization, he had pulmonary edema, which responded to diuresis, digoxin, and initiation of enalapril, which was increased to 10 mg twice daily before dismissal. He tolerated initiation of low-dose carvedilol. Adenosine sestamibi prior to dismissal revealed a fixed anteroseptal defect. On his return one week after dismissal, he reported being physically inactive but denied having angina, dyspnea, or palpitations.

- Medications

Enalapril:	10 mg twice daily
Furosemide:	40 mg once daily
Digoxin:	0.25 mg once daily
Carvedilol:	6.25 mg twice daily
Aspirin:	81 mg once daily

- Vital signs

BP:	110/50 mmHg
HR:	60 bpm, regular

- Physical examination

Lungs:	Clear to auscultation
Cardiac:	JVP normal, heart sounds normal without murmurs
Extremities:	No edema

- Laboratory

Creatinine:	1.7 mg/dL (previously 1.3 on admission and 1.8 on dismissal from hospital)
Potassium:	4.9 mEq/L

- ECG:

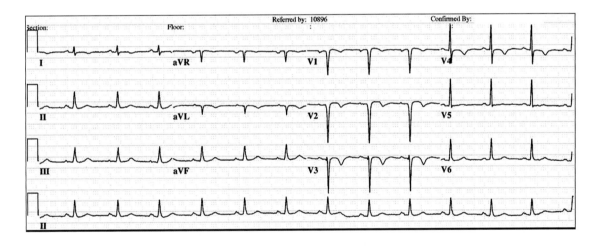

- Echocardiogram:
  Dilated LV with thinning and akinesis of the anterior wall and septum
  EF 15%

The most appropriate medical therapeutic changes at this point include which one of the following?

a. Discontinue treatment with enalapril, start treatment with hydralazine/isosorbide dinitrate

b. Add warfarin

c. Discontinue treatment with enalapril, start treatment with losartan

d. Discontinue treatment with enalapril and metoprolol, start treatment with hydralazine and isosorbide dinitrate

e. Insert ICD now

56. A 68-year-old woman presents with DOE and pedal edema that clears overnight. She has a long history of HTN. She does not have angina. She is a nonsmoker and has normal cholesterol levels.

- Medications
Metoprolol:	25 mg twice daily
Amlodipine:	5 mg once daily

- Vital signs
BP:	170/100 mmHg
HR:	58 bpm, regular

- Physical examination
Lungs:	Clear to auscultation
Heart:	Jugular venous pulse poorly visualized, LV impulse prominent, no murmurs, heart sounds distant
Extremities:	Mild pedal edema

- The ECG and chest radiograph are within normal limits.

- Echocardiography:
  Normal LV size and function, EF 70%, no regional wall motion abnormality
  LV wall thickness 16 mm; LV mass index 175 g/m^2
  LA moderately enlarged
  E/A ratio of the mitral inflow Doppler velocity profile 2.0
  Deceleration time 140 msec
  Isovolumic relaxation time 65 msec
  TR velocity 3.2 m/sec

Which one of the following statements is correct?

a. This patient has heart failure with normal EF
b. This patient has LVH
c. The LV end-diastolic filling pressures are increased
d. All of the above

57. Which of the following answers is correct regarding BNP?

a. Indicates increased ventricular volume and/or wall stress
b. Is not affected by renal function
c. Is elevated in only systolic, but not diastolic heart failure
d. Will always be elevated in heart failure

58. A 72-year-old woman with insulin dependent DM and chronic renal insufficiency is admitted to the hospital with dyspnea at rest, 15-pound weight gain and severe lower extremity edema.

- Vital signs
BP:	165/60 mmHg
HR:	76 bpm, regular
Respiration:	30, moderately labored
Oxygen saturation:	90% on 3 L nasal canula

- Physical examination
General:	Difficulty completing sentences due to breathlessness
Lungs:	Diffuse crackles
Cardiac:	Elevated JVP to 14 cm, regular rate and rhythm, normal heart sounds with 2/6 early-peaking SEM over right upper sternal border
Extremities:	2+ lower extremity pedal edema

- Laboratory
Creatinine:	1.8 mg/dL (at baseline)
Troponin T:	0.09 ng/mL (0.04 ng/mL 16 months ago)
BNP:	1450 pg/mL

- Chest radiograph:

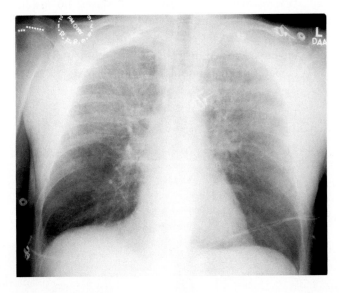

- Echocardiogram:
  EF 70%
  Mild LVH
  Severe biatrial enlargement
  Diastolic filling pattern consistent with pseudonormal pattern

Coronary angiography and left heart catheterization reveal mild diffuse coronary disease, but there was no evidence of hemodynamically significant plaques.

Using a micromanometer catheter, during which phase of diastole is it most appropriate to measure the compliance characteristics of the LV?

a. Isovolumic relaxation
b. Early filling
c. Mid-diastolic diastasis
d. Atrial contraction

59. A 59-year-old man is admitted to the hospital with refractory heart failure, ascites, and lower extremity edema. He has a history of 2 MIs and had coronary artery bypass surgery 10 years ago complicated by several bouts of acute pericarditis shortly thereafter. Two years ago, his EF was 40%. Recent coronary angiography revealed patent grafts. He currently denies anginal symptoms.

- Medications

Lisinopril:	20 mg once daily
Carvedilol:	12.5 mg twice daily
Spironolactone:	25 mg once daily
Furosemide:	120 mg twice daily
Metolazone:	2.5 mg once daily
Digoxin:	0.25 mg once daily
Potassium:	40 mEq once daily

- Vital signs

BP:	90/50 mmHg
HR:	98 bpm, regular

- Physical examination

Lungs:	Clear to auscultation
Cardiac:	JVP reaches angle of jaw, no V waves, no inspiratory decrease, S1, S2 normal, loud early filling sound audible at base and apex
Extremities:	Pitting edema to the level of the umbilicus
Abdomen:	Hepatomegaly (nonpulsatile), ascites

- Laboratory

Creatinine:	1.7 mg/dL
Potassium:	3.9 mEq/L
BNP:	512 pg/mL
Troponin T:	< 0.01 ng/mL
Urinalysis:	no proteinuria

- Chest radiograph:

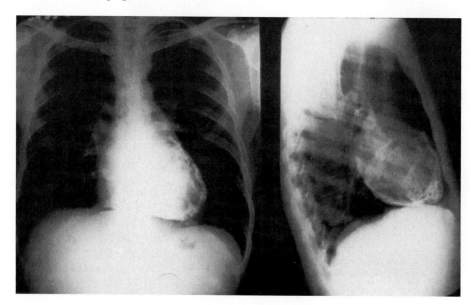

- Echocardiogram:
  Normal RV size and function
  LV is upper normal in size
  Anterior and inferior hypokinesis, no areas of scar
  EF 40%
  Mild mitral valve regurgitation
  Paradoxical septal motion
  IVC and hepatic veins were dilated

Which of the following is the most appropriate next step in management?

a. Hemodynamic monitoring, inotropic therapy, and renal dose of dopamine (2 μg/kg/min)

b. Increase lisinopril, furosemide, and metolazone

c. Add hydralazine and isosorbide dinitrate

d. CT of the chest and surgical consultation

60. Diuretic therapy, particularly the use of loop diuretics, is mainstay therapy for symptomatic heart failure.

Which of the following is **incorrect** regarding loop diuretics in heart failure?

a. Provides the greatest sodium and water excretion of all diuretics

b. Acts on the thick ascending loop of Henle

c. Action is amplified if thiazide diuretic (ie, metolazone) given ~30 minutes prior to loop diuretic

d. Potential side effects include hypovolemia, electrolyte abnormalities (ie, hypokalemia, hypomagnesemia, hypocalcemia) and ototoxicity

e. Does not require higher dosing in renal insufficiency or heart failure

Answers

1. Answer g.

This patient has acute (or chronic) renal failure secondary to taking NSAID, which can reduce renal blood flow and inhibit production of prostaglandins. NSAIDs are known to precipitate heart failure episodes due to alterations in renal function. This leads to sodium retention, increased creatinine, and possibly clinical deterioration. Myocardial ischemia is unlikely as the clinical presentation, and ECG/cardiac bio-markers do not suggest this. Finally, while he does have mitral valve regurgitation, it does not appear severe enough to cause or exacerbate heart failure.

2. Answer d.

Each of these statements is correct. LV relaxation is an *active process* and is accomplished by forcing Ca^{2+} back into the SR via the SERCA pump. It is through Ca^{2+} reuptake into the SR that actin-myosin bridges can be fully separated so that relaxation can occur. Dysfunction of Ca^{2+} reuptake may contribute to diastolic dysfunction.

3. Answer b.

Current assessment of LV *diastolic* function focuses on analysis of ventricular filling patterns by means of Doppler echocardiography. This technique is readily available, relatively easy to perform, lacks ionizing radiation, and is capable of providing important information regarding LV function, cardiac anatomy, and estimated filling pressures. The "gold standard" test remains left heart catheterization. However, since it is invasive, time-consuming, expensive, and not readily available, this test is infrequently performed for these indications. Newer techniques, such as cardiac MRI and strain imaging techniques, are currently being studied, but are not for clinical use as of yet. Finally, while BNP may *aid* in the diagnosis of heart failure, Doppler echocardiography would be the more appropriate choice.

4. Answer d.

This patient has peripartum cardiomyopathy based on clinical presentation. Patients usually present during the last trimester of pregnancy or during the first 6 months postpartum. Pharmacologic management includes ACE inhibitors and beta blockers as well as delivery of the child. The etiology is unknown and 50% seem to recover ventricular function within 6 months of delivery. Recurrent ventricular dysfunction with subsequent pregnancies may occur and the risk of recurrence is greater in women with persistent LV dysfunction.

Since the patient was previously asymptomatic and had no evidence of CV disease, she is unlikely to have AS. Further, neither her physical examination nor clinical presentation is consistent with any of these other diagnoses.

5. Answer b.

The LVEDP volume curve is shifted *up and to the left*, suggesting worsened stiffness (compliance ≈ pressure/volume) and higher filling pressures. Specifically, a shift up and to the left suggests that, for a given volume, the filling pressure is elevated. Note compliance and stiffness are *inversely* related to one another. A shift in the end-diastolic pressure volume curve up and to the left would be expected in diastolic heart failure.

5. (*continued*)

However, a *parallel* shift upward would be more compatible with external forces (ie, pericardial constraint or ventricular interdependence). In most cases of systolic heart failure, the end-diastolic pressure volume curve is shifted rightward (ie, increased ventricular volume).

6. Answer a.

NO is an endogenous endothelial cell-derived relaxing factor that stimulates guanylate cyclase and activates cGMP. NO is a potent vasodilator and its production is impaired in heart failure as well as atherosclerosis. NO synthetase is the enzyme responsible for NO production. Answers **b–e** are incorrect, as data suggest that NO promotes the opposite effects.

7. Answer a.

Patients with isolated cardiac volume overload (ie, mitral or aortic valve regurgitation) typically develop LV enlargement and eccentric hypertrophy. Under these circumstances, the LVEDP–volume relationship shifts *rightward*, so that end-diastolic volume is increased, but filling pressures remain the same. A *leftward* shift in the end diastolic pressure-volume relationship does just the opposite (ie, less volume per given pressure, decreased compliance) and commonly occurs in restrictive cardiomyopathy or heart failure with normal ejection. In most cases of pure valvular heart disease, the speed of LV relaxation is not significantly altered so answer **c** is incorrect.

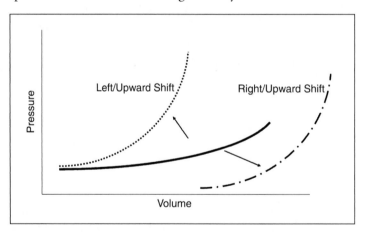

8. Answer e.

The clinical presentation is consistent with hypertensive urgency and AF (rapid ventricular response). However, this patient likely has coexistent heart failure with normal EF. Appropriate management goals include BP and HR control as well as diuresis. Given her advanced diastolic dysfunction, the tachycardia and relative loss of "atrial kick" is also confounding the problem and thus electrical cardioversion would likely be beneficial following TEE (to exclude left atrial thrombi).

9. Answer a.

This patient has evidence of progressive heart failure, orthostasis, and an ECG that reveals *low voltage*. Thus, the most likely diagnosis from the choices is amyloid heart disease. This would need to be confirmed by echocardiography, serum, and/or urine electrophoresis and biopsy (ie, fat aspirate, endomyocardial biopsy, or bone marrow biopsy). The clinical presentation, physical examination, and ECG do not support a diagnosis of HCM, hypertensive heart disease, or mitral valve disease.

10. Answer a.

Each answer choice listed above is a necessary component to evaluate a potential heart donor with the exception of an endomyocardial biopsy.

11. Answer b.

The 3 basic abnormal LV filling patterns are (in increasing order of dysfunction): (1) impaired relaxation, (2) pseudonormal filling, and (3) restrictive filling. Patients with impaired LV relaxation display a reduced proportion of ventricular filling in early diastole due to slow relaxation and increased stiffness. In turn, this decreases the early transmitral pressure gradient and, as a compensatory mechanism, filling at atrial contraction is increased. This is the earliest diastolic abnormality in most cardiac disease states and the least *abnormal* of the 3 filling patterns.

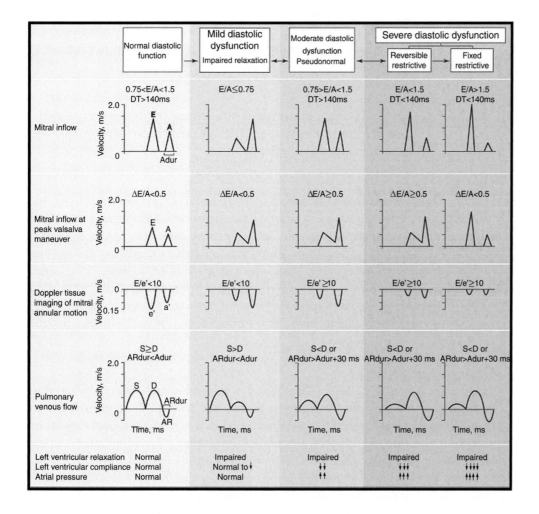

12. Answer b.

Cardiopulmonary receptors are located within the atria, ventricles, coronary vessels, and lungs and are important in neurohumoral control. In *normal* conditions and in response to stretch (ie, pressure or volume overload), these baroreceptors are activated, leading to inhibition of the adrenergic nervous system. However, in *heart failure*, cardiopulmonary baroreceptors are attenuated, leading to impaired inhibition of the adrenergic nervous system; thus, there is vasoconstriction, adrenergic stimulation, and activation of the renin–angiotensin–aldosterone system.

13. Answer a.

This patient appears to have diastolic dysfunction based on clinical presentation (elderly woman with HTN and diabetes) and echocardiography. The Doppler mitral inflow pattern is consistent with abnormal relaxation (ie, grade I diastolic dysfunction). The E/A ratio is < 1.0 and does not change with valsalva maneuver. Further, the tissue Doppler (E′) is mildly reduced, consistent with worsened relaxation. She does not have diastolic heart failure (heart failure with normal EF), as this is a clinical diagnosis based on historical symptoms, physical signs, and chest radiographic evidence of pulmonary edema (Framingham criteria). The most common presenting symptom is exertional dyspnea, since ventricular relaxation is impaired due to poor compliance and increased stiffness. While filling pressures may be normal or near-normal at rest, they are often accentuated with exercise, tachycardia, or increased afterload (ie, systolic HTN). Answer **b** is incorrect since we have no information regarding pulmonary pressures. Finally, although the patient does have multiple CV risk factors for CAD including diabetes, the clinical presentation is not consistent with cardiac ischemia.

14. Answer b.

ACE inhibitors are beneficial in heart failure with reduced EF because these agents have been demonstrated to reduce vasoconstriction, ventricular hypertrophy, and dilatation, as well as mortality and morbidity.

15. Answer c.

He has progressive and severe (NYHA class III) heart failure. Previous evaluation has included coronary angiography, which has revealed normal coronary arteries and therefore repeat coronary angiography is unlikely to contribute much additional information. Similarly, repeat assessment of EF is somewhat unnecessary as it was last checked 2 months ago and is stable. There is no evidence of tachy- or brady-arrhythmias, so a Holter is also unnecessary. However, the most helpful prognostic information will be derived from exercise capacity as assessed by maximal oxygen uptake (VO_2 max). If this is <14 mL/kg/m^2 or < 50% predicted, transplant evaluation may be appropriate.

16. Answer f.

This patient has an EF ≤ 30% with a history of idiopathic cardiomyopathy and thus is a candidate for an ICD. Interestingly, he also has evidence of ventricular dysynchrony (based on prolonged QRS wave from ECG), is NYHA functional class III by symptoms and thus may also be a candidate for cardiac resynchronization using a biventricular pacemaker. However, he is not yet on an optimal medical regimen including beta-receptor (carvedilol) and aldosterone (spironolactone) blockers. To truly meet criteria for resynchronization therapy, one should have "failed" this medical regimen. Increasing digoxin and/or diuresis may also be helpful to improve symptoms, but should be done with caution.

17. Answer b.

This patient has asymptomatic LV dysfunction, likely on the basis of a familial dilated cardiomyopathy. Patients who are "asymptomatic" do not always have normal exercise capacity when tested objectively. This patient should be treated with an ACE inhibitor and beta blocker to help prevent the combined end-point of death and progression to heart failure. Because she is asymptomatic, digoxin and diuretics are *not* indicated. She should definitely have genetic counseling and her first degree relatives (ie, children and siblings) screened appropriately with echocardiography. At this point, with an EF of 30%, only mild to moderate reduction in exercise capacity and lack of symptoms, transplant evaluation and biventricular pacing are premature.

18. Answer b.

On the basis of symptoms, physical examination findings, and chest radiography, this woman has heart failure, which could be due to systolic or diastolic heart failure. One needs to establish the type of cardiac dysfunction before selecting therapy, and echocardiography would be the best test to help make this distinction. Although CAD is possible, in the absence of angina, a noninvasive screening test may be more appropriate than going directly to angiography. Empiric therapy for systolic or diastolic dysfunction is inappropriate, because studies have shown that physical examination and chest radiography are not able to differentiate systolic from diastolic heart failure. At this time, ACE inhibitors have not been shown to have tremendous benefit in diastolic heart failure and, unless there is concomitant HTN as is the case in this patient, should not be part of routine practice. While this patient above would benefit from this medication from a HTN standpoint, echocardiography is still the best next step.

19. Answer c.

Patients with a *restrictive* LV filling pattern typically have a poorly compliant LV and evidence of elevated filling pressures. In these patients, filling occurs predominantly in early diastole and terminates abruptly because of the severe decrease in LV compliance. There is little filling from atrial contraction due to atrial systolic failure. Therefore, a decrease in HR may result in a decrease in CO and worsening of symptoms. In contrast, patients whose predominant pattern is *impaired* LV relaxation frequently benefit from slowing of the HR (assuming the PR interval is not affected) because the slowly relaxing ventricle has more time to fill appropriately. Often, patients with pseudonormal LV filling also benefit from some slowing of the HR, but the response is somewhat variable.

20. Answer d.

Endothelin is a potent vasoconstrictor from direct and indirect (activates angiotensin II) activity on the endothelium. Thus, an endothelin-receptor antagonist would be expected to promote vasodilatation. Thus far, there are no data to suggest a survival benefit in heart failure (ie, LV dysfunction) with or without the presence of pulmonary HTN.

21. Answer e.

This patient likely developed TICM due to AF with rapid ventricular response. Treatment should include anticoagulation, rate and BP control, and an attempt at electrical cardioversion (with TEE, since unknown duration of AF). Thus, all of these answers are correct.

22. Answer c.

National average data demonstrate that the one-year overall survival is 85%, but results are variable from center to center. Posttransplant survival is worse in the elderly population (thus cardiac transplantation is an absolute contraindication if age ≥70 years) and if the donor heart ischemic time is prolonged (ie, >240 minutes).

23. Answer e.

Administration of recombinant BNP (ie, Nesiritide) to patients with heart failure has been well studied. While the natriuretic response to natriuretic peptide infusion is blunted in patients with heart failure as compared to control subjects, the natriuretic peptides are still natriuretic when administered to patients with heart failure. They have potent effects on venous capacitance, resulting in reduction in venous return and reduced filling pressures. Administration of natriuretic peptides to normal subjects results in decreases in CO (mediated by the decrease in venous return) and reflex increases in systemic vascular resistance. However, in heart failure patients, administration of natriuretic peptides decreases systemic vascular resistance and increases CO.

24. Answer b.

The peak oxygen uptake (VO$_2$max) remains the single *best* predictor for transplantation benefit and need. In general, if patients value have under 14 mL/kg/min, they are good transplant candidates. However, recent data suggest that those patients with severely reduced exercise capacity (VO$_2$max ≤ 10 mL/kg/min) derive even greater benefit and thus answer **b** is correct. EF and BNP level provide less accurate predictive assessment. Answer **d** is incorrect since this patient's age (age > 70 years) excludes him from being an acceptable transplant candidate.

25. Answer d.

Arterial baroreceptors act as pressure (ie, mechanoreceptors) sensors and are located at the carotid sinus and aortic arch. They respond to increased stretch (either from higher distending pressure or widened pulse pressure) by increasing the discharge rate of *afferent* nerve action potentials. The impulse travels from cranial nerves 9 and 10 to the medulla oblongata in the brainstem. Then, *efferent* sympathetic or parasympathetic nerves innervate the heart and blood vessels to regulate BP and HR accordingly. In this particular case, an abrupt drop in BP decreased the discharge rate from arterial baroreceptors (answer **d**), and thus the medulla responded by increasing sympathetic and decreasing parasympathetic discharge from *efferent* neurons. To maintain homeostasis, one would expect that BP and HR would increase due to sympathetic discharge. Consider the opposite effect, such as occurs with carotid artery massage, which is known to stretch the carotid baroreceptor. In that scenario, one would expect that HR and BP would decline.

26. Answer 26 a.

This patient remains symptomatic on a good dose of an ACE inhibitors, beta blocker, and diuretic. She also remains quite hypertensive. Although digoxin or more diuretic would be indicated for persistent symptoms, additional vasodilator therapy is most appropriate at this time because of the persistent HTN. A combination of hydralazine and isosorbide would likely be the first option. Given her severe renal insufficiency, one should use great caution in the use of an aldosterone antagonist although under different circumstances it would be the next best choice. Her dose of furosemide is not maximized and if additional diuretic were needed for dyspnea, furosemide should be increased before metolazone initiated. At this time, one could consider CRT since she has NYHA functional class III symptoms, an EF < 35% and a widened QRS. However, her systolic HTN should be corrected before consideration of a device.

27. Answer b.

Longstanding catecholamine excess may result in a dilated cardiomyopathy as opposed to uncontrolled HTN of other causes that leads to LVH. Certainly, the fact that this patient's BP is uncontrolled despite 4 antihypertensive medications should raise a "red flag." This is most likely related to a pheochromocytoma. Renal artery stenosis is another possibility, but less likely since the patient has minimal CV risk factors to cause severe atherosclerosis of the renal arteries and this would also be more likely to cause LVH. Viral myocarditis and amyloid heart disease are unlikely since these conditions should reduce, not increase, BP.

28. Answer c.

Routine assessment for heart transplant recipients includes all of the following with the exception of CT (unless clinically indicated).

29. Answer c.

Repeated hospitalizations are common in patients with heart failure, especially the elderly. Thus, it is critical to ensure that the medical regimen is optimized. She needs much higher doses of ACE inhibitor and diuretic and indeed she does not possess any apparent contraindication to this therapy (ie, hypotension, hyperkalemia, or renal insufficiency). If up-titration of ACE inhibitor results in significant renal insufficiency, treatment could be switched to hydralazine and isosorbide dinitrate. Underdosage of ACE inhibitor and failure to titrate diuretics is one of the most common errors in the management of heart failure and may be responsible for repeated hospitalizations. Since the patient has marked fluid overload, simultaneous increase in diuretics is appropriate, although caution should be used while up-titrating the ACE inhibitor. Amlodipine is not indicated unless BP is still elevated after up-titration of ACE inhibitor. Other important issues in this patient would be salt restriction and compliance with medication. CRT is not necessary for 2 reasons: (1) she is not on maximal medical therapy; and (2) she does not have ECG evidence of dyssynchrony (ie, QRS prolongation).

30. Answer d.

This cardiac biopsy is consistent with moderate grade 2R acute cell mediated rejection. The following is the ISHLT nomenclature for the assessment of rejection from an endomyocardial biopsy.

- Grade 0—no rejection
- Grade 1R, mild—Interstitial and/or perivascular infiltrate with up to one focus of myocyte damage
- Grade 2R, moderate—two or more foci of infiltrate with associated myocyte damage
- Grade 3R, severe—diffuse infiltrate with multifocal myocyte damage, with or without edema, hemorrhage, or vasculitis

Typically, a patient with acute T-cell mediated rejection of at least moderate grade would receive high-dose oral or IV corticosteroids (particularly with hemodynamic compromise). Of note, Grade 1 R rejection is often not treated unless there is evidence of hemodynamic compromise or significant symptoms. While the patient would also likely receive diuresis, it is more important to initiate high-dose steroids first. Importantly, her normal echocardiogram does not exclude LV dysfunction and rejection.

31. Answer d.

(See figure to Answer 11.) There are 3 *abnormal* filling patterns that can be observed echocardiographically and correlate with filling pressures and diastolic abnormalities. The most common pattern observed is *impaired relaxation*, which reflects reduced filling in early diastole and increased contribution of filling by atrial contraction. LV relaxation and compliance are abnormal, but filling pressures are normal at rest. A more advanced pattern of diastolic dysfunction is termed *pseudonormal* as it resembles the normal filling pattern, although diastolic abnormalities are clearly present. Patients with advanced diastolic dysfunction may demonstrate a *restrictive* filling pattern, with vigorous filling in early diastole and little filling at atrial contraction because of atrial failure. This can be either reversible or irreversible, but clearly reflects elevated filling pressures. A *diastolic predominant* pattern has little meaning because it does not specify when diastolic filling is occurring.

32. Answer c.

(See figure to Answer 11.) Patients with the *restrictive* filling pattern typically display abnormally slow relaxation and a severe reduction in LV compliance with marked increases in left atrial pressure. These patients usually have marked reductions in exercise capacity and may have symptoms/signs of pulmonary congestion and enhanced sensitivity to loading conditions (ie, volume or pressure overload). Filling pressures are often elevated in patients with *pseudonormal* relaxation, but is often normal at rest in those with *impaired* relaxation.

33. Answer b.

Nesiritide (recombinant BNP) has been approved for use as a vasodilator in patients with cardiac pulmonary edema and elevated pulmonary capillary wedge pressure. It enhances sodium and water excretion and has been shown to reduce pulmonary capillary wedge pressure as well as BP (at the standard dosing regimen). This agent has *not* been shown to improve survival. In fact, recent reports have suggested that Nesiritide may worsen renal function and survival, but this issue warrants further study.

34. Answer a.

Since hypotension has occurred, but clinical status has improved, the best recommendation is to temporarily stop the Nesiritide infusion and wait for her BP to improve. When this occurs, Nesiritide should be restarted at a lower dose without a bolus. BNP levels are not helpful when Nesiritide is administered as this agent will artificially elevate the level. Initiating dobutamine would not be the best first choice since discontinuing the Nesiritide briefly and lowering the dose may be all that is necessary. Finally, it is not recommended to discontinue the ACE inhibitor during a decompensated heart failure hospitalization.

35. Answer d.

This patient has end-stage dilated cardiomyopathy and acute pulmonary edema. If he was at a transplant center and his hemodynamic condition deteriorated after initiation of inotropic therapy, he should be considered for a LVAD as a bridge to transplantation. There is a clear indication for inotropic therapy in this patient. With his symptomatic hypotension, additional diuretic or ACE inhibitor alone is unlikely to be tolerated or adequate to stabilize his condition. Carvedilol is not indicated for class IV heart failure and would not likely be tolerated at this time without inotropic support. Finally, addition of spironolactone is also unlikely to be tolerated without inotropic support due to severe, symptomatic hypotension.

36. Answer c.

This patient is asymptomatic and has no evidence of hypoperfusion. She has a history of tolerating ACE inhibitors despite low BP. The ACE inhibitor should be restarted at her usual dose and you should reassure the nursing staff. Asymptomatic hypotension is not an indication to reduce the dose of ACE inhibitor. The combination of hydralazine and isosorbide dinitrate offers no advantage here. While one could consider discontinuing furosemide as it may not be absolutely necessary and one should always hope to achieve down-titration of diuretics due to neurohumoral stimulation, the more correct answer is **c** in this scenario. Finally, the patient has NYHA functional class II symptoms and thus does not qualify for a cardiac resynchronization device, although an ICD is indicated due to her cardiomyopathy.

37. Answer c.

This patient is at high risk for CAD since he has multiple CV risk factors, cardiomyopathy, and apparent angina. Thus, coronary angiography should be preferred and non-invasive stress bypassed. A Holter monitor and transplant evaluation are not clinically warranted at this time.

38. Answer d.

This patient has severe LV dysfunction and heart failure without clear evidence of transmural MI. In addition, he has angina and severe three-vessel CAD. Although the major surgical trials excluded patients with severe LV dysfunction, this patient would be best served with CABG. Many surgeons like some confirmation of the presence of a large amount of viable myocardium before deciding to operate in such a high-risk candidate. Thallium imaging, dobutamine echocardiography, PET scanning, and cardiac MRI would be appropriate. Further, medical therapy with an ACE inhibitor and beta blocker would also be warranted.

39. Answer c.

Given the patient's EF, he should have an ICD. However, since he does not have NYHA functional class III or IV symptoms on *maximal medical therapy* and no evidence of *ventricular dyssynchrony*, CRT is not indicated. Asymptomatic, nonsustained VT is not an indication for antiarrhythmic therapy. In the absence of syncope or near-syncope, invasive EP testing is not indicated. The patient has a strong indication for warfarin treatment (previous cardioembolic event and very low EF) so warfarin should not be discontinued.

40. Answer d.

Endothelial cells in the pulmonary vasculature (and systemic vascular endothelium) produce ACE. This enzyme converts angiotensin I to the more potent and active angiotensin II while also promoting the degradation of bradykinin. ACE inhibitor have proved useful in blocking the formation of angiotensin II in heart failure and have demonstrated survival benefit in those with LV systolic dysfunction or failure. Angiotensin II, not ACE, stimulates production of aldosterone and norepinephrine; thus b and c are incorrect.

41. Answer d.

This patient is currently on maximal medical therapy for heart failure but continues to have NYHA functional class III symptoms. Since her EF is <35%, QRS duration is ≥ 120 ms, and is clinically NYHA functional class III, she meets criteria for biventricular pacing (CRT) in addition to ICD. One may consider also increasing her diuretic or trying Nesiritide in the short-term, but CRT ± ICD is the *more* correct answer. Initiation of an ARB is not warranted and may cause more harm since she is already receiving enalapril. Thus far, 2 large randomized clinical trials (CARE-HF and MIRACLE) have shown improvement in cardiac function and structure, exercise capacity, quality of life, and survival with CRT.

42. Answer b.

Overdiuresis before initiating treatment with ACE inhibitors can result in excessive activation of the renin–angiotensin–aldosterone system and hypotension. On physical examination, the patient appears volume depleted, and thus diuretics and isosorbide dinitrate should be held, and perhaps gentle hydration would be helpful. The ACE inhibitor and beta blocker should be continued if possible. The patient is not in cardiogenic shock (clear lungs, no JVP elevation) so there is no need for inotropic therapy. Finally, switching the ACE inhibitor for an ARB at this time is unnecessary.

43. Answer b.

ACE inhibitors and beta blockers are the mainstay treatment of heart failure with reduced EF (HF↓EF) since they improve morbidity and mortality. Aldosterone antagonists improve survival in those with HF↓EF with NYHA functional class III/IV symptoms. Isosorbide dinitrate/hydralazine improves outcomes in HF↓EF, but traditionally has been thought to be inferior to ACE inhibitor. However, recent data suggest the effect of these agents may be more potent in African-Americans. While digoxin improves hospitalization rates and morbidity in HF↓EF, it has no effect on survival so answer **b** is incorrect.

44. Answer b.

Although many factors influence LV diastolic function and filling, they all exert their effect through the transmitral pressure gradient. Understanding the effects of various diastolic properties, such as LV relaxation and compliance, on this gradient is a key to understanding LV filling and diastolic function.

45. Answer b.

Approximately half of the patients with heart failure have a normal EF. These patients are typically older, have a history of HTN, and are more often female. Morbidity and mortality is similar to those patients with HF↓EF. It is exceedingly difficult to distinguish patients with heart failure and reduced or normal EF based solely on clinical grounds. One needs additional testing, such as echocardiography or left heart catheterization, for hemodynamic assessment.

46. Answer d.

While central sleep apnea is common and may occur in those with asymptomatic LV dysfunction, it is clearly associated with severity of heart failure and has implications regarding prognosis. All of the other answers are correct regarding central sleep apnea.

47. Answer d.

(For institutions that do not use Wood units, 1 Wood unit = 80 dynes/sec/cm^{-5}.) To answer this question correctly, one must have an understanding of some *absolute* contraindications to cardiac transplantation. For example, age over 70 and *fixed* pulmonary HTN are 2 particular contraindications. While the patient in answer **d** has marked pulmonary HTN, it is reversed by NO administration, and thus is *reversible*. Therefore, she would not have a contraindication to cardiac transplantation based on published criteria. Of note, transpulmonary gradient is calculated as *mean pulmonary pressure–pulmonary capillary wedge pressure* (a value > 15 mmHg represents an *absolute* contraindication to cardiac transplantation).

48. Answer b.

Endomyocardial biopsy is only supported if a "specific diagnosis is suspected that would influence treatment," but guidelines do not advise this for routine diagnosis. Otherwise, all of the other answers are correct. The following is a list of the initial diagnostic work-up for heart failure that is *strongly* (class I and IIa) supported by ACC/AHA guidelines (2005).

Class I:

- Thorough history (including use of alcohol, illicit drugs, chemotherapy, and NYHA functional class) and physical examination (assess volume status, orthostatic BP, weight, BMI)
- CBC, electrolytes (including calcium and magnesium), glucose, lipid panel, liver function tests, thyroid-stimulating hormone, urinalysis
- ECG
- Chest radiography
- Two-dimensional echocardiogram with Doppler
- Coronary angiogram in patients with angina or significant ischemia

Class IIa:

- Viability testing in patients with known CAD
- Maximal exercise testing with or without measurement of respiratory gas exchange
- In those patients with clinical suspicion, screening for hemochromatosis, sleep-disturbed breathing, human immunodeficiency virus, rheumatologic diseases, amyloidosis, or pheochromocytoma
- BNP in those patients in whom a clinical diagnosis of heart failure is uncertain
- Endomyocardial biopsy when a "specific diagnosis is suspected that would influence treatment." Otherwise, endomyocardial biopsy receives a class III recommendation for routine assessment

49. Answer d.

IV inotropic support has a limited (*and understudied*) role in the management of heart failure. All the above scenarios represent appropriate and reimbursable uses of inotropic therapy.

50. Answer c.

Endomyocardial biopsy remains the only reliable diagnostic method for detection of transplant rejection. Echocardiographic abnormalities such as LV dysfunction may not occur until rejection is more advanced and potentially irreversible. While a CBC and echocardiogram are likely to be ordered, rejection is more reliably detected by biopsy. Coronary angiography would be appropriate in the setting of clinical deterioration or LV dysfunction thought to be secondary to ischemia and transplant vasculopathy.

51. Answer a.

Although many question the use of a beta blocker in patients with COPD, its use is clearly indicated in this patient since he has severe CAD and systolic heart failure. Additionally, it appears that his episodes of recurrent heart failure are likely being precipitated by ischemia. Currently, he is well-compensated hemodynamically and it appears that his COPD is mild, so outpatient initiation of a low dose of a cardioselective beta receptor antagonist could be achieved and careful up-titration would be reasonable, although hospital admission may be advised by some physicians. Nifedipine (or any dihydropyridine) without added beta blockade is not an optimal antianginal choice, especially in the presence of heart failure. EECP may be helpful, but should be considered after adding a beta blocker first.

52. Answer d.

Natriuretic peptides (ANP and BNP) have multiple biologic actions including, *but not limited* to, regulation of myocardial function, antifibrotic and natriuretic inhibition of the renin–angiotensin–aldosterone system, and vasodilatation via smooth muscle relaxation

53. Answer c.

The patient most likely has coronary artery vasculopathy, which is the second most common cause of death after the first year posttransplant. The incidence at 5 years is 30% to 40%. This is often slowly progressive and since the heart is denervated, most patients do not present with typical chest discomfort, but rather with evidence of a silent MI, sudden death, or heart failure. Therefore, most centers recommend yearly coronary angiography for surveillance. Treatment is often disappointing and since lesions are often diffuse and concentric, PCI is often less than ideal. While increasing immunosuppressive agents may halt progression, the risks of infection and malignancy from this approach may exceed the potential benefits. Re-transplantation remains the only definitive treatment. This clinical scenario is not consistent with acute rejection or post-transplant neoplastic disease.

54. Answer d.

This patient has asymptomatic LV dysfunction. Therapies proven to be beneficial include ACE inhibitors, ARBs, beta blockers, and ICD. Aldosterone blockers also have survival benefit, but are reserved for patients with systolic failure who have NYHA functional class III/IV symptoms. While a combination of hydralazine/isosorbide dinitrate provides survival benefit, V-Heft II demonstrated that ACE inhibitors are superior to hydralazine/isosorbide dinitrate. Digoxin and diuretics are indicated primarily only for symptoms and since this patient is asymptomatic, these therapies are unnecessary. Consequently, an ICD is indicated since he has LV systolic dysfunction with an EF < 35%.

55. Answer b.

This patient should be taking warfarin because of the large anterior MI and akinetic wall. He does not need to discontinue taking the ACE inhibitor with the relatively mild increase in creatinine, which is stable on a good dose of ACE inhibitor. Since he has had a recent MI, treatment with the beta blocker should be continued. Since he is at risk for VF or VT, he will be eligible to have an ICD, but studies and guidelines suggest that he should be at least one month out from MI, so answer **e** is incorrect.

56. Answer d.

The echocardiographic findings are entirely consistent with hypertensive heart disease with advanced diastolic dysfunction and chronic increase in LV filling pressures. The patient has concentric hypertrophy as evidenced by increased wall thickness and LV mass index (< 125 g/m^2 is normal). The mitral inflow Doppler shows evidence of increased filling pressures, with increased E/A and short deceleration time. With LVH and normal left atrial pressures, an abnormal relaxation pattern with decreased E/A and prolonged deceleration time is expected. However, the E/A of 2.0 and deceleration time are more consistent with restrictive physiology and indicate reduced LV compliance and increased filling pressures. The left atrial enlargement and mild pulmonary HTN suggest that her filling pressures have been chronically increased. Despite the absence of regional wall abnormalities, one could not assume an absence of epicardial CAD, and further evaluation of that may be appropriate. With these echocardiographic findings and the patient's clinical scenario, a diagnosis of heart failure with normal EF can be established.

57. Answer a.

BNP is activated when there is elevated atrial and ventricular volume and/or wall stress. Glomerular filtration rate is inversely related to BNP concentration and thus elevated values do not always indicate high filling pressures, particularly in patients with renal insufficiency. Studies have shown that BNP is elevated with LV systolic and, to a lesser degree, diastolic heart failure. Finally, BNP may not always be elevated in heart failure. For example, the value may be normal with flash pulmonary edema and is also reduced in obesity.

58. Answer c.

Diastole is broken down into 4 phases: isovolumic relaxation, early filling, diastasis, and atrial contraction. The compliance characteristics of the LV are best measured after relaxation is complete and during a period in which there is little cardiac filling (ie, diastasis). It would be inappropriate to measure LV compliance at the other stages since the ventricle is either filling or contracting and thus changing its volume and/or shape rapidly.

59. Answer d.

"Refractory" heart failure while a patient is receiving effective doses of medications should always prompt careful evaluation and consideration of other factors contributing to the patient's symptoms, especially when the degree of heart failure is out of proportion to the degree of systolic dysfunction. This patient appears to be in right heart failure based on clinical presentation. The presence of significant residual myocardial ischemia has been addressed in this patient, and patent grafts were demonstrated on coronary angiography. This patient likely has constrictive pericarditis since there are pericardial calcifications on chest radiography, evidence on physical examination of probable constriction (pericardial "knock," ascites, elevated JVP), and echocardiographic evidence of probable constriction. This is likely related to his previous cardiac surgery and history of pericarditis. Although additional diuresis will be needed preoperatively, the most appropriate intervention is pericardectomy, following the demonstration of pericardial thickening on CT scanning of the heart.

60. Answer e.

Loop diuretics act on the thick ascending loop of Henle to block sodium and water reabsorption. In renal insufficiency or heart failure, organic acids may accumulate in that location and cause diuretics to be less effective, thus mandating higher dosing or switching to another mode of water removal (ie, diuretic resistance). All of the other statements are correct regarding loop diuretics.

SECTION VI

Valvular
Heart Disease

Matthew W. Martinez, MD

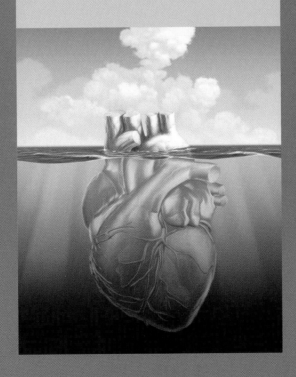

Questions

1. Which of the following would be most likely in a patient with chronic severe MR?

    a. Normal LV cavity size
    b. Dyspnea
    c. EF > 65%
    d. RV lift
    e. Third heart sound

2. Which of the following statements about the natural history of severe AR is true?

    a. Asymptomatic patients with normal LV systolic function develop symptoms of LV dysfunction at a rate of <10% per yr
    b. Symptomatic patients have a mortality rate of <10% per yr
    c. Asymptomatic patients with normal LV systolic function suffer sudden death at a rate of >10% per yr
    d. Asymptomatic patients with abnormal LV systolic function develop symptoms at a rate of <10% per yr

3. Which of the following patients with severe chronic MR is not a surgical candidate?

    a. NYHA functional class III, EF 40%
    b. NYHA functional class I, EF 70%, LV end systolic diameter 35 mm
    c. NYHA functional class II, EF 50%
    d. NYHA functional class II, EF 70%, LV end systolic diameter 42 mm

4. A 45-year-old farmer presents with a history of flushing after eating and diarrhea up to 10 watery stools per day. There has been a 20-lb weight loss over the preceding year. He has also noted a gradual decrease in his exertional tolerance due to dyspnea and wheezing while carrying out his normal daily chores. He denies fever, chills or sweats but has had a decrease in his appetite over the last year. His examination reveals a ruddy complexion. JVP is up to 14 cm with prominent V wave in the venous profile. There is also a loud holosystolic murmur with respiratory variation. The liver is enlarged and pulsatile. There is bilateral lower extremity edema to the knees.

    What would be the next best test to order?

    a. MRI of the chest
    b. TTE
    c. No further testing, reassure and start diuretic
    d. No further testing, start hospice care

Answers to this section start on page 209.

5. A 63-year-old man presents with a heart murmur. He is completely asymptomatic and active. Exam shows carotid delay, single S2, and a 3/6 mid-peaking SEM. TTE shows normal LV size and function, calcified aortic valve, and a mean aortic valve gradient of 52 mmHg with an AVA of 0.8 cm².

   Which of the following is the next best step?

   a. TMET
   b. Right and left heart catheterization with coronary angiography
   c. PABV
   d. AVR after coronary angiogram
   e. Observation with IE prophylaxis

6. An 18-year-old college long distance runner seeks an opinion for approval for track team eligibility. He was told as a child that he had a heart murmur but then underwent precompetition physicals throughout high school without having this brought to his attention again. His is currently asymptomatic.

   On physical examination, his resting pulse rate is 45 bpm and irregular. His BP is 90/50 mmHg. JVP is not elevated. Carotid pulse is normal. S1 and S2 are normal with physiologic splitting. There is a soft early systolic click and a grade 2/6 SEM heard best at the left intercostal space with a soft grade 2/6 decrescendo murmur heard along the LSB and appreciated best with the patient leaning forward with a held expiration. There is a soft early diastolic filling sound (S3) heard at the apex in the left lateral decubitus position. There is no S4. The systolic murmur decreases with Valsalva maneuver. Peripheral pulses are all normal.

   An ECG shows sinus bradycardia with sinus arrhythmia and pauses up to 1 sec in duration with normal QRS morphology. Chest X-ray reveals a slight pectus deformity and the apical impulse is normal.

   I—What would be the next most appropriate step for the evaluation of this athlete?

   a. MUGA
   b. TTE
   c. 24-hr Holter ECG
   d. Stress echocardiography
   e. Chest X-ray

   II—In the above case, in addition to obtaining further diagnostic testing, what other recommendations can be made at this time?

   a. Cardiac surgery consult
   b. EP consult
   c. IE prophylaxis with antibiotics for dental procedures
   d. Reassurance and no further immediate follow-up

7. A 77-year-old man presents with increasing symptoms of dyspnea and chest discomfort on exertion over the past 6 mos. He has NYHA class III symptoms and has had two episodes of near syncope while climbing stairs. No prior cardiac history or risk factors for coronary artery disease.

   On exam:

   The BP is 136/40 mmHg, HR is 75 bpm. His JVP is normal and the carotid upstroke is delayed. The LV impulse is sustained to the left. There is a 3/6 mid-peaking SEM at the base and a 2/6 diastolic decrescendo murmur in the same position. He has a water hammer radial pulse.

A TTE shows a mildly dilated LV cavity with LV EF = 50%. There is mild LVH and LA enlargement. The aortic valve is calcified with a mean gradient of 25 mmHg. AR was described as mild.

I—What would you do now?

a. AVR
b. TMET
c. Cardiac catheterization with aortic valve gradient, CO, aortic root angiogram, and coronary angiography
d. Medical observation

At catheterization the following values were obtained:

■ LV 170/10–15 mmHg, aorta 120/50 mmHg, HR 70 bpm
■ Mean AV gradient 51 mmHg, SEP 250 msec
■ TCO 3.5 L/min, PA saturation 65%
■ Coronary arteries were normal
■ An aortic root angiogram shows LV fills to same density as root in 4 beats

II—What is the calculated AVA?

a. 0.2 cm²
b. 0.5 cm²
c. 0.9 cm²
d. 1.3 cm²

III—What is the severity of AR in this case?

a. Sellers class 1
b. Sellers class 2
c. Sellers class 3
d. Sellers class 4

8. A 23-year-old female with a family history of Marfan syndrome comes to you for prepregnancy counseling. An MRI of the chest is performed and shown below. There is no mitral valve prolapse by echocardiogram, and the patient is asymptomatic.

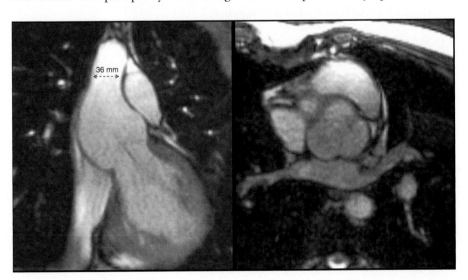

8. (*continued*)

Based on the patient's known family history and investigations, what would you recommend?

a. Avoid pregnancy at this time due to the size of the aorta

b. Proceed with pregnancy, preferably sooner rather than later, due to the size of the aorta

c. Recommend avoiding pregnancy due to the autosomal dominant nature of Marfan syndrome

d. Question the diagnosis of Marfan syndrome and request genetic evaluation

9. A 32-year-old woman has known MS. She is able to exercise daily for 45 min without symptoms. Six months ago she had a TTE that showed a mean gradient of 5 mmHg, MVA of 1.6 cm^2, and a PAP of 30 mmHg. She wants to get pregnant. What would you recommend?

a. Repeat TTE

b. TEE

c. PMBV

d. MVR

e. Proceed with pregnancy with beta blockade as necessary

10. A 67-year-old man develops prolonged chest pain while on a hunting trip. Upon his return home 3 days later he sees his doctor. On examination, there is a new 2/6 apical holosystolic murmur and the ECG shows a new inferior–posterior infarction. Coronary angiography demonstrates proximal total occlusion of the CFX artery without any other significant CAD. Pharmacologic nuclear perfusion imaging demonstrates a fixed inferior defect that does not improve on 24-hr delayed images. A TTE reveals an inferior akinetic zone, EF 52%, intact mitral valve with moderate MR, RVSP 41 mmHg. He is started on aspirin, a statin, an ACE inhibitor, and a beta blocker. He undergoes a rehabilitation level stress test without symptoms, ischemic changes on ECG, or dysrhythmia.

Which of the following next steps is most appropriate?

a. Ask a surgeon to consider him for CABG and MV repair

b. Arrange a 6 wk office visit with prescheduled TTE to reassess his MR

c. Continue with medical therapy

d. Add an ARB to his medical regimen

11. Which one of the following patients needs endocarditis prophylaxis?

a. Patient with isolated secundum ASD having dental extraction

b. Patient with ligated patent ductus arteriosus having cystoscopy

c. Patient with an AVR that is functionally normal, having dental cleaning and scaling

d. Patient with coarctation having cardiac catheterization

e. Patient with primum ASD having TEE

12. A 22-year-old woman presents with a heart murmur in the 12th wk of pregnancy. She never had any prior history of heart disease and is an active person, walking 1–2 miles per day without any limitations. This is her first pregnancy, and there has been no problem with the pregnancy. Her obstetrician noted a heart murmur and has sent her to you for further evaluation. She has no other medical problems.

Her BP is 110/70 mmHg and pulse is 70 bpm and regular. The JVP and carotid upstroke are normal. The lungs are clear. The LV impulse is tapping. The first heart sound is loud. The second heart sound is split with inspiration with a normal pulmonic component intensity. There is a crisp opening snap approximately 80 msec from the second heart sound and a 2/6 diastolic rumble is present with a presystolic accentuation.

A TTE is performed. This shows normal LV size and function with an EF of 60%. The LA is moderately enlarged. There is evidence of MS with diastolic doming of the mitral valve leaflets but they are pliable and noncalcified. The mean gradient across the mitral valve is 8 mmHg and the MVA calculated by diastolic half-time is 1.2 cm^2. There was no MR. PA systolic pressure is calculated to be 40 mmHg.

In this woman who is 12 wks pregnant, what would you do at this point in time?

a. PMBV now
b. PMBV at 20 wks of pregnancy
c. MVR at 20 wks of pregnancy
d. Medical observation with frequent periods of rest daily
e. Right and left heart catheterization with exercise

13. A 27-year-old woman presents 18 wks pregnant with a diagnosis of MS. She has a past history of rheumatic fever as a teenager and was told that she had an abnormality on her mitral valve 10 yrs ago. However, over the last few weeks she has developed mild symptoms of exertional dyspnea. This is her first pregnancy, and she definitely wants to keep the baby. She has no other medical problems.

On examination her BP is 110/70 mmHg and pulse is 90 bpm. The JVP is not elevated and carotid upstroke is without delay. The lungs are clear. The LV impulse is tapping. The first heart sound is loud and the second heart sound is split with inspiration with a mildly increased intensity of the pulmonic component. There is a crisp opening snap present approximately 60 msec from the second heart sound and a 2/6 diastolic rumble is heard at the apex with a presystolic accentuation.

TTE reveals normal LV size and function with a moderate increase in LA size. There is a typical "hockey stick" deformity of MS and the valve leaflets appear to be pliable and noncalcified with no significant subvalvular fusion. The mean gradient across the mitral valve is 10 mmHg and the valve area calculates to 1.1 cm^2 by the half-time method. The PA systolic pressure is calculated to be approximately 36 mmHg.

What would you do at this point in time?

a. Proceed with TEE and if no LA/appendage thrombus then PMBV
b. Advise termination of her pregnancy
c. Try to avoid any intervention for the next 4 weeks with the patient being as inactive as possible; then plan for elective mitral valve operation at 22 to 24 wks
d. Medical therapy to control her HR
e. Closed commissurotomy

14. A 28-year-old woman with a new diagnosis of symptomatic MS is referred to you. After your evaluation you find that she has MS that is appropriate for PMBV. The procedure is planned for the following day. She asks what follow-up if any is necessary after the procedure.

Which of the following do you tell the patient?

a. Advise her that her symptoms will improve slowly over several months
b. Advise her that she needs annual echocardiograms to follow her for recurrence
c. Advise her that she will need frequent visits to see if her symptoms are improving
d. Advise her that after the procedure, a follow-up echocardiogram will be performed as an outpatient 1 wk later
e. You reassure her, after her procedure no follow-up is necessary

15. A 62-year-old woman presents to you with severe class III symptoms of shortness of breath. She has a known history of heart murmur and a past history of rheumatic fever and has had increasing symptoms of shortness of breath for the past 4 yrs.

On examination, her venous pressure is elevated to 10 cm with a V wave and the carotid upstroke has no delay. The LV impulse is slightly enlarged. There is 2/6 holosystolic murmur at the apex with a 2/6 diastolic rumble. An opening snap is present 60 msec from the second heart sound.

The TTE shows normal LV size and function with a moderately enlarged LA. The aortic valve is normal. The mitral valve is thickened and mildly calcified with diastolic doming. There is mild MR by color-flow Doppler. There is MS with a mean gradient of 15 mmHg. The MVA by half-time is 1.9 cm^2.

Based on this information, this patient has:

a. Mild MS and mild MR
b. Severe MS and mild MR
c. Mild MS and severe MR
d. More information is required

16. A 24-year-old woman presents with exertional dyspnea and orthopnea in the 30th wk of her first pregnancy. She has a history of rheumatic fever in childhood and has not had a recent cardiac evaluation. She is currently on no medications.

Physical examination reveals a pulse of 100 bpm with a regular rhythm. The BP is 110/76 mmHg. There is mild JVD. A and V waves are visible. The lungs are clear. Cardiac examination reveals a palpable first heart sound and a parasternal lift. The second heart sound is somewhat increased. There is an opening snap followed by a grade 2/6 diastolic rumble noted at the apex and LSB.

The ECG demonstrates sinus rhythm with LA abnormality.

A TTE is performed and this demonstrates MS with an estimated valve area of 0.9 cm^2. The resting mean gradient across the mitral valve is 14 mmHg. The posterior mitral leaflet is pliable with diastolic doming. Minimal calcification is present. Mild mitral valve regurgitation is noted. The estimated RVSP is 80 mmHg.

I—Which of the following is most appropriate at this time?

a. Institution of HR control, diuresis, and warfarin
b. Open mitral commissurotomy
c. PMBV
d. MVR

The patient is started on medical therapy. She returns with persistent symptoms of dyspnea and orthopnea after 1 wk of therapy. Physical examination demonstrates a HR at 65 bpm. The cardiac examination findings are similar to those previously noted. A limited TTE is repeated. This demonstrates similar mitral valve morphology. The resting mean gradient across the mitral valve is 12 mmHg. The calculated valve area is 1.0 cm^2. The calculated RVSP is 60 mmHg.

II—Which of the following is the most appropriate at this time?

a. Change medical therapy
b. Open mitral commissurotomy
c. MVR
d. PMBV
e. Urgent cesarean delivery

17. A 67-year-old man presents to you with severe CHF. He had a bypass operation 10 yrs ago at which time mild AS was diagnosed. He had done well until the past month when he began to have progressive shortness of breath and now cannot walk across the room before having to stop.

On examination, his HR is 130 bpm and irregular. His BP is 90/60 mmHg. The venous pressure is 20 cm of water. The carotid upstroke is mildly delayed. The LV impulse is displaced to the anterior axillary line and enlarged. The second heart sound is single. A 2/6 SEM is present at the LSB with a mild peak.

The ECG shows AF with a rate of 120 bpm and LV hypertrophy. A chest X-ray shows pulmonary venous congestion and cardiomegaly.

A TTE shows an EF of 20% with regional wall motion abnormalities. The aortic valve is calcified with a mean gradient of 17 mmHg and an aortic valve area of 0.6 cm^2. Coronary angiography performed at home had shown severe three-vessel disease but patent grafts to the LAD, OM, and posterior descending artery.

What would you do at this time?

a. Optimize medical therapy with increasing dosages of ACE inhibitor and diuretics
b. Left and right heart catheterization with CO and coronary angiography
c. Dobutamine Doppler echocardiography
d. Thallium with 24-hr imaging
e. TEE-guided cardioversion

18. A 50-year-old man presents to you with a heart murmur. He has had a history of a heart murmur for the past 20 years but has never had any prior cardiac evaluation. He has gone in for an executive physical and is referred to you for evaluation of the heart murmur. The patient himself is active, plays racquetball twice a week, and jogs 4 days a week. He denies any significant symptoms of shortness of breath, chest pain, or lightheadedness. He does not smoke, does not drink, and has no HTN or diabetes. He is on no medications.

On physical examination, his BP is 130/70 mmHg and pulse is 70 bpm and regular. His JVP is normal and carotid upstroke is 2+ parvus and tardus. The lungs are clear. LV impulse is sustained and localized with a bifid quality. There is a fourth heart sound present. The second heart sound is single. There is a 2/6 harsh SEM at the right upper sternal border with a mid peak. Diastole is clear.

TTE is performed. This reveals normal LV cavity size with a mild increase in LV wall thickness and EF at 60%. There is a calcified aortic valve with restricted opening. The Doppler gradient across the aortic valve is 48 mmHg with a calculated valve area of 0.83 cm^2. The mitral and tricuspid valves appear normal.

18. (*continued*)

What would you do at this point in time?

a. Perform right and left heart catheterization to obtain an accurate measurement of valve gradient and valve area
b. Perform coronary angiography and refer to surgery
c. Trial of ACE inhibitor
d. Medical observation with warning against strenuous physical activity
e. TMET

19. A 53-year-old man presents with a 1-yr history of exertional dyspnea and chest tightness. He has no prior history of cardiac disease, although he was told he had a heart murmur several years ago. He is not limited by these symptoms that occur with a moderate degree of exertion, such as walking up 2 flights of stairs. These symptoms are reproducible and have increased only slightly over the past few months. He has had no rest discomfort. He does not have any other significant medical problems aside from mild HTN. He is on no medications.

On physical examination, his BP is 130/80 mmHg and pulse is 60 bpm and regular. His JVP is normal and carotid upstroke low volume and mildly delayed. The lungs are clear. The LV impulse is sustained and bifid. The first heart sound is normal. The second heart sound is clearly split with inspiration and an audible but decreased intensity aortic component of the second heart sound. There is a fourth heart sound audible. There is a 2/6 SEM at the base with a mid peak which ends at the second heart sound. Diastole is clear.

His ECG shows normal sinus rhythm without any significant abnormalities and specifically no evidence of LV hypertrophy. His chest X-ray shows LV predominance with clear lung fields.

A TTE is performed that reveals normal LV cavity size with normal systolic function and no LV hypertrophy. The EF is 70%. The aortic valve is calcified with a restricted opening and the mitral valve is normal. The mean gradient is 35 mmHg with a valve area of 1.1 cm^2. The aortic root is 52 mm.

Limited coronary angiography is performed that reveals normal coronary arteries.

What would you do with this patient?

a. AVR
b. PABV
c. Dobutamine hemodynamic study
d. TMET
e. Ergonovine challenge

20. A 72-year-old man presents with severe symptoms of shortness of breath and a diagnosis of AS. He underwent CABG 10 yrs ago at which time he was found to have severe three-vessel disease and a moderate depression of LV systolic function. His EF was 35% with a mild degree of AS (mean gradient 10 mmHg). He had a LIMA and two saphenous vein grafts placed. He did well until 2 yrs ago when he began to develop increasing symptoms of shortness of breath. At the time of his presentation, he was in severe heart failure—NYHA class IV.

On examination, his BP was 90/70 mmHg and pulse was 100 bpm and regular. His JVP was elevated to 20 cm of water with a large V wave. The carotid upstroke had very low volume and moderately delayed. The lungs had rales at both bases. The LV impulse was displaced and enlarged. The first heart sound was soft. The second heart sound was single. There was a soft 2/6 SEM at the right upper sternal border with a mid peak that ended at the second heart sound. A loud third heart sound was audible. The abdomen was soft and nontender without masses.

A chest X-ray showed cardiomegaly with pulmonary venous congestion. The ECG showed sinus tachycardia, HR of 100 bpm with high voltage, and loss of anterior forces.

A TTE revealed a severe depression in systolic function with an EF of 20% and multiple regional wall motion abnormalities. The aortic valve was calcified with restricted opening. The mean gradient was 22 mmHg with a valve area of 0.5 cm². Coronary angiography revealed patent grafts with diffuse distal disease.

What would you do at this point in time?

a. Right and left heart catheterization to measure gradient and CO
b. PABV
c. AVR
d. Aggressive therapy for heart failure with ACE inhibitor, diuretics, and beta blocker
e. Dobutamine challenge

21. A 70-year-old man presents to you with progressive symptoms of dyspnea over the past 2 mos. He has a history of implantation of a Carpentier-Edwards AVR 8 yrs ago for severe symptomatic AS. His coronary arteries were normal at the time of the operation. Following the operation, he was able to lead a very active lifestyle without limitations. The exertional shortness of breath has gradually increased but does not limit his lifestyle. He is still able to walk up a flight of stairs without shortness of breath which is about the most activity that he would want to do. He does not have any other past cardiac or medical history.

On examination, his BP is 150/60 mmHg and pulse is 76 bpm and regular. His JVP is not elevated and the carotid upstroke has full volume. The LV impulse is sustained and localized. The first heart sound is normal. The second heart sound is single. There is a 2/6 SEM at the right upper sternal border with an early to mid peak and a 2 to 3/6 holodiastolic decrescendo murmur at the LSB. There is no diastolic rumble or third heart sound audible. He has pulsations in his uvula and a pistol shot pulse in his peripheral pulse examination.

A TTE reveals a mildly dilated LV cavity (end diastolic dimension 58 mm) with a mild increase in LV wall thickness. Overall systolic function is normal with a EF of 60% and no regional wall motion abnormalities. The aortic valve prosthesis is well seated but the cusps are not able to be visualized due to acoustic shadowing. The mean gradient across the aortic valve during systole is 18 mmHg and the LVOT velocity has a TVI of 29 cc. AR is detected by continuous wave Doppler echocardiography but is an eccentric jet so the half-time cannot be measured. The jet occupies <30% of the LVOT. There is flow reversal in the descending aorta with a peak of 0.5 m/sec and holodiastolic. The echocardiographic report describes the valve as normal with mild to moderate regurgitation.

What would you do at this point in time?

a. Right and left heart catheterization with aortic root angiography and coronary angiography
b. TEE
c. Look for other causes of dyspnea
d. Exercise radionuclide angiogram
e. Treat with afterload reducers

22. A 30-year-old man presents with a heart murmur but is completely asymptomatic. He was an athlete in high school and played football and ran track without any

22. (*continued*)

limitations of activity. He was told that he had a very soft heart murmur when he was a teenager and, during an employment physical several years ago, he was told that he had a bicuspid aortic valve with AR. However, he did not follow-up and has had no medical care since then. He went to a family physician for an upper respiratory infection that subsequently resolved and he was found to have a loud heart murmur. Echocardiography revealed severe AR. He has no other significant medical problems and is otherwise active and healthy without symptoms.

On physical examination, his BP is 125/45 mmHg and pulse is 60 bpm and regular. His JVP is normal and carotid upstroke is bounding. The lungs are clear. The LV impulse is displaced and sustained. First and second heart sounds are normal. There is a soft 2/6 SEM at the right upper sternal border with an early peak and a loud 3/6 diastolic decrescendo murmur. A mid diastolic rumble is present at the apex.

TTE is performed. The LV is dilated with a systolic dimension of 45 mm. The EF is 60%. There are no regional wall motion abnormalities. The aortic valve is bicuspid with no significant stenosis but severe AR is present. The descending aorta is interrogated and there is a high velocity flow reversal during diastole.

An exercise radionuclide angiogram test is performed. On the test, he is able to go to 1200 kg/m/min, 95% of his predicted functional capacity. His EF, which was 60% at rest, dropped to 50% at peak exercise.

What is the next step in this patient's management?

a. Right and left heart catheterization with aortic root angiography and coronary angiography
b. Proceed to AVR with an aortic valve homograft
c. Proceed to AVR with a mechanical aortic valve prosthesis
d. Follow-up every 6 mos with echocardiography
e. Follow-up every 12 mos with echocardiography and start ACE inhibitor

23. You have attended a 56-year-old dairy farmer with rheumatic valvular heart disease for many years. Two years ago he had elective replacement of his mitral valve with a St. Jude prosthetic valve and a tricuspid annuloplasty. His dentist calls you for advice regarding endocarditis prophylaxis prior to dental extraction. The patient has never had IE. One year ago he developed a marked urticarial rash associated with bronchospasm following ampicillin administration prior to dental cleaning.

How would you now advise the patient and his dentist?

a. Clindamycin 600 mg orally 1 hr before the procedure
b. Erythromycin stearate 1 g orally before the procedure
c. Amoxicillin 2 g 1 hr before the procedure with steroid and antihistamine coverage
d. Nafcillin sodium 2 g IV 1 hr before the procedure
e. Gentamicin sulfate 0.1 mg/kg IV 1 hr before the procedure

24. A 28-year-old female is referred to you for evaluation of a heart murmur noted during the second trimester of her first pregnancy. The patient has no history of cardiac disease and the murmur has not been heard during medical evaluations in the past. The patient is asymptomatic. CV examination demonstrates a normal apical impulse. The first and second heart sounds are normal. A third heart sound is noted at the apex. A grade 2/6 early- to mid-peaking systolic murmur is audible at the LSB. There is a systolic click present that decreases with inspiration.

Based on the history and physical findings, the murmur is most likely due to which of the following?

a. Bicuspid aortic valve with mild to moderate stenosis
b. A congenitally abnormal pulmonary valve with moderate stenosis
c. A physiologic murmur related to pregnancy
d. Mitral valve regurgitation related to mitral valve prolapse
e. Bicuspid aortic valve with moderate regurgitation

25. Which of he following mechanical prostheses has the highest rate of structural deterioration?

a. Björk-Shiley C-C (convexo-concave) valve
b. Carbomedics valve
c. St. Jude medical valve
d. Medtronic-Hall valve
e. Björk-Shiley standard valve

26. On echocardiographic evaluation of an aortic Medtronic-Hall prosthesis, the following measurements were obtained: LVOT diameter, 1.8 cm; LVOT TVI, 20 cm; and prosthesis TVI, 100 cm.

The EOA is approximately:

a. $0.63\,cm^2$
b. $0.4\,cm^2$
c. $0.5\,cm^2$
d. $0.8\,cm^2$
e. $1.2\,cm^2$

27. A 43-year-old woman had acute onset of shortness of breath and lightheadedness. She had a history of rheumatic fever and subsequent MVR. On physical examination, she was pale and tachypneic. HR was 95 bpm and regular, with a low-volume pulse. BP was 95/44 mmHg. There were bilateral pulmonary rales with associated lower extremity edema and elevated JVP. A new murmur was present.

The next step in your evaluation should be:

a. Cardiac catheterization
b. Cardiac CT
c. TTE
d. TEE

28. Which of the following valves has a built-in leakage volume?

a. Stented heterograft
b. Caged-ball
c. Homograft
d. Bileaflet
e. Stentless heterograft

29. The Ross procedure is:

a. Replacement of a mechanical valve for a bioprosthetic valve in the tricuspid position
b. Transposition of the pulmonic valve into the aortic position
c. Indicated for elderly patients with AS who are poorly compliant with medication regimens
d. Indicated for patients with Ebstein's anomaly

30. Which of the following **least** influences mean gradient for a mechanical prosthesis?

    a. Prosthesis type
    b. Prosthesis position
    c. Prosthesis size
    d. Prosthesis regurgitation
    e. Length of time the prosthetic valve has been implanted

31. A 63-year-old man with a history of aortic valve regurgitation and St. Jude AVR comes to your office for anticoagulation recommendations prior to colonoscopy. He is chronically anticoagulated with warfarin with a goal INR of 2.5. His EF is 35% by echocardiogram.

    Which of the following do you recommend?

    a. Stop his warfarin 10 days prior to the colonoscopy and restart the day after the procedure
    b. Stop his warfarin 3 days prior to the colonoscopy, admit him to the hospital prior to the procedure for heparinization. He should remain in the hospital until the INR is above 2.0
    c. Stop his warfarin now, begin full dose aspirin (325 mg) and perform the colonoscopy in 7 days
    d. Admit directly to the hospital for 10 mg of vitamin K. Once his INR is <1.7, proceed with the colonoscopy. Keep him in hospital until his INR is higher than 2.0
    e. Continue warfarin, but reduce the dose such that the goal INR is now 2.0 and proceed to colonoscopy

32. Which of the following is an indication for IE prophylaxis in a patient undergoing sclerotherapy for esophageal varices?

    a. Previous bacterial endocarditis
    b. Isolated secundum ASD
    c. Previous CABG
    d. Prosthetic knee joint
    e. Cardiac pacemaker

33. First line therapy for native mitral valve endocarditis caused by methicillin-susceptible *Staphylococcus aureus* is:

    a. Nafcillin or oxacillin with gentamicin
    b. Vancomycin
    c. Ceftriaxone
    d. Cefotaxime
    e. Gentamicin alone

34. The most common cause of IE in IV drug users is:

    a. Viridans streptococci
    b. *Enterocuccus faecium*
    c. *Staphylococcus aureus*
    d. *Candida parapsilosis*
    e. *Kingella kingae*

35. A 56-year-old man with bicuspid aortic valve is admitted with fatigue, malaise, and 2 wks of fevers. Over the past few days he has become more lethargic and is

seen by his local physician. On physical exam he is diaphoretic and tachycardiac. His WBC is elevated and his blood cultures are positive after 6 hrs. His chest X-ray shows CHF.

Which of the following is the next best step?

a. A head CT with and without contrast
b. Wait for identification and sensitivities of cultures
c. Surgical consultation for AVR
d. Obtain a TTE to evaluate for paravalvular invasion and abscess

36. Which of the following is true about the treatment of IE?

   a. When enterococci resistant to both penicillin G and vancomycin cause endo-carditis, no medical therapy is reliably effective
   b. Cefazolin may be used to treat enterococcal endocarditis
   c. Oral agents such as fluconazole and itraconazole are the treatment of choice for fungal endocarditis
   d. High-dose IV penicillin alone is effective in curing enterococcal endocarditis caused by penicillin-susceptible enterococci

37. Which of the following is true of Chagas disease?

   a. Most commonly, transmission occurs from the bite of a blood-sucking redu-viid bug
   b. Nifurtimox and benznidazole are useful for treatment of chronic chagasic car-diac disease
   c. Cardiac involvement is a rare complication of Chagas disease
   d. The diagnosis of Chagas disease may be made easily by the isolation of the organisms from blood cultures

38. You are asked for consultation on a 46-year-old farmer with a history of AR. He has had low grade fevers, fatigue, night sweats, and weight loss for 2 mos. He has been to several physicians for evaluation, and a complete workup has not deter-mined an etiology. His echocardiogram shows no vegetations, and previous blood cultures have been negative. His blood cultures again return negative.

Which of the following is a possible cause of the negative cultures?

   a. *Escherichia coli* endocarditis
   b. *Coxiella burnetti*
   c. *Cardiobacterium hominis*
   d. *Strep bovis* endocarditis

39. A 28-year-old homeless man in Seattle, Washington, presents with a 2-mo history of fever and night sweats. Examination is significant for heart murmur compati-ble with aortic insufficiency. Three sets of blood cultures are negative after 48 hrs. The patient has not recently received antimicrobial therapy.

The most likely diagnosis is endocarditis caused by:

   a. *Bartonella quintana*
   b. *Staphylococcus aureus*
   c. *Enterococcus faecium*
   d. *Staphylococcus epidermidi*

40. A 60-year-old man presents for a general medical examination. He is totally asymptomatic, has a normal physical activity but a 3/6 systolic murmur is heard over his precordium, at the base of the heart and at the apex.

I—Among the following diagnoses, which is the **least** likely to produce this murmur?

a. AS
b. MR due to a prolapse of the posterior leaflet
c. MR due to a prolapse of the anterior leaflet
d. VSD
e. HCM

Dynamic maneuvers are performed during clinical examination. The murmur decreases after amyl nitrate and is unchanged after a post-extrasystolic beat.

II—Which of the following is the most likely diagnosis?

a. AS
b. VSD
c. MR
d. Aortic insufficiency
e. HCM with outflow obstruction

III—An echocardiogram is performed and shows the presence of MR. What is the most frequent cause of MR leading to surgery in the United States?

a. Rheumatic disease
b. Mitral valve prolapse
c. IE
d. Mitral annular calcification
e. Ischemic MR

41. A 38-year-old asymptomatic woman comes to see you for evaluation of a murmur. She has a 3/6 systolic murmur heard over the precordium and at the base of the heart. The murmur is preceded by a mid systolic click and is late peaking but ends with the second heart sound. The click moves closer to the first heart sound upon standing.

I—Which of the following is the diagnosis?

a. MR due to a flail leaflet
b. MR due to leaflet prolapse
c. AS due to a pliable bicuspid valve
d. MS with pliable leaflets
d. An "innocent" flow murmur

II—The echocardiogram shows moderate MR. Which of the following is correct?

a. IE prophylaxis is unnecessary
b. The risk of AF is <20%
c. Surgical referral is essential before the regurgitation becomes severe
d. In MR, nifedipine allows safe delay of surgery
e. In MR, ACE inhibitors improve survival

42. You are sending your patient for surgery for MR. The patient asks what to expect postoperatively?

Which of the following statements is true?

a. Postoperative heart failure is unusual
b. Postoperative heart failure can be predicted by preoperative LV EF
c. Postoperative heart failure occurs more often with mitral valve repair than replacement
d. Postoperative heart failure is mostly due to associated CAD

43. Indications for surgery in patients with severe MR include which of the following?

a. Asymptomatic patients without prior history of CHF
b. LV EF < 60%
c. LV end-diastolic diameter ≥30 mm
d. LV end-systolic diameter ≥30 mm

44. A 52-year-old woman is referred for shortness of breath. Her clinical examination shows a 2/6 diastolic murmur along the LSB and a wide pulse pressure. The patient has no signs of heart failure but has a third heart sound and a soft systolic murmur of MR.

In patients with a barely audible diastolic murmur and heart failure, what sign is suggestive that severe AR is the cause of the heart failure?

a. A third heart sound
b. A murmur of functional MR
c. An increased second heart sound
d. A BP of 130/45 mmHg
e. A decreased first heart sound

45. An echocardiogram is performed and it shows the presence of AR.

Which of the following is the most frequent cause of AR leading to surgery in the United States?

a. Rheumatic disease
b. Bicuspid aortic valve
c. IE
d. Syphilis
e. Degenerative aortic valve disease with or without annuloaortic ectasia

46. The echocardiogram shows an ascending aortic aneurysm without dissection.

What clinical sign should have lead to the suspicion of the aneurysm of the aorta?

a. Increased first heart sound
b. Increased second heart sound
c. Systolic HTN
d. Decreased femoral pulses

47. Which of the following is true regarding MR due to ischemic heart disease?

a. An audible murmur is always present if moderate or severe MR is present
b. The mechanism of ischemic MR is mostly a valve prolapse
c. This is more likely to occur after an anterior MI than from an inferior MI
d. The degree of ischemic MR may be overestimated by color flow imaging

48. Which of the following are accepted indications for surgery in patients with severe chronic AR?

    a. LV EF < 60%
    b. LV end-diastolic diameter ≥ 65 mm
    c. LV end-systolic diameter ≥ 45 mm
    d. NYHA class III or greater
    e. Bicuspid aortic valve with ascending aortic diameter of 40 mm

49. A 32-year-old woman presents with gradually increasing DOE for 2 yrs. Her daily activity is now limited. She has a history of rheumatic fever and was told of a heart murmur during an insurance examination at the age of 21 yrs. She has no other medical problems and does not take any medication. On examination the BP was 110/70 mmHg with a pulse of 70 bpm. The JVP and carotid pulse were normal. The LV impulse had a tapping quality. The first heart sound was loud with a normal S2. There was a high-pitched early diastolic opening snap 80 msec from aortic component of S2 and a 2/6 holodiastolic rumbling murmur. Her chest radiograph and ECG are below:

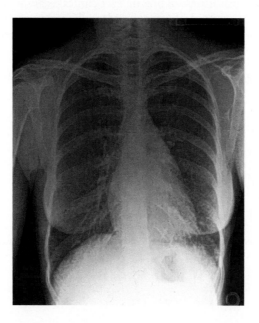

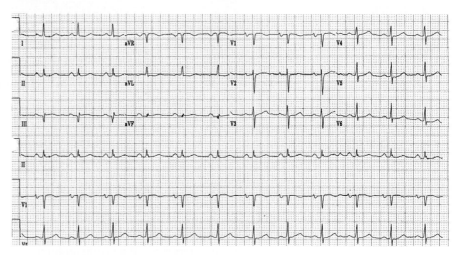

What would you do at this time?

a. Observation only
b. TTE
c. TEE
d. Catheterization of the right and left sides of the heart with exercise
e. Pulmonary angiography

50. Another patient is sent to you for evaluation of dyspnea. A prescheduled exercise echocardiogram is performed. The patient performs only to 50% of her predicted functional aerobic capacity before having to stop because of dyspnea. At peak exercise, the following Doppler signals were obtained:

- Mean transmitral gradient 22 mmHg
- TR velocity 3.8 m/sec
- HR 140 bpm

What would you do at this time?

a. TEE, then PMBV
b. MVR
c. Pulmonary angiography
d. Catheterization of the right and left sides of the heart
e. Treatment with beta blockers

51. A 60-year-old woman has class III symptoms of DOE. She has a long history of a heart murmur (since adolescence) but no symptoms until the last 5 yrs. On examination, she has a loud P_2, a 2/6 holosystolic murmur at the LSB, and a 2/6 long diastolic rumble at the apex. Echocardiography reveals a mildly dilated LV and LA, with an EF of 60%. A heavily calcified mitral valve is present. Doppler transmitral gradient is 20 mmHg.

What would you do next?

a. Coronary angiography, then MVR
b. TEE to look for MR
c. TEE, then PMBV
d. Continuity equation for MVA
e. Catheterization of the right and left sides of the heart

52. A 22-year-old man is asymptomatic but comes for evaluation of a heart murmur. There is a thrill in the carotid arteries, with a 3/6 long SEM in the aortic area with a mid peak. A soft 1/6 diastolic decrescendo murmur is present. TTE reveals moderate LV hypertrophy, with an EF of 65%. There is a normal-appearing 3-cusp aortic valve with mild regurgitation and a 4.5 m/sec jet across the aortic valve on Doppler echocardiography. No systolic anterior motion of the mitral valve is present. A cardiac MRI is obtained and shown below.

52. (*continued*)

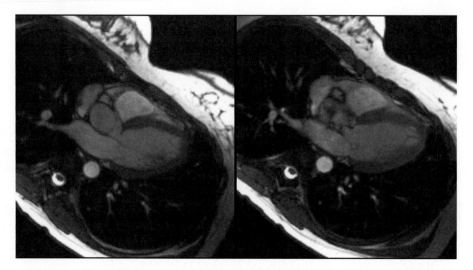

What is the next best step?

a. Catheterization of the right and left sides of the heart
b. Coronary angiogram and AVR
c. Observation, with yearly echocardiography
d. Repeat Doppler echocardiography with amyl nitrite
e. Cardiac surgical evaluation

53. A 57-year-old man is sent to you for evaluation of a new murmur. He is asymptomatic. His physical examination is unremarkable except for a 1/6 SEM without radiation. An echocardiogram is performed prior to your visit. It reveals a preserved LV EF, no LVH and a tricuspid aortic valve with a 20 mmHg gradient across the aortic valve.

What is the next step?

a. TMET evaluation to attempt to elicit symptoms
b. AVR
c. TTE in 3 yrs
d. Catheterization of the right and left sides of the heart
e. Annual echocardiogram

54. A 64-year-old woman has class III DOE. She has known MS from rheumatic heart disease and long-standing HTN. Echocardiography reveals mild LVH with an EF of 65%, a moderately enlarged LA, and a calcified mitral valve. Doppler echocardiography reveals a mean transmitral gradient of 4 mmHg, a MVA of 1.9 cm², and a TR velocity of 4.2 m/sec.

What is the next step in management?

a. Catheterization of the right and left sides of the heart
b. MVR
c. PMBV after TEE
d. Dobutamine stress test
e. Observation with yearly TTE

55. A 27-year-old female is referred to you for evaluation of a heart murmur noted during the second trimester of her first pregnancy. The patient is symptomatic with mild exertion. CV examination demonstrates a normal apical impulse. The first and second heart sounds are normal. A grade 3/6 early- to mid-peaking systolic murmur is audible at the LSB. An early systolic click is present and decreases with inspiration and there is a parasternal heave present. A TTE reveals pulmonary stenosis with a gradient of 46 mmHg.

Which of the following would you recommend?

a. Observe through the pregnancy and perform a Ross procedure when she is post partum

b. Proceed to pulmonary valve replacement now

c. Provide reassurance; this is increased flow across the valve related to pregnancy

d. Proceed to percutaneous valvuloplasty with appropriate shielding of the baby

e. Observe for now and recheck an echocardiogram in 4 wks

56. A 47-year-old male is referred to you for evaluation of a heart murmur noted. His chest radiograph is below.

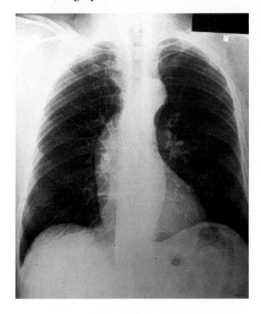

Which of the following is the most likely diagnosis?

a. ASD with Eisenmenger syndrome

b. MS

c. Bicuspid aortic valve

d. Ebstein's anomaly

e. Patent ductus arteriosus

57. A 71-year-old man presents to you with a heart murmur. He has had a history of a heart murmur for the past 20 yrs but has never had any prior cardiac evaluation. He has NYHA class III symptoms. On physical examination, his BP is 134/86 mmHg and his pulse is 70 bpm. His JVP is normal and carotid upstroke is low volume and delayed. There is a 3/6 harsh SEM at the right upper sternal border with a mid peak. The first heart sound is normal and the second heart sound is single. A TTE is performed and the Doppler is on the next page:

57. (*continued*)

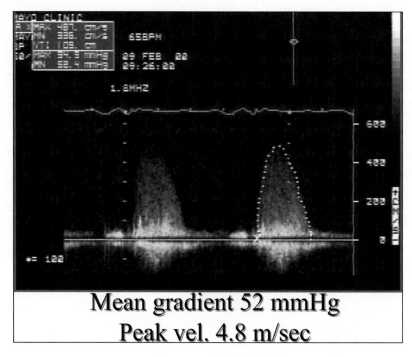

Mean gradient 52 mmHg
Peak vel. 4.8 m/sec

Which of the following would you do next?

a. AVR
b. Coronary angiogram then AVR
c. TET
d. Right and left heart catheterization to determine the aortic valve area

Answers

1. Answer e.
Patients with severe chronic MR should have an enlarged LV. Many of these patients are asymptomatic subjectively and must be assessed by exercise test to determine their level of exercise capacity. The EF, even in asymptomatic patients, can be normal or abnormal. RV dysfunction or pressure overload is variable. Third heart sound indicates chronically elevated end-diastolic volume due to an enlarged ventricle. It coincides with the Y descent of the atrial pressure pulse as well as the end of the rapid filling phase. It is not specific to MR. S3 is an early diastolic event, not end diastolic. It is due to rapid filling of the LV due to enhanced suction in young healthy patients, rapid inflow in restrictive physiology, or rapid inflow due to large regurgitant volume. In the latter the patient may have a rumble as well.

2. Answer a.
Patients with asymptomatic severe AR and normal ventricular function have a low annual risk of developing symptoms, ventricular dysfunction, and sudden death. However, patients will develop symptoms at a rate of >25% per yr after ventricular dysfunction occurs. Furthermore, patients have a >10% per yr risk of mortality after developing symptoms.

3. Answer b.
According to the 2006 ACC/AHA guidelines, patients with symptomatic (NYHA classes II–IV) chronic severe MR should be considered for surgery in absence of severe LV dysfunction (EF < 30% or end-systolic dimension >55 mm). Asymptomatic patients should be considered for surgery if the EF is <60%, the end-systolic diameter is >45 mm, AF has recently started, or there is pulmonary HTN.

In those who are asymptomatic surgery should be performed for severe chronic MR with an LV EF of 30% to 60% and/or end-systolic dimension ≥40 mm. Asymptomatic patients with severe chronic MR and preserved LV function who have new onset AF or pulmonary HTN defined as a PA systolic pressure >50 mmHg at rest or >60 mmHg with exercise should also be considered for surgical intervention.

Lastly, if severe chronic MR is due to a primary abnormality in the mitral valve apparatus and the patient has NYHA classes III–IV symptoms, with severe LV dysfunction (LV EF <30% or end-systolic dimension >55 mm), then surgery could be considered if a mitral valve repair is highly likely.

4. Answer b.
The history is consistent with carcinoid syndrome with cardiac involvement. A TTE can evaluate for valve disease. The tricuspid and pulmonary valves are most commonly involved. However, left-sided valve involvement is possible if there is a PAF or lung metastases. MRI of the chest would not provide any further assistance with the diagnosis.

5. Answer a.

The consensus of the Guidelines Committee is that patients should not have an operation for asymptomatic AS in the absence of critical stenosis, drop in BP during TMET, or LV systolic dysfunction. The committee also recommend performing a TMET to look for ventricular arrhythmias, a drop in BP, or to get an objective measurement of exercise tolerance. Close follow-up and an echocardiogram every year is recommended to identify symptoms and a change in LV function. A hemodynamic catheterization is necessary only to settle a discrepancy of symptoms, echocardiographic findings, or lack of physical findings supporting the diagnosis, or to provide a diagnosis when one needs to clarify different findings. In this case, the exam and findings on echocardiogram are consistent with AS. The current guidelines do not support AVR in those who have asymptomatic AS with preserved LF function. The patient needs appropriate follow-up for changes in clinical status and LV function; therefore, observation alone is not appropriate. Percutaneous balloon valvotomy for AS has a class III indication as an alternative to valve replacement.

6. I—Answer b.

The physical examination described in this athlete is indicative of a bicuspid aortic valve with AR. The clue on physical examination is that this bicuspid aortic valve is the early systolic click or "ejection click." A diastolic murmur is always pathologic and would require further investigation in any subject. In an athlete, a systolic murmur should be further investigated to rule out the possibility of AS, HCM, pulmonic stenosis, and ASD. Nuclear imaging really has no role in the evaluation of murmurs. Chest radiography certainly could offer some clues but would not be definitive.

The sinus bradycardia is common in athletes due to hypervagotonia. The systolic murmur may or may not indicate significant aortic obstruction since many young athletes will have an increase in stroke volume in both the LVOT and RVOT, creating turbulence.

II—Answer d.

This patient has a diastolic murmur that is always abnormal and indicates valvular pathology. Once valvular pathology has been identified, the risk of bacterial endocarditis increases and patients need to follow prophylaxis guidelines. However, the current ACC/AHA 2007 guidelines have changed and no longer include routine IE prophylaxis for patients with bicuspid aortic valves. The current recommendations include IE prophylaxis **ONLY for patients with underlying cardiac conditions associated with the highest risk of adverse outcome from IE**. According to the ACC/AHA guidelines class I indications for valve replacement in severe AR include all patients symptomatic for severe regurgitation regardless of LV systolic function. In those with severe AR who are asymptomatic, AVR is reserved for those with a reduced EF (<50%) or those undergoing CABG, other valve surgery, or aortic surgery. Class IIA indications include those who are asymptomatic with normal LV systolic function (EF >50%) but with severe LV dilatation (end-diastolic dimension >75 mm or end-systolic dimension >55 mm). Class IIB indications include those with moderate AR while undergoing surgery on the ascending aorta or CABG. In addition, it includes those patients that are asymptomatic with severe AR and normal LV systolic function at rest (EF > 50%) with evidence of progressive LV dilatation to an end-diastolic dimension of 70 mm or end-systolic dimension of 50 mm, declining exercise tolerance, or abnormal hemodynamic responses to exercise.

7. I—Answer c.

This gentleman has symptoms out of proportion to the echocardiographic findings. His physical examination is consistent with at least moderate AS and moderate to severe AR. The echocardiogram is discrepant with the clinical information, showing only mild AS and mild AR. Therefore, further evaluation is warranted to determine the true severity of the aortic valve lesion. His symptoms could be explained by concomitant CAD or by an underestimation of the valve disease by echocardiogram. Therefore, further assessment is necessary including evaluation of his coronary arteries. Proceeding directly to AVR or observation alone is not indicated in this patient without further clarification of the diagnosis. TMET in AS is used to elicit symptoms or look for hemodynamic changes (hypotension) with exercise. This patient is already symptomatic; therefore, a TMET will not provide any additional information in this case.

II—Answer b.

The Haake equation can be used. This is the CO $(3.5)/\sqrt{\text{gradient}}$ ($\sqrt{49} = 7$). The calculated AVA is 0.5 cm^2.

III—Answer c.

Grade I Sellers criteria are minimal or no contrast regurgitation into the LV. Grade II Sellers criteria are when the LV fills with contrast after 5 beats with less intensity than that of the aortic root. Grade III Sellers criteria are when the LV fills to the same density of the root but not before 5 beats, and Grade IV Sellers criteria are when the LV fills to the same density as the aortic root within 5 beats, often immediately.

8. Answer a.

The patient has a family history of Marfan syndrome and the MRI shows isolated aortic sinus enlargement which is characteristic of Marfan syndrome. Pregnancy in patients with Marfan syndrome is contraindicated when the aorta is over 40 mm. Beta blocker therapy should be instituted and the patient should be counseled against having a pregnancy at this time. If surgical intervention is performed and the patient has had an excellent result, future pregnancy could be considered. Counseling regarding inheritance of Marfan syndrome would also be appropriate.

9. Answer e.

This patient has only mild MS and is asymptomatic. Therefore, there is no indication for a balloon valvuloplasty or MVR. Most of these patients tolerate pregnancy well. She will need frequent rest during the day, lying in the left lateral decubitus position to avoid compression of the IVC. Beta blockade could be instituted to slow the HR and optimize diastolic filling time if symptomatic tachycardia occurs. Otherwise, she should do well throughout the pregnancy without pulmonary HTN or severe MS. A TEE would not provide any additional necessary information in this case.

10. Answer c.

Patients with ischemic regurgitation are less likely to have a successful mitral repair, and it should be considered only if the regurgitation is severe or if another surgical procedure is required. There are no data regarding the supplemental value of adding an ARB to an ACE inhibitor in the management of MR or post infarction. Digoxin could be added to patients with symptomatic LV systolic dysfunction or for rate control in AF. A follow-up echocardiogram at 6 wks is indicated only if there is a change in his clinical status. The patient is asymptomatic and on appropriate medical therapy; and therefore, continued current therapy is the next best step.

11. Answer c.

Even a patient with a functionally normal prosthetic valve is susceptible to endocarditis and so must be given antibiotic prophylaxis when having dental work. Patients with an isolated secundum ASD do not require routine antibiotic prophylaxis. Patients who have had a ligated patent ductus arteriosus are considered cured and do not require antibiotic prophylaxis. Coarctation of the aorta is a low-risk lesion for endocarditis, and, because cardiac catheterization is a sterile procedure, endocarditis prophylaxis is not required. TEE does not require routine antibiotic prophylaxis. The current ACC/AHA guidelines indicate that **ONLY** patients with underlying cardiac conditions associated with the highest risk of adverse outcome from IE need IE prophylaxis (ie, previous endocarditis, mechanical valve replacement, congenital heart disease with shunt and transplant valvulopathy).

12. Answer d.

This woman has moderately severe MS. However, she is completely asymptomatic and does not have significant elevation of her PA pressure. The majority of patients with asymptomatic or minimally symptomatic MS can have an uncomplicated pregnancy with careful monitoring. Pregnant patients with heart disease should have frequent rest periods during the day, consisting of 20 to 30 mins in the left lateral decubitus position (to avoid the compression of the interior vena cava by the fetus). Patients should be watched closely for the onset of AF and cardioversion should be performed with fetal monitoring should this occur. If the patient were symptomatic before pregnancy, intervention with PMBV would have been appropriate. If she does develop significant symptoms unresponsive to beta blockade, then PMBV could be performed during pregnancy (preferably after 20 wks) with appropriate shielding of the fetus.

13. Answer d.

This patient has a moderately severe MS with mild symptoms at 18 wks of pregnancy. Although her valve is suitable from the morphologic standpoint for either PMBV or closed commissurotomy, most patients with this severity of MS can be safely carried through pregnancy. Therefore, one would not want to subject either the patient or the fetus to a risk of operation if she can be safely carried to term with medical therapy only. Her HR is 90 bpm and the gradient could be significantly lowered with reduction in HR. Therefore, beta blockade would be the treatment of choice in this patient, slowly increasing the beta blocker to try to achieve a resting HR < 70 bpm. This may cause some fetal growth retardation but overall beta blockade even at high doses causes very little permanent effect on the child. If the patient goes into significant heart failure on beta blockade then PMBV, shielding the fetus would be a reasonable option. Surgery with MVR should be performed only if the valve is significantly calcified precluding a safe percutaneous approach, and the patient becomes hemodynamically unstable.

14. Answer d.

Symptomatic improvement occurs almost immediately after successful PMBV. According to the ACC/AHA guidelines a baseline echocardiogram is recommended after the procedure to obtain baseline measurements (post-procedure hemodynamics) and to exclude significant complications (MR, LV dysfunction, or ASD). The echocardiogram should be performed no earlier than 72 hrs after the procedure to allow for the acute changes in atrial and ventricular compliance to stabilize. Otherwise, the half-time in calculation of valve area is unreliable. The management of patients after successful PMBV is similar to that of the asymptomatic patient with MS. With recurrent symptoms, an echocardiogram should be performed to evaluate the mitral valve hemodynamics, PA pressure, and to rule out significant MR or a L-to-R shunt.

15. Answer d.

This patient has symptoms of heart failure and has mixed mild valve disease. There is a discrepancy between the valve gradient and valve area in that the gradient is in the range of "severe" MS but the valve area is in the range of "mild" MS. This is most likely due to concomitant significant MR that is underestimated by the TTE due to acoustic shadowing. However, the half-time may also be erroneous because of the compliance abnormalities. Therefore, either a TEE or the continuity equation can be performed to determine the true severity of MS.

16. I—Answer a.

The patient described in Question 16 has severe mitral valve stenosis but the HR is not well controlled. The initial therapy would be to try to alleviate symptoms with HR control and diuretics. Anticoagulation is appropriate due to the hypercoagulable state of pregnancy. The risk of warfarin is highest during the first trimester. Given the options provided, answer **a** is the best initial step. Other options are not recommended initially in this case.

II—Answer d.

If after appropriate HR control diuresis symptoms persist, PMBV would be carried out if there is no left atrial thrombus or significant mitral valve regurgitation noted by TEE and the valve is deemed amenable to balloon valvuloplasty (based on the degree of leaflet rigidity, severity of leaflet thickening, amount of leaflet calcification, and the extent of subvalvular thickening and calcification). Appropriate abdominal shielding to protect the fetus from radiation will be required.

17. Answer e.

This patient has a "low output, low gradient AS." However, from the history, he had done well until he suddenly went into significant heart failure. The etiology of his heart failure may well be the onset of acute AF that may have caused his CO to decrease. Therefore, before proceeding with any other diagnostic or therapeutic studies, one would try to get him back to normal sinus rhythm with a TEE-guided cardioversion under anticoagulation coverage. One would then reassess his hemodynamics. If his CO increases and his valve area increases without an increase in gradient, then no further intervention is warranted since he most likely does have a mild degree of AS. In this case, a 24-hr thallium would not be helpful at this point in the evaluation.

18. Answer e.

This patient has asymptomatic severe AS. The management of these patients continues to be controversial. It is clear that when a patient with severe AS becomes symptomatic, AVR is indicated to prolong life and relieve symptoms. However, it is still unclear as to what to do with the patient with asymptomatic severe AS. The proponents of early AVR cite the occurrence of sudden death occurring in patients with severe AS. However, overall, the incidence is low, < 1% per year. Since in most institutions the mortality of AVR approaches 3% to 5%, the majority of experts from academic centers feel that patients with severe AS should undergo close observation. The clear indication for operation would be either (*i*) the onset of symptoms or (*ii*) LV

18. (continued)

systolic dysfunction, indicating that the afterload on the LV is severe enough to cause deterioration in myocardial performance.

According to the current ACC/AHA guidelines, a TMET should be performed under *carefully monitored* conditions. This should be performed only in *asymptomatic* patients. This is performed to look for an abnormal BP response or exercise- induced symptoms to assist with decision making for whether to pursue AVR. In centers that can perform an operation with <1% mortality, it might be reasonable to proceed with AVR since AS is a progressive disease and 30% to 40% of patients would require AVR in the next 3 to 5 years.

19. Answer a.

This patient has moderate AS as defined by both the gradient and the AVA. However, the patient also has symptoms that are highly compatible with more severe AS. Although the major indication for AVR is severe symptomatic AS, it has been well documented that the natural history of "moderate" AS is defined by a valve area between 0.7 and 1.2 cm², and as severe AS if the patient is symptomatic. Therefore, one should not make a decision not to operate in a symptomatic patient with AS based upon a "single hemodynamic number." According to the ACC/AHA guidelines, symptomatic moderate AS has a class IIA indication for surgical intervention in those going for surgery on the aorta.

PABV for AS has a class III indication as an alternative to valve replacement; this is not a correct answer. The guidelines indicate that it may be a reasonable bridge to surgery in poor surgical candidates who are hemodynamically unstable or as a palliative measure. These indications were given a class IIB indication. Ergonovine challenge has no role in this patient.

20. Answer e.

This patient represents a "low output, low gradient" AS. The mean gradient is <30 mmHg yet the valve area is calculated to a "critical" range. In these patients it is unclear whether or not this is truly severe AS with the LV dysfunction related to the high afterload on the heart. Alternatively, this may be only mild AS with concomitant severe LV dysfunction in which the ventricle is not able to generate enough force to fully open the valve. Therefore, the "calculated" AVA is smaller than the true AVA. In the former, aortic valve operation should be performed. In the latter, medical therapy for LV dysfunction is indicated.

In order to determine which of these is present, it has been recommended that a challenge with either dobutamine or nitroprusside be performed in order to increase the forward stroke volume. By "normalizing" the CO, the gradient can then be reassessed. If the gradient rises to more than 40 mmHg then severe AS is present and the patient should undergo operation. However, if there is normalization of the CO and the gradient is still <30 mmHg, then this is only mild AS and operation is not warranted.

In addition, dobutamine challenge allows one to assess for contractile reserve as evidence by an increase in stroke volume of 20% or more. The presence of contractile reserve in this patient population has been shown to have lower mortality when undergoing AVR. Although both those with and without contractile reserve benefited from valve replacement, overall mortality was lower in those with contractile reserve.

21. Answer a.

This patient presents with symptoms of shortness of breath and finding of a deteriorating tissue AVR. There is a major discrepancy between the physical findings and the echocardiogram as there appears to be severe AR on examination due to the wide pulse pressure measured. The echocardiogram may not be able to accurately determine the severity of the AR due to the eccentric nature of the jet (making the color flow area determination inaccurate) as well as the acoustic shadowing that may be present.

There are subtle clues that the AR is severe, including the significant elevation of the TVI in the LVOT as well as the reversal in the descending aorta. TEE will most likely not be of additional benefit due to the fact that there is acoustic shadowing covering the LVOT. Aortic root angiography should be performed to confirm the suspicion of severe AR. Despite the fact that the ventricle is not dilated and systolic function is not decreased, this patient should undergo AVR if the AR is severe. Once a bioprosthesis begins to deteriorate there is progressive rapid further deterioration. The LV is most likely not able to dilate because of the pre-existing hypertrophy from the AS. An exercise nuclear study would not be helpful in this patient. Medical therapy will provide no benefit to this patient.

22. Answer d.

This patient has severe AR with preserved systolic function. AR is secondary to a bicuspid aortic valve and has most likely been present for many years. The patient himself is completely asymptomatic, able to exercise to an excellent workload on the exercise test. The indication for operation in AR is either (*i*) the onset of symptoms (class II to class IV), or (*ii*) the asymptomatic patient with LV systolic dysfunction at rest. If LV systolic function is preserved, then close observation is indicated as this indicates that irreversible myocardial fibrosis has not yet occurred. There are some who advocate AVR in an asymptomatic patient with normal systolic function in a markedly enlarged LV, but these are end-systolic dimensions $>25\,mm/m^2$. This patient is well below that limit. The drop in EF during the exercise radionuclide angiogram test in itself is not an indication for operation. However, this does stratify the patient into a higher risk group in whom the probability of the onset of symptoms or LV dysfunction is higher ($>10\%$) than patients who would have no drop in EF with exercise. Therefore, in this patient, follow-up every 6 mos, mainly to look at a measurement of LV systolic function, is indicated. If the patient was able to increase the EF with exercise, yearly follow-up would be appropriate. Medical treatment of severe AR using vasodilators is not currently recommended according to the ACC/AHA guidelines unless needed for hypertension control.

23. Answer a.

This question tests your knowledge of the AHA/ACC guidelines on the administration of antibiotics prior to dental and invasive procedures in patients at risk of IE.

Clindamycin 600 mg orally 1 hr before the procedure is now the treatment of choice for penicillin allergic patients needing endocarditis prophylaxis, even those with prosthetic valves. IV antibiotics are needed only for very high risk patients or those unable to take oral medications. Vancomycin 1.0 g IV or vancomycin combined with gentamicin 1.5 mg/kg IM/IV is used in this situation.

24. Answer b.

A pulmonary valve stenosis murmur is usually best heard of the left upper sternal border as opposed to the right upper sternal border. The murmur often radiates to the left shoulder as well. Pulmonary valve stenosis is commonly associated with a pulmonary ejection click. In addition, the RV may be palpable in a patient with severe pulmonary valve stenosis. There is a decrease in the pulmonary valve click with inspiration, which is the only audible sound on the right side of the heart that decreases with inspiration. This is due to increased volume to the right side of the heart with inspiration, which is thought to cause a bulge in the stenotic valve and partially open the valve. This would decrease the click.

Aortic valve stenosis in a patient in this age group could be most likely related to a bicuspid aortic valve and an ejection click may be noted with this murmur as well. However, the remainder of the exam is more consistent with pulmonary valve disease then aortic valve disease. The aortic outflow murmur is usually best heard over the sternum or aortic area and is usually described as increasing with provocative maneuvers. The murmur of mitral valve regurgitation is usually best heard at the apex and when associated with mitral valve prolapse it is often associated with one or more systolic clicks. Aortic valve regurgitation is a diastolic murmur that does not correlate with the findings described in this patient.

25. Answer a.

The convexoconcave Björk-Shiley valve, especially in the larger annulus sizes, has been associated with an increased risk of in vivo strut fracture. The remaining valves are newer generation valves and have not been reported as having strut fracture related failure.

26. Answer c.

$$\text{EOA} = \frac{\left[\text{LVOT area (cm}^2)\right] \times \left[\text{LVOT TVI (cm)}\right]}{\text{Prosthesis TVI (cm)}}$$

$$= \frac{\pi\, r^2 (cm)^2 \times \left[\text{LVOT TVI(cm)}\right]}{\text{Prosthesis TVI (cm)}}$$

$$= \frac{\pi\, (0.9)^2 \times 20}{100}$$

$$= 0.5 \text{ cm}^2$$

27. Answer c.

TTE should be performed initially and, if adequate views of her prosthetic valve are not obtainable, TEE may be helpful.

28. Answer d.

Bileaflet mechanical valves have a built-in leakage volume that serves to "clean" the leaflet surface and reduce thrombus formation on the valve surface. The other valves listed do not have this feature.

29. Answer b.

An alternative to valve replacement with a mechanical valve or bioprosthesis is the Ross procedure. With this procedure, a pulmonary valve autograft replaces the aortic valve, while right-sided reconstruction is usually performed with an aortic or pulmonary homograft. Strict indications are not established for when to perform a Ross procedure. There are some potential advantages of a Ross procedure that should be considered: (*i*) autologous tissue with documented long-term viability, (*ii*) possible resistance to infection, (*iii*) lack of valve noise, (*iv*) lack of need for anticoagulation. The following are considered to be contraindications to a Ross procedure: (*i*) advanced three-vessel coronary disease, (*ii*) severely depressed LV function, (*iii*) pulmonary valve pathology, (*iv*) Marfan syndrome or other connective tissue disorders, or (*v*) size mismatch between the pulmonic and aortic annulus.

30. Answer e.
In the absence of prosthetic or ventricular dysfunction, the mean gradient across a prosthesis does not change significantly with time since implantation. The type, size, valve position and regurgitant volume have a significant role in the gradient across a prosthetic valve.

31. Answer b.
According to the ACC guidelines, those patients with a bileaflet mechanical AVR with no risk factors (ie, AF, previous thromboembolism, LV dysfunction, hypercoagulable conditions, older generation thrombogenic valves, mechanical tricuspid valves, or more than one mechanical valve) should stop their warfarin 48 to 72 hrs before the procedure (so the INR falls to <1.5) and restarted within 24 hrs after the procedure. Heparin is usually unnecessary. In those patients at high risk of thrombosis (defined as those with any mechanical MV replacement, or a mechanical AVR with any risk factor), therapeutic doses of IV UFH should be started when the INR falls below 2.0 (typically 48 hrs before surgery), stopped 4 to 6 hrs before the procedure, restarted as early after surgery as bleeding stability allows, and continued until the INR is again therapeutic with warfarin therapy. This patient has a mechanical AVR and reduced LV function; therefore, admitting the patient for heparin bridging before and after the procedure is necessary.

32. Answer a.
Certain underlying conditions such as previous bacterial endocarditis are associated with a relatively high risk of IE (ie, previous endocarditis, mechanical valve replacement, congenital heart disease with shunt and transplant valvulopathy). In contrast, other disorders such as isolated ASD, previous CABG, prosthetic joints, and cardiac pacemakers are associated with very low or negligible risk.

33. Answer a.
In methicillin-susceptible staphylococcal endocarditis, a beta-lactam agent is more effective than vancomycin.

The current ACC/AHA guidelines recommend treatment of native valve endocarditis due to methicillin-susceptible *Staphylococcus aureus* with a semi-synthetic penicillin, such as nafcillin or oxacillin. Six weeks of therapy is recommended for all left-sided native valve endocarditis cases. In addition, the use of gentamicin for the first 3 to 5 days of therapy is recommended for synergy.

34. Answer c.
Staphylococcus aureus is the most common cause of IE in injection drug users. Staphylococci and streptococci account for the majority of cases of endocarditis with nearly 75% of all cases having a pre-existing structural cardiac abnormality. *S. aureus* accounts for nearly one third and *S. viridans* accounts for 18% of all cases of endocarditis. Enterococcus accounts for approximately 10% of cases of IE. The

34. (continued)

Haemophilus aphrophilus, Actinobacillus actinomycetemcomitans, Cardiobacterium hominis, Eikenella corrodens, and *Kingella kingae* organisms have been thought to be common etiologies of culture-negative endocarditis. However, these organisms can be easily isolated with current blood culture systems when incubated for at least 5 days. Candida endocarditis is one of the most serious manifestations of candidiasis and is the most common cause of fungal endocarditis. Overall, this is an unusual cause of endocarditis.

35. Answer d.

An echocardiogram is the next step in evaluating this patient. Given his history of bicuspid aortic valve, he is at higher risk for IE. His lethargy may be due to a CNS process and a CT may be helpful. However, given his history, establishing a diagnosis for endocarditis is paramount. There is no need to wait for specific identification. After cultures are obtained, broad spectrum antibiotics should be utilized until a specific organism is identified. Indications for cardiac surgery in patients with endocarditis include heart failure directly related to valvular dysfunction, persistent or uncontrollable infection despite appropriate medical therapy, or recurrent emboli due to the presence of large vegetations. Without a diagnosis, a surgical evaluation is inappropriate. In addition to these indications, relative indications include evidence of perivalvular infection (intracardiac abscess or fistula), a ruptured sinus of Valsalva aneurysm, fungal endocarditis, highly resistant microorganisms, and a relapse after an adequate course of antimicrobial therapy or persistent fevers of more than 10 days after starting empiric therapy.

36. Answer a.

Enterococci have a narrow spectrum of sensitivity and the majority of cases of enterococcal endocarditis are caused by strains of *Enterococcus faecalis*. The AHA guidelines recommend therapy for *E. faecalis* with combination of IV aqueous penicillin G or ampicillin plus gentamicin or, alternatively, combination therapy with vancomycin plus gentamicin if a penicillin allergy is present. When enterococci that are resistant to both penicillin G and vancomycin cause endocarditis, no medical therapy is reliably effective.

37. Answer a.

Trypanosoma cruzi, the etiologic agent of American Trypanosomiasis, or Chagas disease, is transmitted by various species of blood-sucking reduviid bugs. The reduviid bug takes a blood meal and subsequently defecates around the bite site. This results in local irritation and subsequent scratching of the wound site leading to contamination of the wound with the parasites in the feces. Humans are typically bitten on the face while sleeping. Nifurtimox and benznidazole may be useful in the treatment of acute Chagas disease but show minimal usefulness in the treatment of chronic Chagas disease. The diagnosis of chronic Chagas disease is usually made by detecting IgG antibodies that bind to parasite antigens in the serum of patients. Cardiac involvement is very common in Chagas disease and can be seen in all 3 phases of the disease (acute, indeterminate, and chronic). Chronic Chagas disease manifests as a biventricular heart failure, dysrhythmia, and thromboembolism.

38. Answer b.

Culture-negative endocarditis may occur with fungal endocarditis and with slow-growing fastidious organisms such as nutritionally variant streptococci, *Coxiella burnetii* (the causative agent of Q-fever), and *Bartonella quintana*. *Escheria coli* generally is not a cause of culture-negative endocarditis. The *Haemophilus aphrophilus*, *Actinobacillus actinomycetemcomitans*, *Cardiobacterium hominis*, *Eikenella corrodens*, and *Kingella kingae* organisms have been thought to be common etiologies of culture-negative endocarditis. However, these organisms can be easily isolated with current blood culture systems when incubated for at least 5 days. *Streptococcus bovis* bacteremia is associated with colon cancers, not with culture negative endocarditis.

39. Answer a.

Bartonella quintana recently has been associated with endocarditis in homeless persons with alcoholism and in patients in inner-city settings. *Bartonella spp.* are slow-growing gram-negative bacteria that may require a month or longer for culture isolation. *Staphylococcus aureus* is the most common cause of IE in injection drug users. Enterococcus accounts for approximately 10% of cases of IE and the majority of cases of enterococcal endocarditis are caused by strains of *Enterococcus faecalis*. The coagulase-negative staphylococci isolated initially after a surgery/procedure are almost always *Staphylococcus epidermidis*. This is often encountered in pacemaker pocket infections, and the majority are methicillin-resistant and resistant to all beta-lactam antibiotics.

40. I—Answer c.

AS, MR due to a prolapse of the posterior leaflet, and HCM may all produce murmurs that can be heard with equal intensity from the base to the apex. The VSD murmur is heard over the precordium. The murmur of MR due to an anterior leaflet prolapse is typically maximum at the apex and radiating to the axilla following the jet's tract.

II—Answer c.

The murmur of MR decreases with amyl nitrite, which decreases both preload and afterload, but increases with methoxamine and in the left lateral decubitus position and does not change after extrasystole or expiration.

III—Answer b.

The lesion most frequently leading to surgery for MR in the United States is mitral valve prolapse with or without flail leaflet in more than half of the cases. Rheumatic disease represents around 10% of the cases of pure MR and endocarditis, a little less. Ischemic MR is the second lesion leading to surgery for pure MR, representing 20% to 30% of the cases. Mitral annular calcification may be associated with mitral valve prolapse, but isolated, causes most often mild regurgitation.

41. I—Answer b.

In mitral valve prolapse the standing position (by decreasing LV filling) increases the time of systole during which the prolapse is present, bringing the click and beginning of regurgitation earlier in systole. This change is related to the fact that the prolapse and the regurgitation occur at a fixed ventricular volume irrespective of the maneuvers performed. The jet area of MR may increase during exercise because of increased regurgitant volume or velocity.

41. (continued)

Non-ejection clicks (those not associated with the aortic valve) are usually high intensity and are due to sudden snapping of the chordae tendineae of the mitral leaflets as they bow back into the LA. One additional clue is that ejection clicks occur before the carotid upstroke, while non-ejection clicks occur after.

II—Answer a
Endocarditis prophylaxis is unnecessary in patients without underlying cardiac conditions associated with the highest risk of adverse outcome from IE (previous endocarditis, mechanical valve replacement, congenital heart disease with shunt, and transplant valvulopathy). Neither ACE inhibitors nor nifedipine have been shown to have the ascribed effects. According to the ACC/AHA guidelines, surgical intervention for mitral valve regurgitation involves valves that have severe regurgitation only. There is no indication for surgical intervention to prevent progression to severe regurgitation. The risk for AF in patients with severe MR due to flail leaflets who are treated conservatively is >20%.

42. Answer b.
LV dysfunction is the most common cause of heart failure following surgery and can be predicted by LV and EF and end-systolic diameter and prevented in part by valve repair. It is more frequent in patients with incidental coronary disease associated with organic MR but most often occurs in patients without associated coronary disease.

43. Answer b.
Class III or IV symptoms, transient heart failure, or LV dysfunction should lead to prompt consideration of surgery. Severe LV enlargement appears associated with the occurrence of sudden death and does not preclude an excellent postoperative result and therefore is a widely accepted indication of surgery.

According to the 2006 ACC/AHA guidelines, patients with **symptomatic** (NYHA classes II–IV) chronic severe MR should be considered for surgery even in the absence of severe LV dysfunction (EF < 30% or end-systolic dimension >55 mm). **Asymptomatic** patients should be considered for surgery if the EF is <60%, the end systolic diameter is >45 mm, or there is pulmonary HTN (defined as a PA systolic pressure >50 mmHg at rest or >60 mmHg with exercise), or new onset AF.

In those patients who are asymptomatic with preserved LV systolic function (EF > 60%) and an end systolic diameter <40 mm, surgery should not be routinely considered unless a high likelihood of valve repair is present.

44. Answer d.
In patients with heart failure of any cause, an S3, a murmur of functional MR and a soft S1 are commonly observed. An increased S2 is unrelated to the degree of MR. Persistent peripheral signs of AR despite the heart failure, such as bounding arteries, increased BP, differential and decreased diastolic pressure, are particularly suggestive of severe AR.

45. Answer e.
Degenerative disease with dystrophic valves, enlarged annulus, and possibly aortic ectasia is the most frequent cause of surgical AR followed by congenitally abnormal valves.

46. Answer b.
The second heart sound (S2) consists of two components, aortic and pulmonary valve closure sounds. An increased second heart sound may be due to the amplifying effect of an enlarged aorta and is suggestive of an ascending aortic aneurysm in patients with

AR. Increased intensity of the first heart sound occurs when the mitral valve remains widely open at end diastole and then closes rapidly. Clinically this occurs if there is an increased transvalvular gradient (such as MS), an increased transvalvular flow (such as a left-to-right shunt), tachycardia (shortened diastole), or a shortened PR interval. A decreased pulse could be due to variety of clinical problems including arteritis, decreased CO or peripheral atherosclerotic disease.

47. Answer d.

Ischemic MR may be silent, especially in the setting of an AMI. It is considered a negative prognostic sign and is most frequently associated with an in inferior MI. The degree of regurgitation may be overestimated by color flow imaging because it is usually a central regurgitation jet into an enlarged atrium which can lead to spuriously large jets. The etiology is most commonly due to regional remodeling due to apical displacement of papillary muscles and annular enlargement. This entity is difficult to manage both medically and surgically.

48. Answer d.

According to the ACC/AHA guidelines class I indications for valve replacement in severe chronic AR include all patients with symptomatic severe regurgitation regardless of LV systolic function. In those with severe AR who are asymptomatic, AVR is reserved for those with a reduced EF (<50%) or in those undergoing CABG, other valve surgery or aortic surgery. Class IIA indications include those who are asymptomatic with normal LV systolic function (EF > 50%) but with severe LV dilatation (end-diastolic dimension >75 mm or end-systolic dimension >55 mm). Class IIB indications include those with moderate AR while undergoing surgery on the ascending aorta or CABG. In addition, it includes those patients that are asymptomatic with severe AR and normal LV systolic function at rest (EF > 50%) with evidence of progressive LV dilatation to an end-diastolic dimension of 70 mm or end-systolic dimension of 50 mm, a declining exercise tolerance, or abnormal hemodynamic responses to exercise.

49. Answer b.

The figure shows an ECG with left atrial enlargement and a chest X-ray with flattening of the left heart border which is consistent with left atrial enlargement. The physical exam is consistent with mitral valve stenosis but a valve that is pliable (presence of an opening snap). A TTE is the best first step to evaluate a gradient across the mitral valve and whether the valve is suitable for valvulopasty.

50. Answer a.

The exercise study shows exercise-induced severe MS. This question tests your knowledge of the ACC/AHA 2006 guidelines. For evaluation of MS using an exercise evaluation, if the gradient across the mitral valve exceeds 15 mmHg or the pulmonary systolic pressure exceeds 60 mmHg, percutaneous valvuloplasty or mitral valve surgery is indicated. The TEE is indicated to evaluate pre-procedure for a left atrial thrombus and to ensure there is not significant MR. There is no role for a pulmonary angiogram in this patient. A hemodynamic catheterization is necessary only if the diagnosis is in question. At this point a catheterization would only be necessary for treatment of the MS if the valve was appropriate for valvulplasty (pliable valve leaflets, lack of commissural calcification, absence of moderate or greater regurgitation and no left atrial appendage thrombus).

51. Answer a.

The valve is severely stenotic and heavily calcified. Therefore, valvuloplasty would not be appropriate given the risk of mitral valve rupture and subsequent severe MR. Given the age of the patient, evaluation of the coronary arteries and referral for MVR is the best option. There is no other diagnostic evaluation necessary at this point.

52. Answer e.

The figure shows two images of a cardiac MRI with a subaortic membrane/web and documented flow disturbance that would account for the findings on physical exam and TTE. In those with a SEM and gradient on echocardiogram, alternative possibilities should be considered such as supravalvular stenosis (Williams syndrome), subvalvular stenosis, and outflow tract obstruction. A TEE may also have provided anatomic detail as well. Observation may be appropriate after an accurate diagnosis is made.

53. Answer c.

The patient has mild AS by physical examination and echocardiogram. The valve is not bicuspid and his LV and EF is preserved. Therefore, no further assessment and no intervention is necessary. However, according to the ACC/AHA guidelines a follow-up echocardiogram is indicated at 3 to 5 yrs for mild AS, 1 to 2 yrs for moderate AS, and annually for severe asymptomatic AS.

54. Answer a.

There is a discrepancy between the echocardiogram and the patient's NYHA class III symptoms. The echocardiogram indicates only mild to moderate MS which is not enough to explain the symptoms and there is resting pulmonary HTN present. Therefore, more information is needed. Among the answer choices given, the best answer is right and left heart catheterization. The severity of the MS and PA pressures need further investigation. A right heart hemodynamic assessment will also allow for evaluation of the TR velocity. The pressures were out of proportion to the findings on the echocardiogram. There is no indication for surgery or valvuloplasty with the current gradient across the mitral valve. An exercise echocardiogram using supine bicycle may illustrate an exercise gradient of 10 mmHg or higher; this answer choice is not given.

55. Answer d.

The 2006 ACC/AHA guidelines indicate that mild pulmonary stenosis is a benign disease and often does not progress in severity. However, balloon valvotomy is recommended in symptomatic patients with a peak systolic gradient >30 mmHg and in asymptomatic patients with peak systolic gradient >40 mmHg. Observation and a Ross procedure are not appropriate in this patient given the success of percutaneous balloon valvotomy. A follow-up echocardiogram would provide no incremental benefit since her gradient is above the necessary gradient for intervention.

56. Answer c.

The chest X-ray shows a dilated ascending aorta. Although this is not exclusively associated with bicuspid aortic valve, among the answer choices given this is the best answer. Eisenmenger syndrome would have enlarged PAs with peripheral "pruning" due to pulmonary HTN. MS would show an enlarged LA. Ebstein's anomaly classic appearance on chest X-ray is that of a markedly enlarged RV. A patent ductus arteriosus would have an enlarged LV due to volume overload.

57. Answer b.

This patient has symptoms and physical examination findings consistent with severe AS. His echocardiogram Doppler measurements indicate a mean gradient over 50 mmHg. No further assessment of his valve is necessary. According to the ACC/AHA guidelines, this is a class I indication for surgical intervention. At his age and multiple risk factors, preoperative coronary angiogram is indicated. There is no further workup necessary since his history, physical exam, and echocardiogram have the same findings. Therefore, there is no indication for TMET evaluation or hemodynamic assessment.

SECTION VII

Noninvasive Cardiac Imaging

Garvan C. Kane, MD, PhD

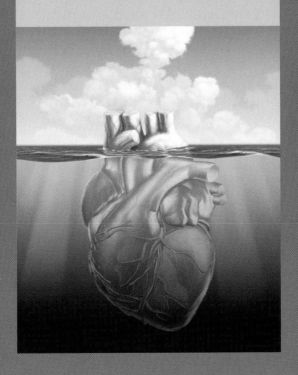

Questions

1. What is the structure identified with an asterisk on this apical two chamber TTE performed for the evaluation of chest pain?

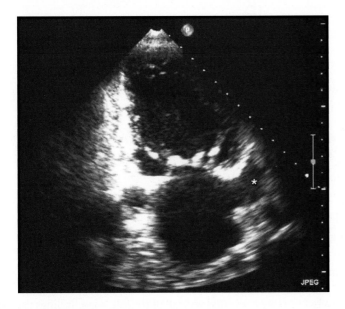

   a. Dilated left lower pulmonary vein
   b. IVC
   c. Aneurysm of the LCX artery
   d. Dilated CS
   e. Left atrial appendage

2. A 50-year-old man is referred to you for an outpatient evaluation of atypical chest symptoms. He has HTN and hyperlipidemia. He walks regularly with his wife and has no orthopedic problems. His resting ECG shows greater than 1 mm nonspecific ST depression in multiple leads.

   Which of the following tests should be performed?

   a. Exercise ECG
   b. Exercise SPECT
   c. Adenosine SPECT
   d. Dipyridamole SPECT
   e. Dobutamine echo

Answers to this section start on page 259.

3. A 55-year-old man has undergone a TMET. He has a normal resting ECG. He walked 7 minutes on the Bruce protocol, achieving 8 METs, 77% predicted functional aerobic capacity. The test was stopped due to angina. The stress ECG showed + 1 mm ST depression in leads V4–V6.

    The patient's Duke treadmill score is:

    a. 12
    b. 5
    c. 0
    d. −6
    e. −11

4. A patient with known CAD reports worsening of his DOE. There is a history of a bipolar psychiatric disorder, and the patient has had many evaluations because of similar complaints, all of which have been negative. You would like to quantitate the patient's exercise tolerance and order a TMET ECG. On the day of the test, you receive a call from the stress laboratory, indicating that the patient has LBBB.

    You would do which of the following?

    a. Cancel the test because you cannot interpret the ECG
    b. Proceed with the test
    c. Change the test to dobutamine echocardiography
    d. Change the test to adenosine thallium test
    e. Decide to perform coronary angiography

5. The findings on this MRI scan are associated with all of the following findings **except:**

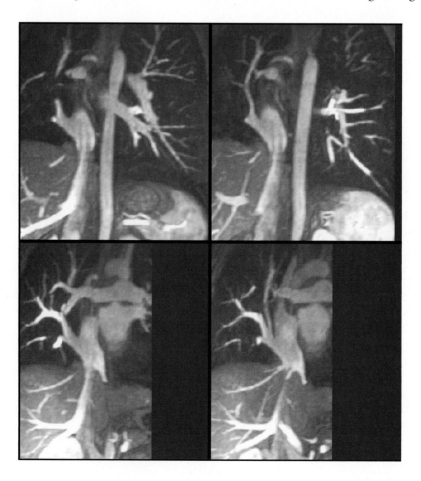

a. RV enlargement
b. Atrial arrhythmias
c. Pulmonary hypoplasia
d. Pulmonary emboli

6. You are performing an adenosine stress study in a 60-year-old woman without known CAD who is referred for chest symptoms. You are 2 minutes into the adenosine infusion at 140 g/kg/min. The patient is experiencing flushing and mild chest pain. The rhythm remains stable and there is no ST segment deviation. Her hemodynamic parameters are as follows:

Time (min)	HR (bpm)	BP (mmHg)
0	68	128/72
1	72	124/68
2	74	122/70

What is the next best step?

a. Increase the adenosine infusion to $280\,\mu g/kg/min$ to achieve a higher double product before injecting the tracer
b. Decrease the adenosine infusion to $75\,\mu g/kg/min$ due to the patient's chest pain and inject the tracer
c. Continue the adenosine infusion at $140\,\mu g/kg/min$ and inject the tracer at 3 minutes
d. Follow by another 3 minutes of adenosine infusion then stop
e. Stop the infusion and wait for the patient's chest pain to subside
f. Administer NTG

7. A 60-year-old diabetic woman is referred for evaluation of heart failure. She had known CAD with prior MIs. Her LV EF is 27% by echocardiography with apical and anterior akinesis and inferior and inferospetal hypokinesis. Her RV systolic pressure is 30 mmHg. Her cardiac medications include ASA, ACE inhibitor, beta blocker therapy, diuretics, and a statin. She is on insulin with satisfactory glycemic control. Her height is 165 cm and weight 75 kg. Her creatinine is 1.4 mg/dL. She is unable to walk up 6 steps of stairs without marked dyspnea and a sensation of chest fullness. Her BP in the hospital has been in the range of 78–85/40–50 mmHg and she has been experiencing lightheadedness. A coronary angiogram is performed and shows severe three-vessel disease with good target vessels. A cardiac surgeon is consulted. He would not consider operation without some objective evidence of myocardial viability.

What is the next best step?

a. Implant ICD
b. Perform a PET rest-stress rubidium-82 study
c. Perform a resting SPECT sestamibi study
d. Perform a resting thallium study with 24-hour views
e. Obtain a cardiac CT for viability

8. A 45-year-old male with fatigue presents for an echocardiogram. The LV end diastolic dimension is 60 mm and the end systolic dimension is 40 mm. What is the EF?

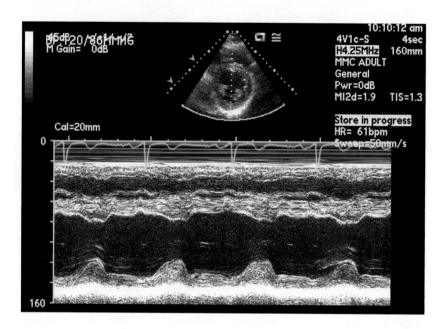

a. 56%

b. 33%

c. 67%

d. 45%

e. 50%

9. A 54-four-year old woman presents with a 6-month history of progressive symptoms of right heart failure. On physical examination the JVP is 16 cm with prominent V wave. There is also a loud holosystolic murmur with respiratory variation. The liver is enlarged and pulsatile. There is bilateral lower extremity edema and evidence of ascites.

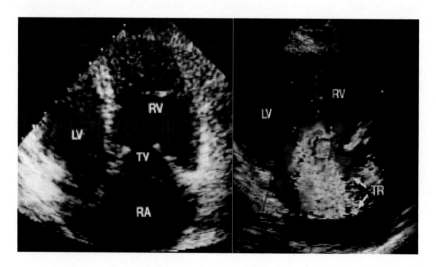

Upon reviewing her TTE, which is the next best diagnostic step?

a. Coronary angiography and right heart catheterization
b. Urine cytology
c. Thyroid function studies
d. 5-HIAA
e. Blood cultures

10. A "biphasic" response of a segment or segments to dobutamine during a stress echocardiogram is interpreted to mean:

a. Ischemia in the territory supported by that artery
b. Infarction in the territory supported by that artery
c. Normal response to dobutamine
d. Ischemia and viability in the territory supported by that artery
e. Indeterminate result

11. An elevation in which pressure is most likely to be associated with pulmonary congestion and clinical symptoms?

a. LA mean pressure
b. LV developed pressure
c. LA A-wave pressure
d. LVEDP
e. PA mean pressure

12. A 65-year-old male was admitted with an AMI and received thrombolytic therapy 3 days ago. The resident is called to evaluate new onset hypotension. The patient is more short of breath and diaphoretic, BP 80/40 mmHg, pulse 123 bpm. Arterial saturation is 93%. She believes she hears a new murmur, is having difficulty characterizing it. A bedside TTE is obtained.

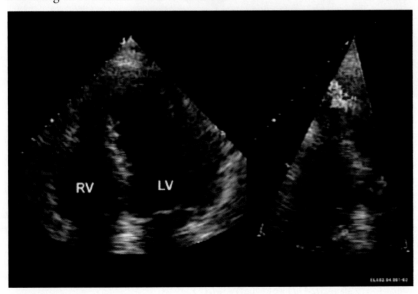

The study indicates:

a. A ruptured ventricular septum with L→R shunt
b. Cardiac tamponade
c. A pseudoanerurysm of the LV
d. A ruptured papillary muscle and severe MR
e. A large pulmonary embolism with RV enlargement

13. Patients with this finding on echocardiography are also likely to have:

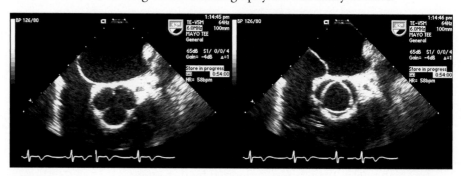

a. A VSD
b. Anomalous pulmonary venous drainage of the right upper pulmonary vein
c. A PFO and a higher risk of stroke
d. An ASD
e. Patent ductus arteriosus

14. The diastolic echocardiographic frame was obtained, and is most consistent with:

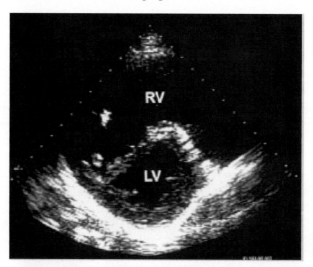

a. Right-sided pressure overload
b. Cleft mitral valve
c. VSD
d. ASD
e. Septal wall infarction

15. A 70-year-old man comes to your practice for evaluation of recurrent chest pain. He is very active, walks 2 miles a day, but has noticed early chest pain within 6 minutes, which he is able to "walk through." He stopped smoking 10 years ago after a 100-pack-year history of cigarettes. His family history cannot be elicited because he was adopted. He does not have HTN, and his cholesterol level is increased at 230 mg/dL (LDL, 140 mg/dL).

You perform a stress test, in which the patient achieves 130% of his predicted functional aerobic capacity. The test was stopped because of 3 mm of ST-segment depression at peak exercise. The patient did notice angina at approximately 4 minutes into the test; however, the symptoms subsided with continued exercise. His peak HR was 105 bpm and his BP response was normal. The ST-segment depression started in the inferior and lateral leads at 2.5 minutes into the exercise.

According to your epidemiologic data, the pretest likelihood of disease in men of this age with angina is approximately 95%. Assuming a test sensitivity of 70% and a test specificity of 50%, you conclude, with a certainty level of 90% or more, that:

a. A negative test would have been helpful to rule out CAD

b. The chance that the patient has no disease if the test would have been negative is approximately 20%

c. There is a greater chance of a false-positive than false-negative test in this patient

d. The patient should have been sent directly for coronary angiography

e. A positive test is useful to confirm CAD

16. Which of the following conditions are **not** typically associated with the lesion found on TTE?

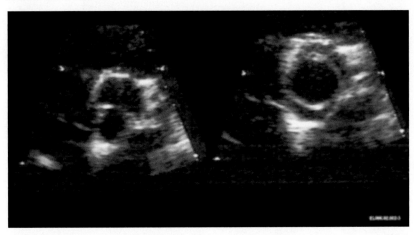

a. Coarctation of the aorta

b. AS

c. Patent ductus arteriosus

d. Thoracic aortic dissection

e. All of the above are associated

17. A 50-year-old woman has left shoulder discomfort that she notices when she climbs stairs, walks uphill, or becomes upset with her children. The discomfort generally resolves within one or two minutes after she stops the activity. Her resting ECG showed nonspecific ST- and T-wave abnormalities, with less than 1 mm of ST-segment depression. The patient had a TMET and exercised for 6 minutes on a Bruce protocol to a HR of 130 bpm and a BP of 155/70 mmHg. She stopped because of severe chest heaviness and left shoulder pain. The exercise ECG did not show any ST-segment depression.

Which of the following statements is **correct** about this patient's Duke treadmill score?

a. It is not clinically meaningful because the treadmill score applies only to patients with normal resting ECGs

b. It is not clinically meaningful because the treadmill score applies only to men

c. It is calculated as −2 and places the patient at intermediate risk for subsequent cardiac event

d. It is calculated as +2 and places the patient at low-to-intermediate risk for subsequent cardiac events

e. It is calculated as +6 and places the patient at low risk for subsequent cardiac events

18. Calculate the MVA.

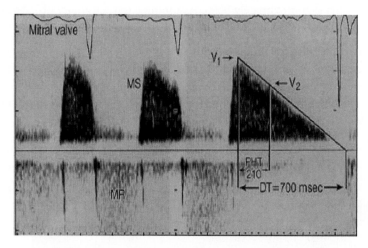

   a. 1.1 cm²
   b. 2.0 cm²
   c. 1.5 cm²
   d. 0.5 cm²
   e. Cannot calculate with information available

19. A patient with which of the following pacing devices can be safely placed in an MRI scanner?

   a. DDD, not pacemaker-dependent
   b. VVI, not pacemaker-dependent
   c. ICD
   d. None of the above
   e. All of the above

20. A 42-year-old woman presents for the evaluation of shortness of breath. What is the most likely diagnosis?

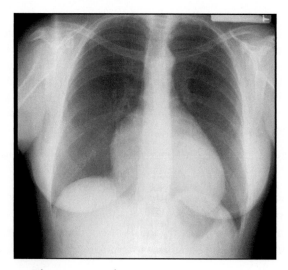

   a. Ebstein anomaly
   b. Primary pulmonary HTN
   c. Partial anomalous pulmonary veins (Scimitar syndrome)
   d. ASD
   e. No obvious cardiac disease on chest radiograph

21. Which statement about cardiac MRI is true?

    a. Prosthetic heart valves heat excessively from radiofrequency exposure during MRI
    b. Prosthetic valves cause image artifact that prevents adequate visualization of most other cardiac structures
    c. Placed in the wrong position, ECG electrodes often burn the patient's skin during MRI scanning
    d. Pacemaker wires may heat excessively in an MRI scanner
    e. MRI visualizes coronary calcium well

22. A 72-year-old female patient is referred to you for the evaluation of exertional chest pain. She is an ex-smoker. You refer her for an exercise sestamibi MPI test. She exercises for 3 minutes on the Bruce protocol before stopping because of chest pain. Her HR increased from 56 bpm at rest to 94 bpm at peak exercise. Her ECG is nondiagnostic secondary to resting ST depression. Representative stress (*left*) and rest (*right*) images on short-axis (*upper*), vertical long axis (*middle*), and horizontal long axis (*lower*) views are shown below.

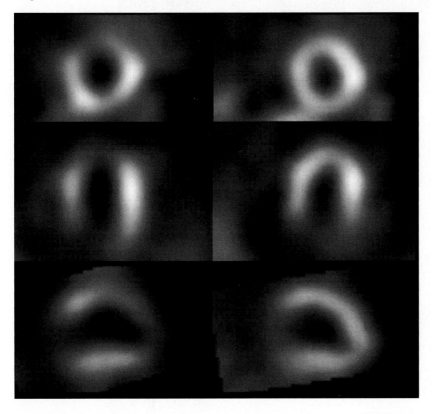

Which of the following conclusions are correct?

    a. Coronary angiography will likely indicate a high grade stenosis of the LAD
    b. Coronary angiography will likely show occlusion of the LAD
    c. Findings are most consistent with breast artifact
    d. Technically, the study is inadequate, as the patient did not reach an adequate HR

23. Which stress test variable is associated with the **worst** prognosis in patients after AMI?

    a. Inability to exercise
    b. ST segment depression in the inferior leads in patients with anterior infarction
    c. A hypertensive response to exercise
    d. Pseudonormalization of T waves in the infarct leads
    e. Delayed HR recovery ratio (persistently elevated HR in the recovery period)

24. Calculate the maximal instantaneous LVOT gradient.

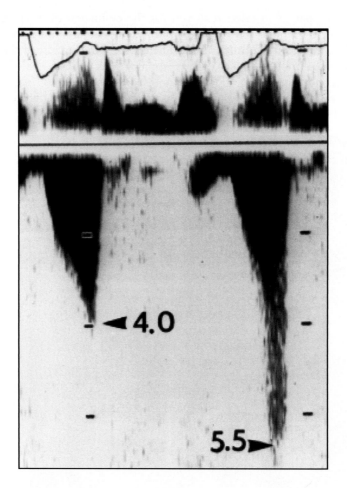

    a. 16 mmHg
    b. 31 mmHg
    c. 64 mmHg
    d. 121 mmHg
    e. 22 mmHg

25. Which of the following mitral annular velocities suggests constrictive pericarditis?

    a. 5 cm/sec
    b. 7 cm/sec
    c. 15 cm/sec
    d. 50 cm/sec
    e. 1 m/sec

26. Which of the following is true concerning the assessment of perioperative risk with noninvasive stress imaging in patients undergoing noncardiac surgery?

    a. Percutaneous intervention reduces perioperative risk of MI in patients with a high risk dobutamine stress echocardiogram
    b. SPECT MPI identifies the need for cardiac treatment in high-risk patients
    c. Percutaneous revascularization has been shown to reduce risk of perioperative death in patients with high-risk myocardial perfusion stress imaging
    d. Results of preoperative stress MPI have not been found to be associated with outcomes in the perioperative period
    e. All patients undergoing noncardiac surgery should receive beta blockers regardless and so should not undergo preoperative stress imaging

27. All the following factors would predispose a 63-year-old male patient undergoing coronary angiography to contrast-induced nephropathy **except:**

    a. Use of low osmolar iodinated contrast agents
    b. CHF
    c. DM
    d. Chronic kidney disease
    e. Multiple myeloma

28. A 65-year-old female presents for evaluation of DOE. She has NYHA class II functional limitation. As part of the evaluation a TTE is obtained. This shows the LV EF = 55% and the following data:

    ■ LVOT diameter 2.0 cm
    ■ Mitral annulus diameter 4.0 cm
    ■ LVOT TVI (pulsed wave Doppler) 20 cm
    ■ Peak aortic velocity (continuous wave Doppler) 1.2 m/sec
    ■ Mitral valve TVI (pulsed wave Doppler) 10 cm

    Based on these facts, you would recommend:

    a. Mitral repair or replacement
    b. Aortic valve repair
    c. AVR
    d. ACE inhibition
    e. Reassurance and serial follow-up

29. Based on the following echocardiographic data, which of the following physical examination findings should you expect?

    ■ LVOT diameter 2.0 cm
    ■ LVOT TVI (pulsed wave Doppler) 30 cm
    ■ Mitral annulus diameter 4.0 cm

29. (*continued*)

- Peak LVOT velocity (pulsed wave Doppler) 1.5 m/sec
- EF 60%
- Peak aortic velocity (continuous wave Doppler) 2.5 m/sec
- Mitral valve TVI (pulsed wave Doppler) 5 cm

a. Absent A2
b. Opening snap
c. Diastolic decrescendo murmur
d. Large V wave
e. Low pulse pressure after PVC

30. Which of the following is **not** an appropriate indication for the use of stress MPI as the initial test in patients with chest pain?

a. Ventricular paced rhythm
b. Rest ECG ST-segment depression greater than 1 mm
c. Female sex
d. LBBB
e. Prior percutaneous or surgical coronary revascularization

31. A 65-year-old woman presents with new onset dyspnea for an echocardiogram. She has a history of a mitral prosthetic valve placed 7 years ago for rheumatic valve stenosis. A routine study six months ago was unremarkable. Which of the following new medications likely explains what has happened?

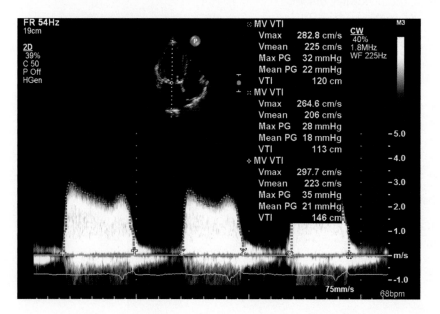

a. Oral ciprofloxacin antibiotic for a lower urinary tract infection
b. Herbal supplementation started to reduce bone loss
c. Ibuprofen for back pain
d. Iodinated contrast for a CT scan
e. Tylenol for headache

32. Each of the following is an appropriate indication for the use of either stress MPI or stress echocardiography as the initial test in patients with chest pain **except:**

   a. Rest ECG ST-segment depression greater than 1 mm
   b. Pre-excitation on the rest ECG
   c. Previous revascularization with PTCA or surgery
   d. Inability to exercise
   e. LBBB

33. For which of the following is TEE **least** often necessary?

   a. Degree of prosthetic MR
   b. Diagnosis of prosthetic valve endocarditis
   c. Differentiation of perivalvular from transvalvular regurgitation
   d. Degree of prosthetic AR
   e. Measurement of tilting-disk opening angle

34. Which of the following modalities are reasonable methods of assessing LV EF in a patient with AF?

   a. First-pass radionuclide angiography
   b. Cardiac MR
   c. Left ventriculography
   d. Cardiac CT
   e. MUGA

35. Which of the following is **not** an important factor in the selection of pharmacologic stress agent (adenosine or dobutamine)?

   a. Ventricular paced rhythm
   b. Chronic theophylline therapy
   c. Asthma
   d. Second-degree AV block
   e. Left axis deviation

36. A 38-year-old woman is referred for the evaluation of new onset systemic HTN. Her renal artery angiogram is shown here.

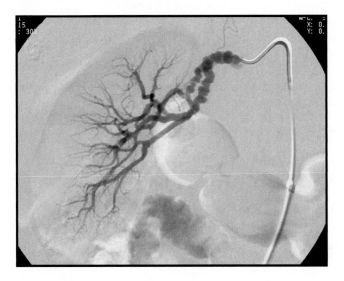

36. (*continued*)

Which of the following statements is true?

a. Percutaneous renal artery intervention has little potential for cure of HTN
b. The identification of this process should prompt use of aspirin, beta blockers, and aggressive treatment with HMG-CoA reductase inhibitors
c. Coronary angiography is indicated in the absence of symptoms due to the high prevalence of concomitant coronary disease
d. Unlike in children, this process is more common in women than in men
e. HTN due to unilateral disease is mediated through a renin-independent mechanism

37. A 50-year-old patient is referred to your practice for a general cardiac evaluation. He does not complain of any angina; however, he is physically inactive and deconditioned. His cardiac risk factors include a strong family history of CAD at younger than 60 years, he is a current smoker at a low level (5 cigarettes a day), he has stage I HTN, and his LDL is 160 mg/dL. You elect to perform a stress test in which the patient achieves 4.5 minutes on a Bruce protocol (approximately 60% of his predicted functional aerobic capacity). The peak HR increases to 110 bpm, and there is a hypertensive BP response of 220/100 mmHg. The patient does not experience angina; however, the test was stopped because of general fatigue and DOE. The ECG tracings indicate no evidence of ischemia.

In your experience, the ECG stress test has a sensitivity of 70% and a specificity of 50% for hemodynamically significant CAD. You will accept a 90% level of certainty of the presence or absence of disease. You also assume a likelihood of 50% that the patient has significant CAD (pretest probability).

You can thus conclude:

a. Given the current sensitivity and specificity, a negative test result will confirm the absence of disease
b. There is a greater probability of a false-negative than a false-positive result in the patient
c. Increasing the test specificity to 90% would reduce the risk of a false-positive result
d. There are more false-positive than true-negative results
e. Increasing the specificity to 90% would markedly reduce the probability of a true-negative test

38. The physiologic significance of a coronary artery lesion can be assessed in the cardiac catheterization laboratory by:

a. Quantitative coronary angiography
b. IVUS
c. Coronary flow reserve to intracoronary adenosine
d. Angioscopy
e. Response to IV methergine

39. A 66-year-old woman with a history of hyperlipidemia and diabetes presents for the evaluation of dyspnea. Her HR is 66 bpm and her systolic BP is 214/90 mmHg. Her

LV size on TTE is normal. Her LV EF is 59%. This is her mitral inflow pattern:

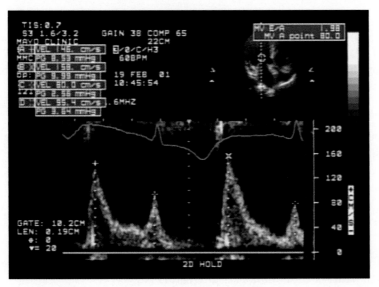

Which is the finding most consistent with the echocardiogram?

a. AF
b. Normal diastolic function
c. Third heart sound on auscultation
d. Fourth heart sound on auscultation
e. Significant AS

40. Which of the following statements is true concerning SPECT MPI?

a. A stress perfusion defect reflects a focal stenosis rather than diffuse atherosclerosis
b. A mild perfusion defect on a SPECT myocardial perfusion study denotes an increased risk for future cardiac mortality
c. SPECT MPI has been shown in *women* to have incremental prognostic value over clinical and exercise variables
d. The occurrence of post stress dilation of the LV denotes multivessel coronary disease, even if the perfusion defect is localized only to one coronary distribution
e. Adenosine stress is preferred in women undergoing SPECT MPI to reduce the incidence of breast artifacts observed with exercise stress SPECT

41. A 68-year-old male presents for the evaluation of NYHA class III exertional dyspnea with progressive fatigue and edema. His past history is significant for a two vessel CABG 10 years ago. He has not had recurrence of his angina symptoms. He also has longstanding rheumatoid arthritis with a past history of "rheumatoid lung." His current medications include: furosemide 60 mg BID, metoprolol 25 mg BID, potassium 20 mEq daily, and hydrochloroquine 200 mg once daily.

On physical examination his BP is 97/70 mmHg, pulse of 90 bpm, JVP elevated to 20 cm of water with rapid descents. He has a regular heart rhythm with normal S1 and S2, with a grade 1/6 SEM at the LSB that peaked early in systole. No diastolic sounds. The abdomen was markedly distended with shifting dullness and a fluid wave. The lower extremities showed 2–3+ pitting edema below the knees and normal pulses.

Chest X-ray revealed bilateral pleural effusions and normal heart size. The ECG showed sinus rhythm with occasional premature atrial contractions and nonspecific

41. (continued)

ST-T wave changes. His Hgb was 11.5 g/dL, WBC 6.4 × 10³/mm³, and platelet count 255,000. Sodium was 135 mg/dL, potassium 3.8 mg/dL, and creatinine was 1.8 mg/dL. An adenosine sestamibi scan revealed a first pass EF of 55% with no evidence of infarction or ischemia. The ECG obtained during the pharmacologic stress test was negative for ischemia.

Which of the following best confirms the diagnosis in this patient?

a. Echocardiography demonstrating markedly enhanced RV filling and decreased LV filling with inspiration
b. CT revealing pericardial thickening
c. Elevated erythrocyte sedimentation rate
d. Chest X-ray demonstrating pericardial calcification
e. Repeat physical examination specifically looking for pulsus paradoxus

42. Which of the following echocardiographic parameters does **not** predict adverse outcomes in patients with pulmonary arterial HTN?

a. Presence of a pericardial effusion
b. An elevated RV index of myocardial performance or Tei index
c. IVC dilatation
d. Diastolic septal shift
e. Maximum TR velocity

43. Which one of the following heart valves is considered more ferromagnetic than the others and therefore presents a hypothetical risk of dislocation or heating during MRI scanning of the heart in a patient with suspected valve dehiscence?

a. Starr-Edwards pre-6000 series (caged ball)
b. St. Jude (bileaflet valve)
c. Bjork-Shiley (tilting disk valve)
d. Medtronic-Hall (tilting disk valve)
e. Porcine bioprosthesis

44. A patient is referred to your practice for review of a TMET. On review of the resting exercise, you notice that LV hypertrophy by voltage criteria is present. You then evaluate the stress ECG that has been performed.

Which of the following statements is **not** correct?

a. The stress ECG is positive for ischemia if 2 mm or more of horizontal or downsloping ST-segment depression is present at 0.08 sec after the J point
b. The stress ECG is positive for ischemia if 1 to 2 mm of additional horizontal or downsloping ST-segment depression is present 0.08 sec after the J point
c. The stress ECG is negative for ischemia if less than 1 mm of additional ST-segment depression is noted
d. The stress ECG is negative for ischemia if there is pseudonormalization of an inverted T wave which occurs without ST-segment depression
e. The stress ECG is nondiagnostic for ischemia if 1 mm or more of ST-segment elevation occurs in a lead in which there are preexisting pathologic Q waves present

45. The most important cardiac properties to determine when assessing LV diastolic function are:

    a. LV contractility and LV relaxation
    b. LV and LA compliance
    c. LV relaxation and LA compliance
    d. LV compliance and LV viscoelastic properties
    e. LV contractility and LA compliance

46. The following end diastolic frame was obtained in a 55-year-old patient undergoing a TTE for the evaluation of dyspnea. What is the structure most likely indicated with the asterisk?

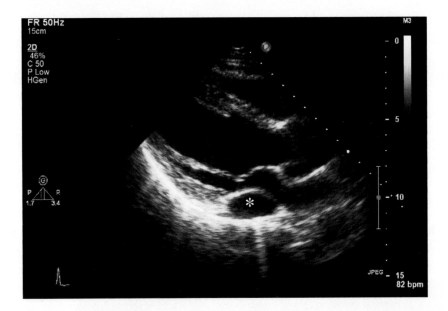

    a. Left atrial appendage
    b. Descending thoracic aorta
    c. Pericardial cyst
    d. CS
    e. Hiatal hernia

47. Concerning the measurement of LV index of myocardial performance by TTE, all of the following are true **except:**

    a. LV index of myocardial performance measurement is relatively independent of systemic BP
    b. LV index of myocardial performance provides a composite measurement of systolic and diastolic function
    c. LV index of myocardial performance measurement requires an adequate signal of MR
    d. LV ejection time is inversely proportional to the severity of systolic function
    e. LV index of myocardial performance measurement is independent of the severity of MR

48. Based on the pretest probability of CAD, noninvasive stress imaging is best indicated for the diagnosis of obstructive CAD in which patient?

    a. A 45-year-old man with typical angina and a LBBB on ECG
    b. A 50-year-old asymptomatic woman with an LDL of 140 mg/dL on digoxin
    c. A 45-year-old woman with atypical anginal chest pain and a normal resting ECG
    d. A 30-year-old woman with typical angina and 1 mm resting lateral ST segment depression
    e. A 75-year-old woman with typical angina and a pacemaker

49. Concerning agents used in stress imaging, which of the following is **false**?

    a. Unlike chest pain, ECG changes occurring with adenosine are highly suggestive of coronary disease
    b. Dobutamine stress echocardiography is indicated in patients with LBBB due to the frequency of false positive septal and apical wall motion abnormalities seen with exercise stress echocardiography
    c. Adenosine is contraindicated in patients with heart block or asthma
    d. AF more commonly complicates dobutamine stress rather than exercise or adenosine
    e. Adenosine is the preferred pharmacologic stress agent in a patient with VT

50. The following Doppler profile obtained from the descending thoracic aorta on TTE imaging demonstrates which of the following?

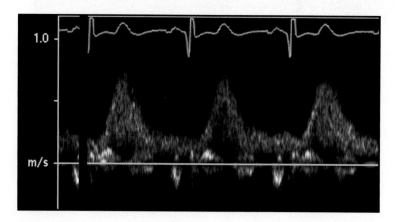

    a. Normal aortic profile
    b. Aortic valve regurgitation
    c. Coarctation of the aorta
    d. AS
    e. Aortic aneurysm

51. A 54-year-old male patient with NYHA class III heart failure on metoprolol and lisinopril undergoes an adenosine sestamibi. Representative stress (*left*) and rest (*right*) images on short-axis (upper), vertical long-axis (*middle*), and horizontal long-axis (*lower*) views are shown below.

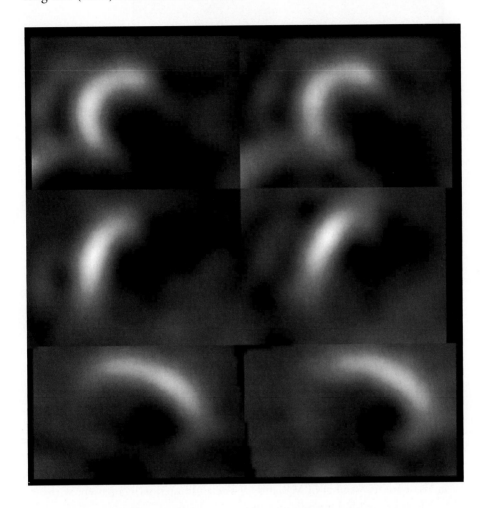

Which of the following is **false?**

a. Images suggest prior MI with little if any ischemia

b. Delayed images at 24 hours will help in the assessment of myocardial viability

c. An infarct size quantitated at 47% of the myocardium would be in keeping with the a calculated LV EF of 33%

d. Gated SPECT images would likely demonstrate inferior wall akinesis

e. Adenosine is not contraindicated in patients on beta blockers

52. A 32-year-old woman presents for the evaluation of exertional dyspnea. The findings on this chest radiograph would be most consistent with which of the following?

52. (continued)

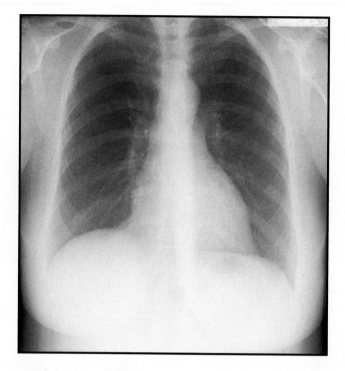

a. Ebstein anomaly
b. Idiopathic dilated cardiomyopathy
c. Pulmonary arterial HTN
d. Left atrial myxoma
e. Right phrenic nerve paralysis

53. Which of the following is **not** an indication for performing a TTE in a patient with MR?

a. Baseline assessment of MR and LV size and function in a patient with a newly documented holosystolic murmur
b. One-year follow-up of LV status in a patient with moderate MR who is now short of breath
c. One-year follow-up in a patient with mild MR, normal LV size and function, and no clinical change
d. One-year follow-up of LV status in a patient with asymptomatic severe MR
e. Four-month follow-up to assess cardiac status in a patient with MR and a change in symptoms

54. You are asked to evaluate a 78-year-old woman admitted from the ED to the ICU with hypoxia and hypotension whose BP has not responded to an IV infusion of dopamine. 12-lead ECG shows sinus tachycardia with 1 mm anterolateral ST segment depression. The chest X-ray is shown on the next page:

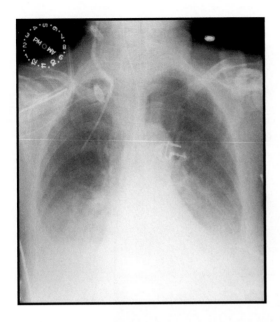

Which is the next best step?

a. Start IV vasopressin or norepinephrine for presumed septic shock in the setting of ARDS

b. Insert a PA (Swan-Ganz) catheter to help guide medical management

c. Insert an aortic balloon pump and consider emergent coronary angiography

d. Obtain an emergent TTE to assess LV systolic function

e. Obtain a CT scan of the chest

55. Which of the following is **not** a high-risk finding in stress MPI?

a. LV cavity dilatation following stress

b. An increase in thallium lung uptake with stress

c. A focal mild to moderate fixed defect in the apex

d. A defect size greater than 25% of the LV myocardium

e. A Duke treadmill score of −16 with a mild anterior perfusion defect with stress

56. Which of the following statements about exercise is **false**?

a. The inability to perform an exercise test is a bad prognostic sign

b. Exercise is the stress technique preferred for use with imaging of myocardial perfusion

c. The ability to complete four METS of exercise predicts a low-risk of cardiac events during most non-cardiac surgical procedures

d. Functional (exercise) capacity does not provide any prognostic information when the results of exercise MPI are taken into account

e. The achievement of 85% of age-predicted maximal HR is not a preferred end-point for exercise testing

57. This Doppler signal was obtained from a pulmonary vein in a 55-year-old patient undergoing TTE:

57. (*continued*)

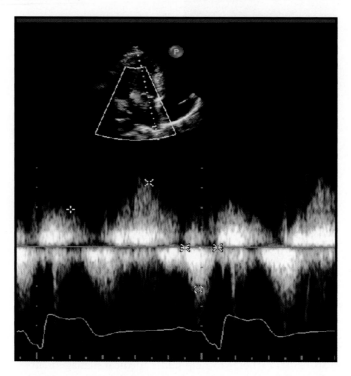

Which of the following findings is most likely to be present in this patient?

a. AF
b. Elevation in mean left atrial pressure
c. Primary pulmonary HTN
d. Pulmonary vein stenosis
e. Normal exercise capacity

58. An 80-year-old woman with chest pain and dyspnea is noted on TTE to have an EF of 25% and restricted aortic valve leaflet motion. Here are the Doppler profiles from her LVOT [pulse wave (*left*) and continuous wave (*right*)]. Assume a normal sized LVOT diameter.

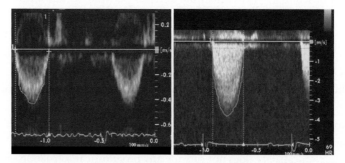

Concerning a potential diagnosis of AS, what should be the best next step?

a. Refer for dobutamine stress echocardiography to separate significant AS from apparent valvular stenosis due to low output
b. Refer for a TEE
c. Consult a cardiac surgeon
d. Refer for left heart hemodynamic catheterization
e. Likely AS, but not severe; plan on medical management and further investigation of symptoms

59. A 65-year-old man undergoes stress echocardiography. He has several CV risk factors, a history of PAF, and atypical chest pain. His medications are digoxin, aspirin, and niacin.

He exercises 8 minutes on the Bruce protocol, and his HR increases from 72 to 126 bpm and BP increases from 120/70 to 152/60 mmHg. He stops because of fatigue and has no chest pain. The exercise ECG is nondiagnostic because of the digoxin effect.

The echocardiographic images were interpreted as follows:

Wall segment	Rest	Stress
Anterior	Normal	Hypokinetic
Septum	Normal	No change
Lateral	Normal	Hyperdynamic
Inferior	Hypokinetic	Hypokinetic
LV EF	55%	55%

The most likely coronary artery anatomy at angiography is which of the following?

a. LAD, occluded; RCA, occluded
b. LAD, 80% stenosis; RCA, 80% stenosis
c. LAD, occluded; RCA, 80% stenosis
d. LAD, 80% stenosis; RCA, occluded
e. LCFX occluded

60. A 65-year-old woman with iron deficiency anemia (Hgb, 10.2 g/dL) complains of fatigue. She has no cardiac symptoms. She has a grade III/VI SEM. A TTE shows normal LV size and function and an EF of 70%. The aortic valve is calcified and there is trivial AR.

The following hemodynamic data was obtained:

- HR: 70 bpm
- BP: 140/90 mmHg
- LVOT diameter: 2.2 cm
- LVOT velocity: 1.4 m/sec
- LVOT TVI: 30 cm
- Aortic velocity: 3.5 m/sec
- Aortic TVI: 75 cm
- TR velocity: 2.4 m/sec

Your next recommendation to the patient is which of the following?

a. Consultation with a cardiac surgeon
b. Left and right heart catheterization, with coronary angiography
c. Repeat echocardiography in 6 to 12 months
d. Exercise thallium stress test
e. Tranesophageal echocardiogram

61. The following statements regarding technetium are correct **except:**

a. Technetium has a higher energy than thallium
b. Given the higher energy profile relative to thallium, technetium poses a higher radiation risk to the patient at an equivalent dose to thallium
c. Technetium is generated in a cyclotron
d. The half-life of technetium is longer than that of thallium
e. Technetium has a less-uniform energy profile than thallium

62. Which of the following statements regarding radionuclide angiography is correct?

   a. Diastolic function can not be assessed since ECG gating is required
   b. Heparin can interfere with radionuclide imaging
   c. Pharmacological stress testing combined with radionuclide angiography is preferred in patients with LBBB over MPI
   d. The presence of a pacemaker precludes the use of radionuclide angiography
   e. Exercise radionuclide angiography presents all coronary artery territories equally

63. A 45-year-old female (156 cm, 82 kg) undergoes radionuclide testing. She reports chest pain lasting for 45 to 80 min, constant, non-radiating. She is uncertain about the relationship of her symptoms to exercise but has experienced episodes at rest.

   Which of the following is correct?

   a. A positive MPI stress test would not establish the diagnosis of CAD
   b. Thallium is preferred over technetium because of its superior imaging characteristics
   c. A pharmacological MPI stress test versus an exercise MPI stress test would make the test more specific
   d. A test should be terminated when the patient has exercised to 85% of her maximal predicted HR
   e. The test should be terminated if the ECG shows ≥ 2 mm ST depression in the absence of symptoms

64. A 78-year-old asymptomatic man presents for follow-up 4 years following CABG. As part of his evaluation he underwent TTE:

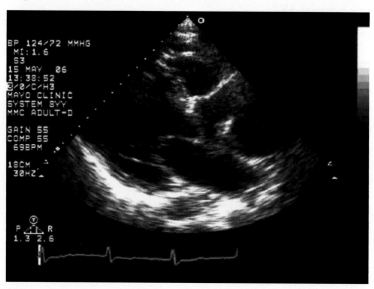

   All of the following factors are associated with the finding **except:**

   a. Associated AVR at the time of CABG
   b. Systemic HTN
   c. Aortic atherosclerosis
   d. The use of off-pump bypass grafting

65. Which of the following statements regarding pharmacological stress testing is true?

    a. Dipyridamole causes more side effects in patients than adenosine

    b. High level dobutamine radionuclide angiography (20–40 mcg/kg/min) is useful to assess viability in patients with known LV dysfunction

    c. Side effects caused by adenosine, but not dipyridamole, and can be reversed with theophylline

    d. Adenosine results in a larger increase of blood flow than dipyridamole or dobutamine

    e. Dobutamine radionuclide angiography is useful to assess CAD in patients with LBBB

66. A 45-year-old man is referred for a TTE for the evaluation of hemoptysis, dyspnea, and chest pain.

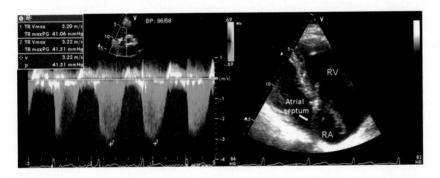

Which of the following are correct?

    a. The absence of tachycardia implies a good prognosis

    b. Management options include calling a surgeon

    c. The findings of an elevated peak TR regurgitant velocity are likely unrelated to the findings on the displayed 2D images

    d. Anticoagulation is contraindicated

    e. Elevations in cardiac biomarkers, such as troponin, have little prognostic information in this case

67. A 65-year-old male patient with HTN and diabetes is referred to your practice for preoperative assessment of cardiac risk prior to peripheral vascular surgery. You elect to perform an adenosine sestamibi. The patient does not indicate any symptoms. The BP drops by 20 mmHg from baseline but returns to normal within 1 min after the cessation of the adenosine infusion. Representative stress (*left*) and rest (*right*) images on planar projection (*upper*) and short-axis (*lower*) views are shown on the next page:

67. (*continued*)

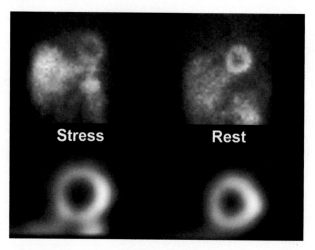

Which of the following statements is correct?

a. The drop in BP is clinically worrisome
b. The absence of symptoms is reassuring
c. The absence of markedly reversible defects is reassuring
d. The findings on imaging denote a high risk
e. A coronary angiogram would have better defined the functional significance of the coronary artery lesions

68. A patient with known idiopathic cardiomyopathy is referred to you for assessment of LV function. An echocardiogram and a radionuclide angiogram at rest had been performed as part of a study with an LV EF by echo of 17% and by radionuclide angiography of 20%. A year later, a repeat echocardiogram and radionuclide angiogram on follow-up exam are done. An echocardiographic LV EF of 25% is now reported and a radionuclide angiogram LV EF of 15%. You are asked to comment on these findings.

Which of the following conclusions is correct?

a. There is significant improvement in his LV function
b. The LV function is about the same
c. Further deterioration of his LV function has occurred
d. The presence of regional wall motion abnormalities would refute the diagnosis of idiopathic dilated cardiomyopathy
e. Additional parameters would not be helpful in further risk stratification

69. A 52-year-old patient (168 cm, 131 kg) is referred with symptoms of Class III dyspnea. The patient is a smoker, sedentary, and has significant COPD and hyperlipidemia. You want to assess the LV function to distinguish between a possible respiratory or cardiac reason for his dyspnea.

Which of the following statements is **not** correct in this setting?

a. TTE will probably yield unsatisfactory images
b. First-pass sestamibi is helpful, especially if 30 mCi are used to improve photon statistics
c. The heart volumes measured and images by radionuclide angiography are affected by body habitus and are likely to be smaller than in a normal-weight person
d. Radionuclide angiography is challenging because of the patient's COPD
e. EBCT would be the imaging modality of choice in this patient

70. Select the best statement regarding radionuclide angiography.

    a. Exercise radionuclide angiography is performed with a camera in the antero-posterior or lateral position

    b. The LAO position is always at 45 degrees, similar to coronary angiography

    c. Determination of EF by radionuclide angiography requires a regular rhythm and is best with a low-energy all-purpose collimator

    d. There is little inter-individual variation in the determination of ventricular volumes

    e. Determination of EF by radionuclide angiography is very discriminate in hyperdynamic ventricles

71. All of the following conditions can produce an artifactual defect in the inferior segments on MPI **except:**

    a. Partial volume effect

    b. Diaphragmatic attenuation

    c. Motion artifact

    d. Obesity

    e. Adjacent tissue uptake (liver/loop of bowel)

72. MRI of the heart is **contraindicated** in which of the following clinical situations?

    a. Presence of a Bjork-Shiley mitral valve prosthesis

    b. Presence of a Carpentier-Edwards mitral valve prosthesis

    c. Intracoronary stent

    d. Cerebral aneurysm

    e. AV sequential pacemaker

73. Which of the following radiopharmaceuticals is used for PET scanning and does **not** require the presence of an on-site or nearby cyclotron?

    a. Nitrogen-13 ammonia

    b. Oxygen-15 water

    c. Rubidium-82

    d. ^{18}F FDG

74. A 57-year-old woman presents for the evaluation of insidious exertional dyspnea. Here is a clip from her TEE:

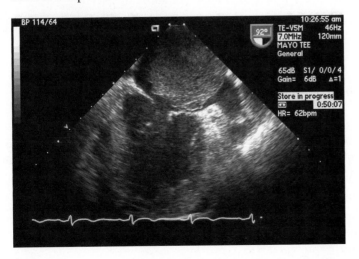

74. (*continued*)

Which of the following is most likely?

a. Myxoma
b. Papillary fibroelastoma
c. Pericardial cyst
d. Hypernephroma
e. Thrombus

75. Which of the following is true when MPI using thallium-201 is compared with PET?

a. They provide images of similar quality in all patients
b. They provide for quantification of absolute regional myocardial blood flow
c. They have similar applicability in defining myocardial viability
d. Imaging can be done without the need for an on-site cyclotron
e. Unlike Tc-99 m sestamibi, thallium provides equivalent imaging quality to PET in obese patients

76. A 75-year-old male smoker with long-standing HTN is brought to the ED after a motor vehicle accident. There is concern for cervical spine trauma, and he is in a cervical collar. He has abdominal pain and nausea. Although his oxygenation is adequate, the patient is confused and thrashing about. Sedation is necessary, an orotracheal tube is inserted for airway protection, and the patient is mechanically ventilated.

The BP is 190/100 mmHg, the HR is 95 bpm, and the pulse is bounding in the right brachial artery but less prominent in the left brachial artery. His complexion is ruddy, but the femoral and peripheral pulses are not palpable and the extremities are cool.

A portable chest radiograph shows hyperlucent lung fields that are generally clear and proper placement of the orotracheal tube. Heart sounds are soft and best appreciated in the subxiphoid area. There are no murmurs. An ECG shows LV hypertrophy and diffuse T-wave inversion but no ST-segment elevation. Baseline serum chemistry values are normal. He has no allergies.

Which imaging modality is best to evaluate for aortic dissection?

a. A two-dimensional TTE
b. A two-dimensional TEE
c. MRI of the thorax and abdomen
d. CT examination of the chest and abdomen with and without contrast
e. Percutaneous aortography

77. Some metallic medical devices may dislocate or heat in the magnetic field of MRI. Which of the following metallic devices is generally regarded as a **contraindication** to MRI scanning of the heart?

a. Prosthetic hip
b. St. Jude heart valve
c. Cerebral aneurysm clip
d. Ureteric stent
e. Dental fillings

78. A coronary calcification score of 100 Hounsfield units on an Imatron-CT scan in an asymptomatic 50-year-old man indicates all of the following **except:**

   a. The calcification is likely located in the proximal coronary arteries
   b. The patient is in the 75th percentile (more calcium than 75% of men his age) for coronary calcification
   c. Occlusion of at least one coronary artery is likely
   d. Risk factor modification might slow progression of coronary calcification
   e. There is no role for a stress imaging test based on these results

79. A patient with renal failure (creatinine, 3.4 mg/dL) and thrombocytopenia (platelet count, 35,000 mm^3) presents to you with a pericardial effusion. He is hemodynamically stable. You are concerned about a paracardiac malignancy and would like to characterize the pericardial effusion further.

   What would be the best method of evaluating this possibility?

   a. TEE
   b. EBCT
   c. MRI
   d. Pericardial tap
   e. TTE

80. A 45-year-old patient with diabetes who weighs 330 pounds and has an EF of 24% and known three-vessel CAD by coronary angiography presents to you complaining of shortness of breath despite intensive medical treatment. The cardiac surgeon is skeptical that LV function would improve after CABG because a non-exercise 24-hour thallium study showed predominantly fixed perfusion defects.

   Which of the following studies would you order to pursue the possibility of myocardial viability further?

   a. Low-dose dobutamine echocardiography
   b. PET with ^{18}F FDG
   c. PET with FDG and nitrogen-13-labeled ammonia
   d. PET with carbon-11-palmitate
   e. None of above; if 24-hour thallium imaging does not demonstrate myocardial viability, none of these tests are likely to be helpful

81. Adenosine PET with rubidium (^{82}Rb) would be a reasonable test in which of the following clinical situations?

   a. A fixed anterior wall defect on stress thallium imaging in a woman with silicone breast implants
   b. Normal results of adenosine thallium test in a patient with recurrent chest pain
   c. Normal results of exercise thallium test in a patient with recurrent chest pain
   d. LV dysfunction (EF, 25%) in a patient with suspected hibernating myocardium
   e. A 58-year-old obese woman with chest pain whose exercise capacity is limited by severe asthma

82. Which test is appropriate for assessing LV viability and the likelihood of functional recovery with revascularization in a patient with systolic ventricular dysfunction?

    a. Positron emission CT with ^{18}F FDG and nitrogen-13 labeled ammonia
    b. Rest, 24-hour thallium study
    c. Low-dose dobutamine echocardiography
    d. Cardiac MRI
    e. All of the above

83. You placed a metallic Palmaz-Schatz stent in the proximal LAD coronary artery in a patient one month ago. Now you are asked by a colleague in neurology whether the patient can undergo nonemergency MRI of the head, scheduled for today. You should answer:

    a. Only if the MRI scanning is an emergency procedure
    b. Ideally, never perform MRI for this patient
    c. Imaging can be done in 6 months, when the stent is completely endothelialized
    d. Yes, go ahead and image today
    e. Head MRI is safe, but thoracic MRI is contraindicated

84. Which of the following imaging methods has a clinically acceptable sensitivity in the diagnosis of proximal pulmonary emboli?

    a. CT
    b. Radionuclide angiography
    c. TEE
    d. Contrast TTE
    e. All of the above

85. Compared with EBCT, radioisotope perfusion-ventilation scanning performed for the diagnosis of pulmonary embolus:

    a. Has low specificity for pulmonary emboli
    b. Readily detects right heart thrombus
    c. Is more likely to be of intermediate probability in COPD
    d. Is hazardous in a patient with renal failure
    e. Should be avoided in patients with severe pulmonary HTN

86. A 45-year-old woman with ankle edema and clinical findings of right heart failure presents to you for the first time. She immigrated to the United States from Vietnam 10 years ago. Her medical history is unremarkable except for a family history of tuberculosis.

    The heart sounds are quiet, and the lungs are clear.

    Frontal chest radiography is normal. ECG shows low voltage in the limb leads but is otherwise unremarkable. A TTE is inconclusive because of poor acoustical windows.

    The single most useful test in this situation is:

    a. PET with ^{18}F FDG
    b. Cardiac MRI
    c. EBCT
    d. TEE
    e. Holter monitor

87. A 65-year-old man with a known ascending thoracic aortic aneurysm (5 cm) and a bicuspid aortic valve is being followed on a yearly basis by a referring physician. The most recent TTE shows an increase in the diameter of the aneurysm to 5.8 cm. The patient is referred to you for further evaluation. You want to confirm the results of the echocardiogram.

You should consider ordering:

   a. CT
   b. MRI with contrast (Magnevist)
   c. TEE
   d. Any of the above

88. A 33-year-old woman presents to your practice with recurrent chest pains. The episodes last several hours, are mostly constant, and there is no radiation of the pain. They occur with and without exercise. Risk factors in the patient include CAD in her father at the age of 78. She does not have HTN, does not smoke, has a normal lipid profile, and does not have DM.

   A stress test is performed. The patient exercised for 12 minutes on a Bruce protocol, achieving more than 100% of her predicted functional aerobic capacity at a peak HR of 156 bpm. She did not experience any angina or DOE. The ECG tracing shows 1 mm of horizontal ST-segment depression beginning at 4 minutes into the exercise and at a HR of 96 bpm. At peak exercise, the ST segments in leads V2-V6 are horizontally depressed 3 mm from the isoelectric line.

Which of the following statements is true?

   a. A positive test result is a good predictor of hemodynamically significant CAD in this patient
   b. There is a higher chance for a false-positive result than a true-positive result in this patient
   c. The test would be a good predictor of coronary disease if its specificity was 80%
   d. There is a higher chance for a false-negative result than a false-positive result in this patient
   e. For safety reasons, the test should have been stopped at 1 mm of ST-segment depression in the fourth minute of exercise

89. The following findings on stress ECG are considered nondiagnostic for MI **except:**

   a. >1 mm of ST-segment elevation in the presence of existing Q wave
   b. ≥2 mm of ST-segment depression in the presence of LV hypertrophy by Sokoloff (voltage) criteria
   c. ≥1 mm of ST-segment depression in leads V1–V3 in the presence of right bundle branch block
   d. ≥1 mm of ST-segment depression in the presence of digitalis
   e. ≥1 mm of ST-segment depression in the presence of Wolff-Parkinson-White syndrome

90. The following criteria are absolute indications for termination of an exercise test **except:**

   a. Moderate to severe angina
   b. Increase in nervous symptoms (ataxia, dizziness, near syncope)
   c. Cyanosis or pallor
   d. New chest pain
   e. Subject's desire to stop

91. A 60-year-old man is referred to your practice with a new weight loss. You diagnose a gastric ulcer on endoscopy, which persists despite adequate medical treatment. Gastric surgery is recommended. The patient also has a history of CAD, treated with CABG approximately 3 years ago. The patient still smokes, but he exercises on a daily basis, walking approximately 3 miles a day in a little under an hour. He denies any shortness of breath or angina.

Before approving him for operation, from a cardiac perspective you would recommend which of the following?

a. A symptom-limited exercise test
b. Resting echocardiography
c. An exercise thallium test
d. Sending patient directly to operation
e. Coronary angiography

92. On echocardiographic evaluation of an aortic Medtronic-Hall prosthesis, the following measurements were obtained:

- LVOT diameter 20 mm
- LVOT TVI 20 cm
- Prosthetic TVI 100 cm
- HR 80 bpm

The EOA is:

a. $0.4 \, cm^2$
b. $0.6 \, cm^2$
c. $0.8 \, cm^2$
d. $1 \, cm^2$
e. $2 \, cm^2$

Answers

1. Answer e.

The clip demonstrates a dilated left atrial appendage in the setting of a dilated LA, likely reflecting a chronic elevation in left atrial pressures.

2. Answer b.

For the diagnosis of obstructive CAD, stress perfusion imaging or stress echocardiography is preferred when the ECG cannot be interpreted, or when the patient cannot exercise. This patient's resting ECG shows greater than 1 mm ST depression. The stress ECG will be nondiagnostic in such cases, and greater than 1 mm resting ST depression is an ACC/AHA Guidelines class III indication for performing an exercise test without imaging for the diagnosis of obstructive CAD. Exercise capacity is a powerful predictor of both all-cause and cardiac mortality. It provides prognostic information that is incremental to imaging findings. Exercise is, therefore, always the preferred stress technique in conjunction with perfusion imaging in those who are able to exercise and who do not have LBBB or paced rhythm on their resting ECG.

3. Answer d.

Duke treadmill score = exercise time $-(5 \times$ ST deviation$) - (4 \times$ angina index$)$

The angina index is: no angina (0); angina during test (1); angina stopped test (2) eg, $7 - (5 \times 1) - (4 \times 2) = -6$

Patients with a low-risk Duke treadmill score (>4) have an annual mortality of less than 1%. Patients with an intermediate score have an annual cardiac mortality of between 1% and 3%, and patients with a high risk score (< -10) have an annual mortality of 3% or greater.

4. Answer b.

This question addresses the exercise tolerance of the patient, *not* the diagnosis of CAD, which has been established. Optimally, you would like to know whether the LBBB is new in onset, but this information is not available. Because the diagnosis has been established, you do not necessarily need to rely on the ECG information. Dobutamine echocardiography would be similar to an exercise thallium test, in that it would also be subject to false-positive regional wall motion abnormalities. An adenosine thallium test would aid in establishment of the diagnosis, but this is not the goal of the test. Coronary angiography does not assess the functional significance of a lesion. In this situation, assessment of the exercise tolerance and the hemodynamic factors (HR and BP response) provides valuable information to objectify the symptoms in this patient.

5. Answer d.

Scimitar syndrome is a rare congenital cardiac anomaly defined by an anomalous right pulmonary vein draining the right lung to the IVC, typically associated with a hypoplastic right lung. RV volume overload predisposes to RV dilation and atrial arrhythmias.

6. Answer c.

Adenosine is a vasodilator that increases coronary blood flow 3 to 5-fold independent of HR and BP at the standard infusion rate of 140 μg/kg/min. Up-titration of the infusion is therefore not required and may have significant adverse effects such as AV block and hypotension. The duration of the adenosine infusion is 6 minutes, with injection of the perfusion tracer at 3 minutes. Chest pain is reported frequently as a side effect and is not usually significant for ischemia. ECG changes with adenosine are infrequent but suggest underlying severe CAD.

7. Answer d.

The patient appears to be a reasonable candidate for bypass surgery: she is fairly young, has mild renal impairment, and good target vessels. An ICD should be deferred until three months post revascularization with reassessment of the clinical condition and LV systolic function. A PET rest-stress rubidium-82 study does allow an assessment of stress-induced ischemia and myocardial viability. However, a PET perfusion-metabolism (viability) study with FDG would be superior for detection viability but a PET viability study was not among the answer choices. In addition, because of unstable hemodynamics, a stress study should be avoided. Sestamibi does not have clinically significant redistribution and would underestimate the extent of myocardial viability. A resting thallium study with 24-hour views is the best option among the answer choices. Thallium undergoes a complex process of redistribution over time, allowing ischemic areas to normalize, and is suitable for the assessment of myocardial viability.

8. Answer a.

56%. Where LVEDD = LV end diastolic diameter, and LVESD = LV end systolic diameter, LV EF by M-mode is calculated by:

LV EF = [(LVEDD)^2 − (LVESD)^2]/(LVEDD)^2 × 100
Here LV EF = [(60)^2 − (40)^2]/(60)^2 × 100 = 56%

9. Answer d.

The echocardiogram clearly shows thickened and retracted tricuspid leaflets. Color images and physical exam were consistent with severe TR. The valve leaflet morphology suggests a drug related (ie, erogotamines or diet drugs, which usually affect left valves more than right valves) or a systemic illness such as hypereosinophillia or carcinoid. This illness seems to be targeting the right-sided valves; this is classically carcinoid syndrome and the diagnosis can be clinched by measuring urinary 5-HIAA.

10. Answer d.

The "biphasic" response to dobutamine during a stress echocardiogram refers to the improvement of function in an area of resting regional akinesis (essentially no wall motion at rest) at low dose dobutamine, followed by deterioration of function or ischemia in that same region at a higher rate pressure product, inferring that that area, if revascularized, should avoid an ischemic event in the future. A region of akinesis that remains akinetic infers infarction. A region of akinesis that improves at high dose infers recruitment of what functioning fibers remain, but not ischemia.

11. Answer a.

Pulmonary congestion correlates best with mean LA pressure. An elevation in LVEDP is frequently associated with an elevation in mean LA pressure, however would not be associated with pulmonary congestion in the absence of elevation in LA pressure.

12. Answer a.
Evident on the two-dimensional imaging is a subtle defect in the ventricular septum, made clear by the color flow imaging.

13. Answer c.
Approximately 20% of patients with atrial septal aneurysms have a PFO. Therefore, if one identifies an atrial septal aneurysm, it is important to carefully look for PFO, particularly if the patient has suffered a neurological/embolic event. This can be done transthoracically by detailed subcostal evaluation with color Doppler and contrast (agitated saline) injection. If clinically indicated, TEE can help to further evaluate the septum.

14. Answer d.
Diastolic septal flattening is suggestive of volume overload of the RV, such as is seen in severe TR or ASD. Systolic flattening is indicative of pressure overload on the RV, which is seen in significant pulmonary HTN. Systolic and diastolic flattening (flattening of the septum throughout the cardiac cycle) can be seen in the combined volume and pressure overload.

15. Answer d.
This patient probably should have been sent directly for coronary angiography. The fact that the patient is able to exercise after the initial onset of ischemia is not helpful diagnostically. The pretest likelihood of significant coronary disease of 95% makes the probability that no significant disease is present, even if there was a negative stress test (true negative ÷ true negative + false negative), extremely low (8%). The probability of disease even with a negative test is still 92%, indicating that a negative test would not be helpful in this case. One can easily determine that the incidence of disease in this patient group is the predominant factor in the diagnostic strategy. The high workload achieved indicates a good prognosis but not the absence of disease.

16. Answer e.
Bicuspid aortic valve is estimated to occur in 1% to 2% of the general population, making it the single most common congenital cardiac anomaly. Factors commonly associated with bicuspid aortic valve include coarctation of the aorta, AS, AR, patent ductus arteriosus, aortic dilatation, and risk of dissection.

17. Answer c.
The Duke treadmill score has been well validated in patients with nonspecific ST- and T-wave abnormalities and in women. In this case, it is calculated as 6 (minutes on the Bruce protocol) minus 4 times the angina score (which would be 2 in the case of limiting angina). Therefore, the Duke treadmill score is −2, and this places the patient at intermediate risk for subsequent cardiac events.

18. Answer a.
The MVA obtained by the pressure half-time method is MVA = 220/PHT. In this case, $220/210 = 1.1 \, cm^2$.

19. Answer d.
It is generally accepted that, ideally, no patient with a pacemaker or ICD should be placed in an MRI scanner.

20. Answer a.

Note the cardiac enlargement with a rounded contour of the cardiac silhouette, consistent with right chamber enlargement. Also note a relatively small aortic arch.

21. Answer d.

Prosthetic heart valves are not known to heat excessively during MRI. Although valves cause image artifact, it is generally localized around a valve, and the chambers of the heart and the ascending aorta can be readily seen. Although it is possible to burn a patient with an ECG electrode, this is rare. Pacemaker wires have been shown to heat during in vitro studies; because pacemaker generators are considered a contraindication to MRI, the clinical significance of this finding is unclear. Temporary pacemaker wires placed at cardiac operation should be removed before MRI is performed.

22. Answer a.

This study is markedly positive. Despite relatively normal perfusion at rest, following a low work rate, and at a low HR, there develops evidence of a large perfusion defect involving the apex, septum, and anterior and anterolateral segments with post stress dilatation. These findings suggest a high grade lesion in the LAD.

23. Answer a.

One of the strongest negative predictors in patients, including those post MI, is the inability to exercise. While a hypotensive response to exercise is a negative predictor, a hypertensive response has not consistently been shown to be negative.

24. Answer c.

The signal on the left is the true LVOT velocity. The signal on the right is contaminated by MR, which has a much higher velocity. Peak gradient is estimated using the formula $4V^2$.

- 1 m/sec—4 mmHg
- 2 m/sec—16 mmHg
- 3 m/sec—36 mmHg
- 4 m/sec—64 mmHg
- 5 m/sec—100 mmHg

25. Answer c.

An elevated/high normal velocity of the mitral annulus is typical for patients with constrictive pericarditis. Velocities greater than 20 cm/sec are not seen in adult patients.

26. Answer b.

In selected patients, preoperative stress testing provides prognostic information and helps risk-stratify patients; however, there is no data indicating that PCI reduces event rate perioperatively. While beta blockers have benefits for patients undergoing noncardiac surgery at medium to high risk for cardiac events, there is no role for indiscriminate use in all surgical patients as, in a low-risk cohort, adverse events may outweigh any benefits.

27. Answer a.

All the above are recognized factors that predispose to contrast-induced nephropathy. Other factors include contrast volume, hypotension, and volume depletion. Use of low osmolar iodinated contrast likely is associated with a reduction in the incidence of contrast nephropathy.

28. Answer a.

This patient has severe mitral valve regurgitation. Based on the echo data, we know that she does not have aortic valve stenosis as the peak velocity is only 1.2 m/sec. This equates to a peak AV gradient of less than 6 mmHg ($4 \times [1.2]^2 = 5.8$). You can calculate the effective SV across the LVOT and the effective mitral inflow SV:

$$SV_{LVOT} = Area_{LVOT} \times TVI_{LVOT} = 3.14 \times (2.0\,cm/2)^2 \times 20\,cm = 62.8\,cc$$
$$SV_{MV} = Area_{MV} \times TVI_{MV} = 3.14 \times (4.0\,cm/2)^2 \times 10\,cm = 125.6\,cc$$

(Remember, you measure diameters, but to calculate area you must convert that to a radius.) So, this means that there is more flow coming into the ventricle across the mitral valve than is leaving the ventricle through the LVOT. The extra mitral inflow is due to mitral valve regurgitation (flow is leaving the ventricle through both the LVOT and MR):

$$SV_{MV} = MR + SV_{LVOT}$$
$$MR\ volume = SV_{MV} - SV_{LVOT} = 125.6 - 62.8 = 62.8\,cc\ of\ MR$$

Therefore, this is severe regurgitation in a patient with dyspnea. Mitral valve operation should be considered.

29. Answer c.

From the data, you can calculate that the peak AV gradient is $4 \times (2.5)^2 = 25$ mmHg, so there is clearly not severe AS. Another clue to this is that the aortic valve dimensionless index $V_{LVOT}/V_{AV} = 1.5/2.5 > 0.5$. Severe AS is present if this ratio is less than 0.25. The next step is to calculate the stroke volume across the LVOT and across the mitral valve:

$$SV_{LVOT} = Area_{LVOT} \times TVI_{LVOT} = 3.14 \times (2.0\,cm/2)^2 \times 30\,cm = 94\,cc$$
$$SV_{MV} = Area_{MV} \times TVI_{MV} = 3.14 \times (4.0\,cm/2)^2 \times 5\,cm = 63\,cc$$

This means there is more flow going out of the LV across the LVOT than is coming in through the mitral valve. The only other way for blood to get into the ventricle would be aortic valve regurgitation:

$$SV_{MV} + AR = SV_{LVOT}$$
$$AR\ volume = 94 - 63 = 31\,cc\ (AR)$$

You would expect a murmur of AR on examination. Absent A2 would be found in severe AS, opening snap in MS, large v-wave in MR, and decreased pulse pressure after PVC in HCM.

30. Answer c.

Stress perfusion imaging is preferred when the ECG cannot be interpreted, the patient is unable to exercise, or the patient has already had revascularization. However, the exercise ECG remains a useful initial test in women. Many women have a low pretest likelihood and do not require further testing if the TMET results are negative. Although women are more likely to have "false-positive" TMET results because of their lower disease prevalence, this does not negate the value of a negative TMET.

31. Answer b.

Her trans-prosthetic mitral valve gradient is now in the order of 18 mmHg, suggesting valve obstruction—potentially thrombosis. One has to be cognizant that, while the majority of medications either do not affect or increase the INR, an increase in ingested vitamin K may lower the INR and predispose the patient to prosthetic valve thrombosis unless the warfarin dose is changed. Vitamin K is a common component of herbal supplements designed to reduce bone loss.

32. Answer e.

Either exercise myocardial perfusion imaging or exercise echocardiography is appropriate in the patient with resting ST segment depression greater than 1 mm, pre-excitation on the resting ECG, or previous revascularization with PTCA or surgery, assuming the patient can exercise. In a patient who is unable to exercise, either dobutamine echocardiography or adenosine or dipyridamole myocardial perfusion imaging is appropriate. However, in patients with LBBB, adenosine or dipyridamole myocardial perfusion imaging is preferred to dobutamine echocardiography.

33. Answer d.

The amount of prosthetic AR usually can be assessed accurately with TTE.

34. Answer c.

All of the answer choices, apart from left ventriculography, require an overall regular rhythm to facilitate data acquisition.

35. Answer e.

Oral dipyridamole, theophylline therapy, asthma, and second-degree AV block are all contraindications to the use of adenosine. Ventricular arrhythmias are a contraindication to the use of dobutamine. The presence of left axis deviation is not a contraindication to the use of any of these pharmacologic stress agents.

36. Answer d.

Among adults, FMD is more common in women, with a prevalence 2 to 10 times higher compared to men. There does not appear to be a female predominance in children. Renal artery FMD should be considered, particularly in women under the age of 50 who develop severe or refractory HTN, a sudden onset of HTN before the age of 30 or an otherwise unexplained rapid deterioration in BP control. FMD of the renal arteries is bilateral in 35% to 50%, and among those with bilateral disease, nearly half have extra-renal involvement.

37. Answer c.

The problem of test sensitivity and specificity is common, regardless of the evaluating test chosen for a specific diagnosis. One always needs to be aware of the pretest likelihood of disease, which in this case is approximately 50%. This means that half of the test population will have true disease and half will not. Thus, you can easily calculate the proportions of test subjects, given the power of your test, that would be in each category (false-positive and negative, true-positive and negative). From these calculations, it is apparent that the probability of disease despite a negative stress test is 38%, given the specificity indicated initially. Increasing the specificity of the test to 90% would reduce the false-negative rate to 25%, still below the acceptable certainty level of 90%.

38. Answer c.

IVUS provides additive anatomical information over coronary angiography, but neither give any information on physiology. The differences in coronary flow with and without the vasodilator adenosine provide information on the hemodynamic significance of an indeterminate lesion.

39. Answer c.

The mitral inflow pattern shows a restrictive pattern of E velocity twice that of the A velocity. There is also mid diastolic flow. Both findings are consistent with an elevation in LV filling pressures, severely abnormal diastolic function, and the presence of a third heart sound on physical examination. A normal late diastolic A wave indicates normal atrial contractility. A fourth heart sound is a late diastolic filling sound that corresponds to a prominence of the A wave commonly seen in less severe diastolic function—a delayed relaxation pattern.

40. Answer c.

Stress perfusion imaging is unable to distinguish the mechanism of reduction in coronary flow. A mild perfusion defect is associated with an increased risk of future MI but not cardiac death. While post stress dilation of the LV suggests a significant ischemic response, it may occur with single vessel disease (although typically indicates a larger area at risk). Modality of stress does not affect the degree of soft tissue attenuation artifacts.

41. Answer a.

This patient had constrictive pericarditis due to longstanding rheumatoid arthritis. The diagnosis was confirmed by characteristic changes on echocardiography. Constrictive pericarditis results in fixed cardiac volume with respiratory dependent preferential filling of one ventricle over the other. Constrictive pericarditis should be expected when signs and symptoms of heart failure are out of proportion to the degree of systolic dysfunction (if present) or valvular heart disease. In this patient, it was important to exclude ischemia. Each of the other answer choices are often present in constrictive pericarditis, however are absent or nonspecific in a significant number of patients.

42. Answer e.

All the above factors have been demonstrated to be associated with adverse outcomes in patients with PAH except the peak TR velocity.

43. Answer a.

The risk of displacement of the Starr-Edwards pre-6000 series valve is hypothetical. This valve shows more magnetism than any other implanted valve, but it is still quite small. All other bioprosthetic and mechanical valves can be imaged in an MRI system. Artifact occurs around the valve, making it impossible to assess the structure of the valve with MRI.

44. Answer b.

Review of the literature indicates that stress ECGs that show LV hypertrophy by voltage criteria only (not fulfilling Estes criteria for the diagnosis of hypertrophy) can be interpreted like a regular stress ECG, with the caveat that horizontal or downsloping ST-segment depression of 1 to 2 mm is considered nondiagnostic but suggestive of ischemia. Horizontal or downsloping ST-segment depression of 2 mm or more indicates that the stress ECG is positive. Conversely, ST-segment depression of less than 1 mm or pseudonormalization of an inverted T wave is still considered negative for ischemia. ST-segment elevation in the presence of existing Q waves is a special case in which the ECG has to be interpreted as nondiagnostic.

45. Answer d.

LV contractility is not directly related to LV diastolic function. Properties that impact diastolic function are the compliance and viscoelastic properties of the LV. LA compliance does not provide direct information on LV diastolic function.

46. Answer d.

This echocardiogram demonstrates a dilated CS. Common causes of a dilated CS include a persistent left SVC, an anomalous connection of the left pulmonary veins to the CS or increased right atrial pressure eg, due to pulmonary HTN or TVR. While direct focused imaging frequently will identify a persistent left SVC, an alternative strategy involves echocardiographic imaging while agitated imaging contrast material is injected into a vein in the left arm and visualizing opacification of the CS prior to seeing contrast in the RV (see figure below).

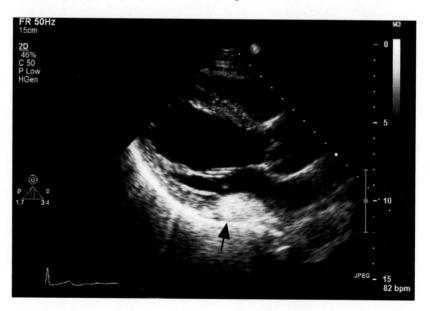

47. Answer c.

LV index of myocardial performance is a Doppler-derived global index of myocardial performance incorporating a measure of systolic and diastolic function. It is relatively independent of HR, systemic BP and the degree of mitral valve regurgitation. It is calculated based of timing measurements taken from the mitral inflow and LV outflow Doppler profiles.

LV index of myocardial performance = ([Mitral valve closure to opening time] minus the [Ejection time]) divided by the (Ejection time).

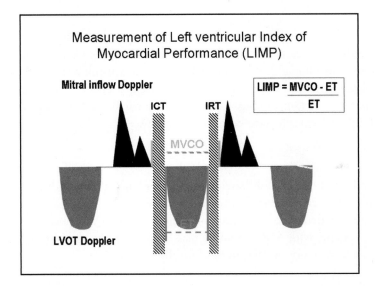

48. Answer d.

Noninvasive stress testing is best indicated in patients with an intermediate pretest probability of disease. The addition of an imaging modality to stress is best indicated in patients in whom an exercise ECG will be nondiagnostic for ischemia, eg, LBBB, ventricular pacing, greater than 1 mm of resting ST segment depression. A man over the age 40 (A) and a woman over the age of 60 (E) with typical angina have a high pretest probability for coronary disease and all things being equal should be referred for coronary angiography directly for the diagnosis. A 50-year-old asymptomatic woman has a very low pretest probability for disease and does not warrant further investigation. A 45-year-old woman with a history of atypical chest pain also has a low pre-test probability of disease and may not require a stress test. With a normal resting ECG a stress ECG would be the preferred initial modality. Despite her young age, the symptoms of typical angina, even in a 30-year-old woman, place her at an intermediate risk of coronary disease, increased further by the presence of resting ST segment depression. Given that she would have a nondiagnostic stress ECG a stress imaging study is appropriate.

49. Answer b.

The frequency of false positive studies with dobutamine stress is as frequently seen as with exercise; a vasodilator stress agent such as adenosine or dipyridamole is indicated in such cases.

50. Answer c.

Persistence of forward flow in diastole suggests the presence of aortic coarctation or patent ductus arteriosus. Aortic valve regurgitation should be suspected if reversal of flow was present in diastole (on this tracing would be indicated by a signal below the baseline).

51. Answer b.

Images show a large, dense infarction involving the lateral and inferior walls of the LV. Repeat images 24 hours after thallium injection, based on redistribution characteristics of thallium in myocardium, is useful in the assessment of viability. However, sestamibi has different properties, and repeat imaging is not useful for assessment of viability.

52. Answer d.

The chest X-ray is normal. The characteristic finding on chest X-ray of Ebstein anomaly is an enlarged "water-bottle" heart. The overall heart size is normal suggesting the absence of Ebstein anomaly or idiopathic dilated cardiomyopathy explaining the dyspnea. There is no RV enlargement or prominence of the PAs to suggest PA HTN and no elevation of the right hemidiaphragm to suggest phrenic nerve paralysis. Patients presenting with left atrial myoma typically have normal chest X-rays.

53. Answer c.

Echocardiography is indicated to establish baseline parameters in patients with MR that has not been previously characterized. Patients with severe MR should have yearly assessment of their ventricular size and function even in the absence of a change in their clinical status. Patients with MR should be reassessed echocardiographically whenever there is a change in symptoms felt to be clinically relevant.

54. Answer e.

The chest X-ray demonstrates that the tip of the central venous catheter (presumably understood to have been placed in the right internal jugular vein) is located out of the normal location of the SVC, concerning for either a venous perforation or an extravascular placement. A chest CT is required to evaluate for the above and exclude a pneumothorax (although not obviously evident on chest X-ray). The hypotension refractory to dopamine could be related to a hemothorax or simply the fact that the dopamine is likely being infused extravascularly.

55. Answer c.

Dilation of the LV that occurs following stress identifies a high risk cohort as does an increase in lung uptake with thallium. Focal defects that are fixed do not denote a high risk unless the defect is significant in severity and degree of distribution.

56. Answer d.

Exercise capacity is a very powerful predictor of both all-cause and cardiac mortality. It provides information that is clearly incremental to imaging. For that reason, exercise is always the preferred stress technique. The inability to perform an exercise test has been associated with an adverse prognosis in several studies. Although 85% of age-predicted maximal HR is commonly used as an end point for exercise testing, symptom-limited end points clearly are preferred because of the known variability in maximal HR in an individual patient.

57. Answer b.

The tracing shows clear systolic and diastolic atrial inflow signals with late diastolic reversal of flow into the pulmonary vein indicative of normal atrial contractility. There is predominance of flow in diastole (twice that of systolic velocity) consistent with an elevation in left atrial pressure. Primary pulmonary HTN would have a normal Doppler pattern (systolic predominant) and pulmonary vein stenosis would have increased flow velocities. A patient with an elevation in mean atrial pressure would most likely have an impaired exercise capacity.

58. Answer c.

Despite a low EF and low CO (low LVOT TVI in the absence of tachycardia), the peak aortic velocity is very high (>3.5 m/sec). In fact her peak aortic velocity is close to eight times her peak LVOT velocity (a ratio over 4 suggests severe AS). In a symptomatic patient, surgery is the best treatment for severe AS regardless of EF. No further testing to characterize the aortic valve is indicated.

59. Answer d.

The exercise test was an adequate stress. The anterior wall and septum had an "ischemic response" to stress suggesting a high grade LAD stenosis. The inferior resting wall motion abnormalities suggest infarction. Only the lateral wall had a normal stress response.

60. Answer c.

The data are consistent with mild to moderate AS, with an AVA of 1.3 cm^2

$AVA = \pi(r_{LVOT})^2 \times (TVI_{LVOT})/(TVI_{AV})$
$AVA = 0.785\ (Diameter\ _{LVOT})^2 \times (TVI_{LVOT})/(TVI_{AV})$
$AVA = 0.785 \times (2.2)^2 \times (30/85)$
$AVA = 1.3\ cm^2$

Note CO is upper limit of normal

$= SV \times HR$
$= [(Area_{LVOT}) \times (TVI_{LVOT})] \times 70$
$= [0.785 \times (2.2)^2 \times 30] \times 70$
$= 114 \times 70$
$= 7980\ mL/min$

61. Answer a.

Thallium and technetium are the two most commonly used isotopes in Nuclear Cardiology tests. Technetium has a higher energy with a characteristic 140 keV photon peak. It is eluted from the stable molybdenum-99 compound that has a half-life of 66 hours and is easily transported. In contrast, thallium-201 is generated from a cyclotron facility and then transported as a finished product. The energy profile of technetium is not only higher but is also more homogeneous since the thallium radio decay process has a marked variability in photon energy with the majority ranging from 69 to 83 keV but other, particularly lower, energy peaks are also present. The higher energy signature in technetium also allows better penetration and transmission through tissue, thus, the residual radiation in a patient is markedly less for technetium than it is for thallium, so larger doses can be used to improve imaging characteristics, without endangering the patient.

62. Answer b.

Diastolic function can be well assessed with radionuclide angiography. To enhance accuracy a different mode of gating has been employed, increasing the gating cycle to 64 rather than the conventional 32 frames for better cycle resolution. This of course enhances the time necessary to obtain the images to achieve the required photon statistics, but diastolic function analysis has been established as a valid tool with radionuclide angiography. Pharmacological stress testing is indeed the preferred choice in patients undergoing radionuclide testing for the diagnosis of CAD. However, the problem with LBBB is a significant change in contraction pattern, which can unpredictably change with additional exercise. Radionuclide angiography is based on the assessment of regional wall motion and thus is not the optimal test for assessing patients with LBBB. The presence of a paced rhythm does not preclude the use of radionuclide angiography, particularly if the patient is paced at a stable rhythm and is capable of achieving a HR plateau after adjustment during the various stages of exercise. Pacemakers are often programmed to emulate this physiological response to exercise while increasing the HR according to

62. (continued)

breathing or motion pattern. Exercise radionuclide angiography is usually performed with a camera in a modified LAO position for maximal separation of the RV and LV. This projection over-represents the circumflex coronary artery with two segments, the LAD also with only two segments, and the RCA with one segment (inferoapical), thus constituting a skewed pattern for the assessment of the coronary artery territories. Heparin has been shown to interfere with the labeling of red blood cells with technetium. It is fairly rare but occurs in approximately 5% of the patients requiring retagging of the red blood cells under special precautions.

63. Answer a.

The patient described above presents a clinical dilemma. As a 45-year-old female, she has a low pretest likelihood of CAD. Thus she is, per se, not a good candidate for exercise testing or imaging. The chance is that a positive test would represent a false-positive test rather than a true-positive. In women of this age group, a pharmacological stress test would increase the sensitivity but would not increase the specificity. Thus, the predictive accuracy of a negative test is similar for exercise or pharmacological testing. The test should not be terminated when the patient has exercised to 85% of her maximal predicted HR due to the significant variability in HR response in the individual patients and also it should not be terminated if the ECG shows more than 2 mm ST depression unless it is accompanied by other clinical criteria (signs of reduced perfusion, hemodynamic compromise, hemodynamically significant dysrhythmia). In a female of her size (moderately obese given her height), sestamibi should be chosen due to its superior imaging characteristics.

64. Answer d.

Chronic proximal thoracic aortic dissection uncommonly complicates CABG (12–16 per 10,000 procedures). Typically it will be identified 3 to 4 years postoperatively. The etiology may be related to injury from cross-clamp. Other factors associated with its occurrence include long-standing HTN, atherosclerosis and/or dilatation of the aorta. Rates are up to 4 times higher in patients who have concomitant aortic valve surgery.

65. Answer d.

Adenosine results in a larger increase of coronary blood flow than dipyridamole or dobutamine. Dipyridamole with its slower onset and slower cessation is usually better tolerated in patients than adenosine. The side effects of both agents can be reversed with theophylline, although because adenosine has a very short half life, usually stopping the infusion is sufficient, should adverse reactions develop. High dose dobutamine (20–40 mcg/kg/min) is useful to establish the diagnosis of CAD. In contrast, low dose dobutamine (5–10 mcg/kg/min) is utilized to assess viability in patients with LV dysfunction. LBBB creates a dyssynergic contraction pattern and the use of dobutamine stress would only enhance these abnormalities, often unpredictably. Thus, it is not helpful in distinguishing a coronary origin for the regional wall motion abnormality.

66. Answer b.

There is echocardiographic evidence of pulmonary HTN (trans-tricuspid gradient of 41 mmHg) with right atrial and ventricular enlargement. There is also a large mass in the RA with a shape that is consistent of a venous cast. The composite findings are consistent with acute thromboembolic disease with a clot in transit. Options include anticoagulation and consideration of thrombolytics or surgical embolectomy. Insufficient data about the patient is given to decide on which of these next steps are appropriate.

67. Answer d.

Adenosine stress testing is helpful in patients whose exercise capacity is limited by orthopedic, neurological, or peripheral vascular problems. Symptoms can be misleading, since a number of patients complain about headaches, flushing, dyspnea, as well as chest discomfort, which is most likely noncardiac. Also, the absence of symptoms does not indicate the absence of disease. A drop in BP is common with adenosine because of peripheral vasodilation and can be usually ameliorated if necessary with a small amount of saline or Ringer lactate infusion. The key feature in the scan is the marked post stress dilatation. The clinical background always needs to be considered in the interpretation of scans. In a patient with marked CV risk factors, the likelihood of disease is high and the absence of a markedly reversible defect in the presence of significant post stress dilatation is worrisome for significant, equally distributed disease in which the extent of reversibility underestimates the true extent of CAD. Despite coronary angiography being helpful for delineating the coronary stenosis, it cannot assess the functional significance of coronary artery lesions.

68. Answer c.

The key to this question lies in the imaging characteristic of each technique. Assessment of LV function by echocardiography is based on the inward motion of the myocardium and wall thickening. In a large, hypocontractile ventricle the inward motion is minimal and significant variance in the determination of LV function can easily occur. In contrast, radionuclide angiography is based on count statistics. In a large ventricle with poor function, the end diastolic and end systolic counts are very high. Thus, high quality determination of LV function can be obtained in patients who are in stable sinus rhythm. Conversely, in hyperdynamic ventricles, the markedly exaggerated inward motion allows excellent discrimination at excellent LV function by echocardiography, whereas the low count density in end systole may lead to a slight exaggeration of LV function by radionuclide angiography. A drop in 5 EF points by radionuclide angiography at this level is a significant change in his LV function. Even in patients with known idiopathic cardiomyopathy and absent CAD, segmental wall motion is not homogeneous. The inferior and inferolateral segments, possibly due to the diaphragmatic buttressing, appear to contract better than the remaining segments. This does not indicate CAD but is a common finding in this disease state. Additional parameters like diastolic function are useful parameters to further aid in risk stratification.

69. Answer c.

This question pertains to the choice of optimal test in a challenging patient who is severely obese with significant COPD. TTE will most likely be hampered by both the body size and the significant COPD, which of course is not a problem for isotope transmission. The tissue attenuation in this markedly obese patient, however, would make the heart appear smaller due to both distance to the detector as well as tissue attenuation. A first pass, sestamibi is potentially helpful. However, if significant LV dysfunction and/or RV dysfunction would be present, the bolus may be of inferior quality and thus result in erroneous measurements. EBCT is not readily available and would also suffer from attenuation given the patient's size.

70. Answer c.

A full resting radionuclide angiography is performed in three positions: the anteroposterior, a LAO equivalent, and a lateral position. The LAO position is always adjusted for optimal alignment of the septum orthogonal to the imaging plane to best discriminate

70. (continued)

between RV and LV function. Cranial tilt is sometimes needed and thus a standard LAO projection is usually not used. Radionuclide angiography is strictly based on count statistics and does not rely on the presumption of a certain contraction pattern or volumetric determinations. Even though there is little intra-individual variation in the ventricular volumes, body habitus, weight, position of the heart in the thoracic cavity, and, thus, distance to the detector are critical parameters that are difficult to account for in the clinical setting. Thus, there is significant inter-individual variation. An accurate assessment of LV function is only possible if the patient is in regular rhythm. Use of low energy all purpose collimator provides optimal counts; improved resolution from a high-resolution collimator is not critical. Determination of LV EF by radionuclide angiography is excellent in discriminating hypo- but not hyperdynamic ventricles. This is because the high count density at both end diastole and end systole results in superior quality images to a hyperdynamic ventricle, which has low counts at end systole.

71. Answer a.

There are several conditions that can cause reduced uptake in the inferior wall. The most notable is diaphragmatic attenuation due to body habitus, such as obesity. A motion artifact can also contribute to reduced inferior uptake though this is most likely accompanied by reduced uptake in the contralateral wall. Adjacent tissue uptake, most notably in the liver and bowel, are also responsible for reduced uptake in the inferior segments and need to be carefully recognized. Partial volume effects occur when tissue rarification is present, which is common at the apex with its clonal shape. This does not play a significant role in the inferior portions particularly at the base and mid-ventricular level where diaphragmatic attenuation is usually noted.

72. Answer e.

Mechanical cardiac valves, the C-ring support structures for tissue valves, and coronary stents are made of nonferrous material and are not contraindications to MRI. However, if there is a question of valve dehiscence, then MRI is relatively contraindicated. Permanent and temporary pacemakers and ICDs are contraindications.

73. Answer c.

Although rubidium comes from a parent compound, strontium-82, which requires a cyclotron for production, rubidium can be generated at a remote site using a portable generator. While technetium-99 m also does not require a cyclotron, it is used in SPECT imaging but not PET.

74. Answer a.

Myoxomas are the most common cardiac tumor and typically arise from the atrial septum in the LA. When small they may present with embolic events, when large (as in this case) the tumor can obstruct the mitral valve mimicking mitral valve stenosis. This patient had a transmitral valve gradient of 22 mmHg. Papillary fibroelastomas are small tumors present typically on valvular surfaces with frondlike projections. A pericardial cyst has a characteristic echocardiographic appearance located outside the cardiac chambers. Hypernephroma is a contiguous tumor arising out of the renal vein through the IVC into the RA.

75. Answer d.

Thallium-201 is a weak radioactive compound, and image quality is not universally excellent, especially in obese patients. Additionally, thallium "scatters," and positrons do not. Thus, imaging with PET is superior for obese patients. Thallium cannot be used to define absolute myocardial perfusion, although it can be used to define relative differences in perfusion between regions. Although some data suggest that thallium can be used to define myocardial viability using reinjection/scanning methods, it is generally accepted that PET, if available, is more applicable for defining myocardial viability using FDG. Because rubidium-82 can be generated with a portable device, all PET scanning need not require an on-site cyclotron. Because thallium has a sufficiently long half-life, it can be stored locally for several days before its use.

76. Answer d.

A TTE examination, especially in a patient with COPD, is inadequate to examine the aorta. A TEE examination is contraindicated if there is a possibility of cervical damage or unknown esophageal or gastric conditions. MRI is not possible in acutely ill patients or patients requiring mechanical ventilation. The most rapid means to assess the entire aorta in a patient with no allergy to contrast media is CT.

77. Answer c.

A prosthetic hip is made of titanium or cobalt-chromium alloy and has no significant ferromagnetic properties. It does not heat and is not significantly magnetic. It may create a large image artifact in the hip on MRI. The St. Jude valve and ureteric stent are also made of nonferromagnetic materials and can be scanned with MRI. They may produce a small image artifact. Although most likely safe, cerebral aneurysm clips should be tested in a magnet before implantation. Made of nonferromagnetic materials, shaping during manufacture can induce some magnetism, and the clip may torque in an MRI scanner. Also, because displacement of an aneurysm clip could be fatal, it is imperative to confirm that the metal used is indeed nonmagnetic, as indicated on the device package insert. A patient's operative record also should confirm that the aneurysm clip used is rated nonferromagnetic. While usually unaffected by the magnetic field dental fillings may distort images of the facial area or brain.

78. Answer c.

Often, the calcium is located in the proximal coronary arteries. Normal calcium scores have been established at Mayo Clinic for sex and age. This patient has more calcium than 75% of men his age. A significant (50% diameter narrowing) stenosis is likely (sensitivity and specificity 85%), but severe CAD occurs with higher scores (>400). Although further research is required, the calcium score likely can be modified by aggressive risk factor modification.

79. Answer c.

TEE does not completely visualize structures around the heart, where one might expect to see a malignancy. EBCT requires a contrast agent, and this may worsen the patient's renal function. Like EBCT, MRI has a wide window of view and is useful for the detection of paracardiac masses but does not require nephrotoxic contrast. While not prohibitive the low platelets greatly increase the risk of a diagnostic pericardial tap in this patient.

80. Answer c.

PET may show myocardial viability where the rest thallium study does not. Viability detected at rest indicates resting ischemia (hibernation) and suggests that revascularization would improve LV function. Low-dose dobutamine infusion may recruit additional myocardial contraction despite resting ischemia and also suggests that LV function will improve with revascularization. However, in this obese patient with very

80. (*continued*)

poor LV function, PET is the better viability test. Because a mismatch in perfusion and glucose metabolism indicates hibernation, both FDG and nitrogen-13-labeled ammonia images must be obtained.

81. Answer a.

Artifacts may occur with standard thallium and sestamibi (Cardiolyte) perfusion imaging. Attenuation correction is performed with PET, and artifact from breast and diaphragm is less common. PET is unlikely to detect significant CAD in patients with a normal stress thallium study. 82Rb is a perfusion agent, and if taken up it indicates viability, just as thallium uptake does. However, metabolic activity detected with ^{18}F FDG is required for the diagnosis of true hibernation on PET scanning.

82. Answer e.

All of the tests can show hibernation and serve as useful guides for revascularization in patients with LV dysfunction. FDG uptake in an area of reduced perfusion on the ammonia image, redistribution of thallium at 24 hours after injection at rest, and contraction of a hypokinetic segment with low (5 to 10 mcg/kg/min)-dose dobutamine all indicate probable myocardial hibernation.

83. Answer d.

Patients with coronary artery stents can be safely imaged in an MRI scanner. A small artifact occurs in the coronary artery. There is no evidence of significant heating. Some manufacturers recommend that MRI be withheld in patients with stents for varying periods of time. Practically, these recommendations are unneeded, and MRI is safe immediately after stent placement.

84. Answer a.

TEE does not adequately visualize all of the proximal PAs. An exogenously administered echocardiographic contrast agent enhances visualization of PAs, but the acoustical window is frequently inadequate in this region.

85. Answer c.

A report indicating a high probability for the presence or absence of pulmonary embolus on perfusion- ventilation lung scanning is about as reliable as EBCT. However, CT is not significantly affected by lung disease, and therefore a report of intermediate probability for pulmonary embolus is much less likely by EBCT. Unfortunately, CT requires a contrast agent, which is toxic in patients with renal failure.

86. Answer c.

The patient probably has calcific constrictive pericarditis secondary to tuberculosis. PET does not visualize the pericardium. Cardiac MRI is an excellent method of examining the pericardium, but it does not detect calcium. EBCT is also very good for visualizing the pericardium, and calcium is readily seen. In this patient, the frontal chest radiograph did not show the calcium. Calcium can be readily appreciated on TEE, but not in the small amounts sometimes seen in constrictive pericarditis.

87. Answer d.

All the tests listed provide good visualization of the ascending aorta. TEE may overall be the least reliable, although in experienced hands it should be as good as CT and

MRI. An MRI study should include contrast images for visualization of the lumen and standard spin echo images to visualize the wall of the aorta.

88. Answer b.

This situation represents the classic problem of combining the power of a test with the incidence of disease in the population. On the basis of the patient's age and sex and the absence of strong risk factors, she has a low risk of hemodynamically significant CAD—probably 10% or less. Because the incidence of CAD is expected to be very low in this patient, a true-positive test is less likely than a false-positive test. Thus, a positive test result would not be a good indicator for CAD. Increasing the test specificity to 80% would only modestly increase its positive predictive value, still not sufficient to make it a reliable diagnostic test. Diagnostic stress testing should, in general, be a symptom-limited test, and modest changes in ECG tracings should not lead to termination of the test.

89. Answer b.

ST-segment elevation in the presence of existing Q waves cannot be interpreted as indicating ischemia, particularly in the presence of voltage criteria for LV hypertrophy. In contrast, ST-segment depression greater than or equal to 2 mm in the presence of LV hypertrophy by voltage criteria alone is interpretable as a positive exercise test. Answers **c**, **d**, and **e** are similar to the previously published guidelines, in which the ST-segment changes in patients taking digitalis, the anteroseptal leads in patients with concomitant right bundle branch block, and the ECG of patients with Wolff-Parkinson-White syndrome cannot be accurately interpreted with respect to myocardial ischemia.

90. Answer d.

Moderate to severe angina, an increase in nervous system symptoms, signs of poor perfusion, and a subject's desire to stop are all absolute indications for terminating the exercise test. Increasing chest pain, however, is only a relative indication and needs to be judged in the presence of other accompanying factors, such as ECG changes, changes in the hemodynamic response to exercise, and increasing dysrhythmia.

91. Answer d.

This question relates to preoperative exercise testing. You are asked to assess the risk of a perioperative cardiac event in this patient. Certain key features help make the decision. This patient has stable, asymptomatic CAD. Despite his persistent risk factors, he is able to exercise well without symptoms. His bypass procedure was only 3 years ago, which is in favor of patency of the coronary grafts, although his smoking is worrisome. In the absence of angina or heart failure, the patient's perioperative risk is low and largely determined by the risk of the gastric procedure and not his CAD, per se.

92. Answer b.

$$
\begin{aligned}
\text{EOA} &= (\text{LVOT area} \times \text{LVOT TVI})/\text{Prosthesis TVI} \\
&= [(\text{LVOT diameter}^2 \times 0.785) \times \text{LVOT TVI}]/\text{Prosthesis TVI} \\
&= [(4 \times 0.785) \times 20]/100 \\
&= [3.14 \times 20]/100 \\
&= 0.628\ \text{cm}^2
\end{aligned}
$$

SECTION VIII

Cardiac Pharmacology

Garvan C. Kane, MD, PhD

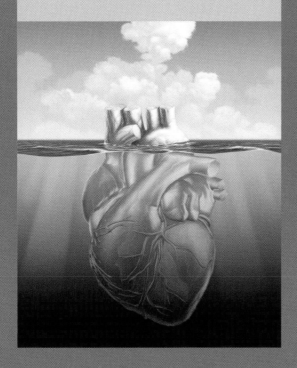

Questions

1. Drug side effects may be controlled most effectively by minimizing risk factors and:

    a. Measuring drug levels
    b. Adding therapy to control side effects
    c. Increasing the number of medications
    d. Increasing the dose
    e. Increasing the frequency of administration

2. Which of the following agents would give the following hemodynamic effect, illustrated in the diagram of pressure-volume relationship, as moving from the continuous line (baseline) to the dotted line?

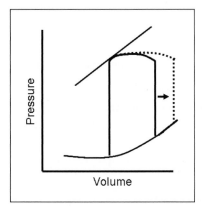

    a. Vasopressin
    b. Dobutamine
    c. Bumetanide
    d. Saline
    e. Epinephrine

3. Which of the following medications increases insulin sensitivity?

    a. ACE inhibitors
    b. Thiazide diuretics
    c. Calcium channel blockers
    d. Beta blockers
    e. Nitrates

4. Which of the following is **not** a common cause for adverse drug events in the elderly?

    a. Increased number of concomitant medications
    b. Noncompliance
    c. Prescription error
    d. Increased volume of distribution
    e. Cognitive decline

Answers to this section start on page 297.

5. A 55-year-old man with a mechanical mitral valve presents with an acute STEMI. His INR is 3. Coronary angiography reveals an occluded LAD artery. Prior to proceeding with emergency PCI, which of the following should be done?

   a. Intravenous heparin
   b. Abciximab
   c. No additional anticoagulant
   d. Subcutaneous enoxaparin
   e. Bivalirudin

6. The following drugs are associated with the following teratogenic effects, **except:**

   a. Lithium and Ebstein's anomaly
   b. Warfarin with facial and CNS abnormalities
   c. ACE inhibitors and oligohydramnios
   d. Heparin and osteoporosis
   e. Beta blockers and growth retardation

7. High-first-pass metabolism is important for many reasons, **except:**

   a. SL NTG administration avoids first-pass metabolism
   b. Impaired liver perfusion decreases dosing requirements
   c. Some medications do not achieve therapeutic effectiveness when given orally
   d. Lidocaine dosing is dependent on first-pass
   e. Oral medications require significantly lower doses compared with intravenous doses

8. Most complications of cardiac drugs can be classed generally as:

   a. Dose-dependent
   b. Allergic
   c. Drug-drug interactions
   d. Dose-independent only
   e. Idiosyncratic

9. Renal insufficiency impacts the use of the following beta blockers, **except:**

   a. Nadolol
   b. Metoprolol
   c. Sotalol
   d. Acebutolol
   e. Atenolol

10. Complications of procainamide typically **exclude:**

    a. Excessive (>50% over baseline) prolongation of QRS interval
    b. Heart block
    c. HTN
    d. VT
    e. Rash

11. The risk of myositis, myopathy, or rhabdomyolysis is greatest with which drug combinations?

    a. Gemfibrozil plus pravastatin while taking digoxin
    b. Gemfibrozil plus pravastatin while taking itraconazole
    c. Gemfibrozil plus ketoconazole
    d. Pravastatin plus beta carotene while taking itraconazole
    e. Gemfibrozil plus pravastatin while taking aspirin and clopidogrel

12. The clinical significance of drug-drug interactions may be most dependent on the:

    a. Method of administration
    b. Magnitude of the therapeutic window
    c. Volume of distribution
    d. Half-life of the metabolite
    e. Drug dose

13. All of the following are effects of loop diuretics, eg, furosemide, **except** which of the following?

    a. Hypomagnesemia
    b. Ototoxicity
    c. Hypercalcemia
    d. Venodilation
    e. Loop diuretics are the most effective diuretic agents

14. Which of the following agents increase cardiac contractility through a mechanism other than an increase in intracellular cAMP?

    a. Milrinone
    b. Epinephrine
    c. Dobutamine
    d. Levosimendan
    e. Dopamine

15. Which of the following statements regarding the action of inotropes is true?

    a. Beta-1 receptor activation is responsible for dobutamine-induced vasodilatation
    b. Milrinone acts on beta-1 receptors to increase inotropy
    c. Isoproterenol activation of alpha receptors may increase systemic BP
    d. The chronotropic effects of dopamine are mediated through action on beta-1 receptors
    e. Epinephrine primarily stimulates alpha receptors

16. Grapefruit juice increases the bioavailability of which of the following drug(s)?

    a. Simvastatin
    b. Nifedipine
    c. Sildenafil
    d. Cyclosporin A
    e. All of the above

17. A 65-year-old man with a history of HTN, hyperlipidemia, and alcoholic cirrhosis is admitted to the coronary care unit with chest pain and an acute ST elevation anterior MI. You are called to assess for frequent premature ventricular complexes followed by sustained monomorphic VT, which is not associated with symptoms or hypotension. He weighs 75 kg.

    Which of the following will you recommend at this time?

    a. Oral amiodarone 800 mg BID
    b. Intravenous lidocaine 100 mg bolus, followed by 1 mg/min infusion
    c. Intravenous lidocaine 100 mg, followed by 75 mg bolus in 5 minutes, and then 3 mg/min infusion
    d. Intravenous bretylium 750 mg bolus, followed by 2 mg/min infusion
    e. ICD implantation

18. Regarding adverse effects with ACE inhibitors, all the following occur, **except:**

    a. Cough and angioedema with enalapril
    b. Proteinuria with captopril
    c. Hyperkalemia with perindopril
    d. Neutropenia or rash with enalapril
    e. Teratogenicity with lisinopril

19. An 82-year-old woman with HTN and chronic renal failure (serum creatinine 3.5 mg/dL) is referred to you for the management of PAF. She has no other risk factors for coronary atherosclerosis and has well-preserved ventricular function. Her ECG is essentially normal, with a QTc interval of 400 msec.

    Which of the following drugs will be suitable for her rhythm management?

    a. Sotalol 120 mg BID
    b. Dofetilide 500 mcg BID
    c. Amiodarone 200 mg QD
    d. Procainamide 1 gm TID
    e. Propafenone 150 mg TID

20. A 60-year-old man with long standing HTN and PAF is referred to you for initiation of amiodarone. Which of the following medication(s) that the patient is currently taking will **not** require dosage adjustment?

    a. Digoxin
    b. Warfarin
    c. Labetalol
    d. Enalapril
    e. Both c and d

21. Quinidine, a stereoisomer of quinine initially derived from the bark of the cinchona tree, has been used for decades for AF. It was originally discovered by a Danish merchant seaman with AF who took quinine for malaria prophylaxis during trips to India. He noted his pulse was regular while in India but irregular at home. Cinchonism describes tinnitus and hearing loss with quinidine excess.

    Which of the following is **not** a side effect associated with quinidine use?

    a. Constipation
    b. Thrombocytopenia
    c. Granulomatous hepatitis
    d. Myasthenia gravis
    e. Torsades de pointes VT

22. Which of the following drugs used at therapeutic levels is most likely to increase the pacing threshold?

    a. Amiodarone
    b. Flecainide
    c. Sotalol
    d. Procainamide
    e. Digoxin

23. Dofetilide blocks which of the following ion channels/receptors?

    a. IK_R potassium channel
    b. Calcium channel
    c. K_{ATP} potassium channel
    d. Sodium channel
    e. Beta receptor

24. Flumazenil (select true answer):

    a. Will antagonize the respiratory depression of morphine
    b. Will antagonize the sedative effects of midazolam
    c. Is so long acting that resedation is not possible
    d. Is safe in patients taking daily benzodiazepines
    e. Has a peak effect 90 minutes after administration

25. Which of the following needs close observation during loading with dofetilide?

    a. Pulse rate interval
    b. QRS interval
    c. QT interval
    d. HR
    e. BP

26. Drug A is more potent than drug B. The potency of a drug helps predict:

    a. Maximal effect obtainable
    b. Likelihood of side effects
    c. Elimination half-life
    d. Dependency of effect on concentration
    e. Selectivity

27. Digoxin used in combination with amiodarone, propranolol, or verapamil can cause:

    a. Torsades de pointes
    b. Pericarditis
    c. AV block
    d. Eosinophilia
    e. None of the above

28. Concerning beta blockers, which of the following is **incorrect**?

    a. Beta blockers are less effective in reducing coronary events in hypertensive men who smoke
    b. Propranolol is contraindicated in patients with severe depression
    c. Selective beta blockers should be avoided in patients with peripheral vascular disease
    d. Beta blockers should be avoided in patients with significant asthma
    e. Propranolol and bisoprolol doses should be reduced in patients with low plasma proteins

29. A 56-year-old man with longstanding CHF faints at home and is brought to the ED. The patient appears to be in no distress, and his vital signs are normal. There are no physical signs of an exacerbation of heart failure. The patient has been treated with digoxin 0.125 mg per day, furosemide 40 mg BID, and quinidine 300 mg BID for many months. He has also been prescribed terfenadine 60 mg BID for chronic rhinitis. One week before collapsing, he was prescribed erythromycin 500 mg TID for bronchitis. An ECG shows nonspecific ST and T wave changes and anterior Q waves consistent with MI that was unchanged from previous tracings. The QT interval corrected for HR is 0.44 ssec.

    The most likely cause of the patient having fainted is:

    a. Digoxin toxicity due to potassium depletion
    b. Digoxin toxicity due to a digoxin-quinidine interaction
    c. Torsades de pointes caused by an interaction between quinidine and erythromycin
    d. Torsades de pointes caused by an interaction between terfenadine and erythromycin
    e. Torsades de pointes caused by an interaction between terfenadine and quinidine

30. A 72-year-old patient presents with an ACS and receives aspirin, unfractionated heparin, and clopidogrel. He undergoes successful PCI. His creatinine is 2.8 mg/dL. Two days later he has a painful swollen left leg and a US confirms a deep venous thrombosis. His platelet count has fallen from 300,000 to 100,000. The best next step is to:

    a. Stop heparin and start enoxaparin and warfarin
    b. Stop heparin and start warfarin
    c. Stop heparin and start lepirudin
    d. Stop heparin and start Argatroban
    e. Start warfarin and repeat platelet count the next day

31. The dose of digoxin should be adjusted downward with all of the following drugs, **except**:

    a. Verapamil
    b. Amiodarone
    c. Quinidine
    d. Propafenone
    e. Captopril

32. Each of the following statements about the antiarrhythmic agent disopyramide is true, **except:**

   a. It can accelerate or slow the sinus node rate depending on serum concentration and underlying sinus node disease

   b. The mean elimination half-life of disopyramide is 8 to 9 hours, and is prolonged in the presence of renal, hepatic, or heart failure

   c. It is effective in reducing the frequency of spontaneous ventricular ectopy and in preventing the recurrence of ventricular and pre-excited supraventricular arrhythmias

   d. It should not be combined with mexiletine because of an opposing effect on repolarization

   e. It is useful in the treatment of neurally-mediated syncope

33. Which of the following agents would give the following hemodynamic effect, illustrated on the diagram of pressure-volume relationship, as moving from the continuous line (baseline) to the dotted line?

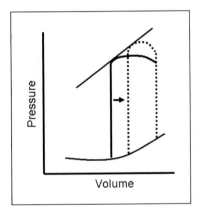

   a. Propranolol
   b. Milrinone
   c. Phentolamine
   d. Phenylephrine
   e. Saline

34. Which of the following drugs is **not** associated with a dose-dependent risk of torsades de pointes?

   a. Sotalol
   b. Ibutilide
   c. Terfenadine
   d. Quinidine
   e. Thioridazine

35. All of the following statements about lidocaine are true, **except:**

    a. Lidocaine has little effect on the electrophysiological properties of atrial myocardial cells or on conduction in accessory pathways

    b. In the absence of severe LV dysfunction, clinically significant adverse hemodynamic effects from lidocaine are rarely noted

    c. Patients treated with an initial bolus of lidocaine followed by a maintenance infusion may experience transient excessive plasma concentrations of the drug 30 to 120 min after therapy is begun

    d. The elimination half-life of lidocaine in patients with uncomplicated MI is 2 to 4 times that in normal subjects

    e. Lidocaine toxicity is increased in patients with MI and heart failure

36. ACE inhibitors have which of the following actions?

    a. Increase degradation of bradykinin

    b. Decrease degradation of bradykinin

    c. Increase production of bradykinin

    d. Increase kallikrein production

    e. Impair the conversion of prekallikrein to kallikrein

37. A 70-year-old woman with AF is admitted with nausea, yellow vision, and a regular ventricular rhythm at 70 bpm. She has been on 0.25 mg/day of digoxin and the plasma level is 3.2 ng/ml. The half-life for digoxin for her is 1.6 days. She has normal renal function.

How long should she hold her digoxin to reach a therapeutic level of 0.8 ng/ml?

    a. 8 days

    b. 2 days

    c. 4.8 days

    d. 2.4 days

    e. 3.2 days

38. Which of the following factors about dobutamine is **false?**

    a. Dobutamine does not stimulate dopaminergic receptors and therefore has no selective effects on renal blood flow

    b. Paradoxical bradycardia with dobutamine has been linked to significant RCA stenosis

    c. Unlike milrinone, chronic infusion of dobutamine is associated with an improvement in survival in heart failure patients, although at the expense of pro-arrhythmia

    d. Dobutamine has little effect on alpha-adrenergic receptors

    e. The typical hemodynamic response to dobutamine is mild hypotension mediated through acting on beta-2 receptors in the periphery

39. The most potent vasoconstrictor is:

    a. Bradykinin

    b. Endothelin

    c. Acetylcholine

    d. PAI-1

    e. Adenosine

40. Which of the following statements is **false**?

    a. Nitroprusside is an endothelial-independent vasodilator
    b. NTG dilates the microcirculation
    c. NO regulates matrix synthesis and smooth muscle migration
    d. Nitrates have an antiplatelet activity
    e. Nitrate-induced orthostatic hypotension is more commonly in the elderly

41. Response to which agent can be used to measure endothelial function?

    a. Methergine
    b. Ergonovine
    c. Acetylcholine
    d. Adenosine
    e. Endothelin

42. A drug administered by the intravenous route has which of the following bioavailabilities?

    a. 0
    b. 1
    c. >1
    d. <1
    e. Variable, depending on specific drug

43. Methemoglobinemia, associated clinically with dyspnea, cyanosis, and low oxygen saturations, has **not** been associated with which of the following agents?

    a. Sodium nitroprusside
    b. Well water
    c. Sildenafil
    d. Benzocaine
    e. Iphosphamide chemotherapy

44. Which of the following is true concerning digoxin?

    a. Digoxin is indicated for patients with stage B heart failure in sinus rhythm
    b. Digoxin toxicity is associated with profound mesenteric dilatation
    c. Digoxin effects are increased with low muscle mass
    d. Hemodialysis is warranted in digoxin toxicity refractory to Digibind
    e. Digoxin increases the pacing threshold

45. Therapeutic uses of calcium channel blockers include all of the following **except**:

    a. Angina pectoris
    b. Pulmonary HTN
    c. Migraine headaches
    d. Right-sided heart failure
    e. HCM

46. Concerning metoprolol, in which of the following conditions will the difference in plasma concentration following oral versus parenteral administration be the **smallest**?

    a. CHF
    b. Chronic renal failure
    c. Cirrhosis of the liver
    d. Malabsorption syndromes
    e. COPD

47. Which of the following is true?

    a. Hyperthyroid patients typically require more warfarin due to effects on vitamin K
    b. Lepirudin is indicated for patients with HIT in the setting of renal failure
    c. Alteplase has a fast onset of action with a prolonged duration of action
    d. Higher doses of heparin are typically required in pregnancy
    e. Thrombolytics are contraindicated in patients with right-sided intracardiac thrombi

48. The efficacy of a drug is best described by the:

    a. Maximal effect of the drug
    b. Median effective dose
    c. Dissociation constant of the drug receptor-complex
    d. Clearance of the drug
    e. Volume of distribution

49. The treatment of procainamide overdose should include:

    a. Potassium chloride
    b. Isoproterenol
    c. Magnesium
    d. Sodium lactate
    e. Dopamine

50. Which of the following drugs has the effects on the cardiac action potential demonstrated in this figure as drug X?

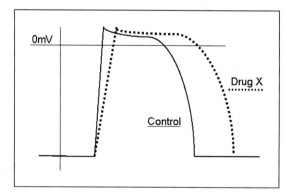

    a. Quinidine
    b. Adenosine
    c. Mexiletine
    d. Flecainide
    e. Dofetilide

51. Which of the following agents is **least** likely to cause hyperkalemia?

    a. Spironolactone
    b. Amiloride
    c. Captopril
    d. Ethacrynic acid
    e. Losartan

52. Which of the following combinations of drug with adverse effect is correct?

    a. Minoxidil and alopecia
    b. Methyldopa and hemolytic anemia
    c. Bisoprolol and tachycardia
    d. Hydralazine and cyanide toxicity
    e. Prazosin and urinary retention

53. Side effects of NTG include:

    a. Raynaud syndrome due to reflex peripheral vasodilatation
    b. Methemoglobinemia
    c. cGMP-mediated excessive vasodilatation with concomitant sildenafil
    d. Edema
    e. Bradycardia

54. Which of the following agents may exacerbate angina pectoris?

    a. SL NTG
    b. Labetalol
    c. Verapamil
    d. Hydralazine
    e. Lisinopril

55. Which of the following agents would give the following hemodynamic effect, illustrated on the diagram of pressure-volume relationship, as moving from the continuous line (baseline) to the dotted line?

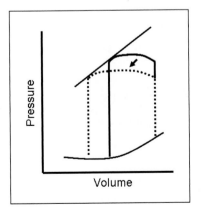

    a. Saline
    b. Furosemide
    c. Enalaprilat
    d. Dobutamine
    e. Dopamine

56. Which antiarrhythmic agent is best employed to treat digoxin-induced rhythm disturbances?

    a. Magnesium
    b. Potassium
    c. Lidocaine
    d. Amiodarone
    e. Quinidine

57. Which of the following therapies does **not** have proven survival benefit in patients with low EF heart failure?

    a. Carvedilol
    b. Enalapril
    c. Spironolactone
    d. Candesartan
    e. Digoxin

58. Hepatic clearance is important for all of the following, **except:**

    a. Sotalol
    b. Propranolol
    c. Metoprolol
    d. Labetalol
    e. Amiodarone

59. A 60-year-old man with AF and rapid ventricular response is treated with a drug that slows AV node conduction. Drug A in a dose of 10 mg produces a similar reduction in ventricular rate as 100 mg of Drug B. This indicates that Drug A is:

    a. More efficacious than Drug B
    b. Less toxic than Drug B
    c. More potent than Drug B
    d. Has a shorter duration of action than Drug B
    e. More selective than Drug B

60. All of the following are correct about beta blockers, **except:**

    a. Metoprolol is a selective beta-2 adrenergic receptor antagonist
    b. Nadolol is water soluble and renally excreted
    c. Pindolol has intrinsic sympathomimetic activity
    d. Propranolol is also a sodium channel blocker
    e. Sotalol is also a potassium channel blocker

61. You have recently started 150 mg TID of propafenone to suppress recurrences of PAF in a 40-year-old Caucasian man. He has a structurally normal heart and there is no history of any medical problems. He returns after 3 days of initiation of propafenone with new onset wheezing and shortness of breath. On examination he has prolonged expiration with rhonchi over both lung fields. Heart sounds are normal with a regular rhythm. ECG shows sinus bradycardia with a first degree AV conduction delay.

    What is the most likely reason for his symptoms?

    a. He has acute renal failure with elevated plasma level of propafenone
    b. He is a rapid metabolizer of propafenone, with an elevated plasma level of 5-hydroxypropafaone
    c. He is a slow metabolizer of propafenone, resulting in an elevated plasma level of propafenone
    d. 5-hydroxypropafenone is causing bronchoconstriction
    e. He is a rapid acetylator with an elevated level of NAPA causing bronchoconstriction

62. All of the following are correct about diuretics, **except:**

    a. Thiazide diuretics may exacerbate hyperuricemia and impotence
    b. Ethacrynic acid may be used safely in a patient with a sulfonamide allergy
    c. Thiazide diuretics are a rare cause of pancreatitis
    d. The coadministration of digoxin and spironolactone increases the occurrence of gynecomastia
    e. Thiazide diuretics may cause hypokalemia and hypocalcemia

63. Which of the following agents is most efficacious in the conversion of acute AF into sinus rhythm?

    a. Metoprolol
    b. Digoxin
    c. Amiodarone
    d. Diltiazem
    e. Esmolol

64. Concerning bosentan, used in the treatment of pulmonary arterial HTN, which of the following is correct?

    a. Unlike treprostinol, bosentan is relatively safe in pregnancy
    b. Bosentan is rarely associated with hepatic dysfunction
    c. Bosentan is contraindicated in patients with renal insufficiency
    d. Bosentan is a specific antagonist of the ET-B receptor
    e. Bosentan affects the efficacy of estrogen-based contraceptives

65. Which of the following factors increases hepatic drug metabolism and, hence, reduces drug bioavailability?

    a. Ciprofloxacin
    b. Verapamil
    c. Erythromycin
    d. Heart failure
    e. Tobacco use

66. Which of the following agents may exacerbate gout?

    a. Lisinopril
    b. Simvastatin
    c. Niacin
    d. Bumetanide
    e. Gemfibrozil

67. Which of the following agents is **not** the correct antidote for the listed overdose/toxicity?

    a. Glucagon for a beta blocker overdose
    b. Calcium for a calcium channel overdose
    c. Methylene blue for cyanide toxicity
    d. Esmolol for a caffeine overdose
    e. Digoxin antibodies for digoxin overdose

68. Which of the following agents/therapies is **not** associated with the development of LV systolic dysfunction?

    a. Thyroid hormone
    b. Ethanol
    c. Bleomycin
    d. Radiation
    e. Adriamycin

69. Which of the following agents **decrease** action potential duration?

    a. Adenosine
    b. Mexiletine
    c. Dofetilide
    d. Amiodarone
    e. Digoxin

70. The mechanism of action of niacin is:

    a. Lipid hydrolysis by lipoprotein lipase
    b. HMG-CoA reductase inhibition
    c. Reduction of VLDL secretion by the liver
    d. Enhanced clearance of triglyceride-rich lipoproteins
    e. Bile-acid binding resin

71. The following have the potential for drug-drug interactions **except:**

    a. Erythromycin and quinidine
    b. Phenobarbital and calcium channel blockers
    c. Ibuprofen and lisinopril
    d. Sildenafil and dobutamine
    e. Lovastatin and warfarin

72. Distribution of drugs to skeletal muscle:

   a. Depends on the unbound drug concentration gradient between the blood and the muscle
   b. Has no effect on half-life
   c. Is not associated with the solubility of the drug in muscle
   d. Is decreased for drugs that are weakly bound to plasma proteins
   e. Is independent of blood flow to skeletal muscle

73. What best describes a drug that inhibits the action of a drug at its receptor by occupying those receptors without activating them?

   a. Partial agonist
   b. Pharmacologic antagonist
   c. Noncompetitive antagonist
   d. Physiologic antagonist
   e. Agonist

74. Intravenous administration of which agent (X) gives the effects on BP and HR as illustrated in the diagram?

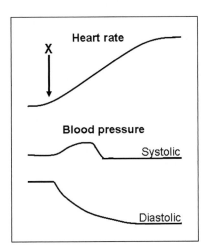

   a. Epinephrine
   b. Norepinephrine
   c. Dopamine
   d. Isoproterenol
   e. NTG

75. The following are true for aspirin, **except:**

   a. Aspirin is indicated in combination with warfarin in patients at high risk for mechanical valve thrombosis
   b. Clopidogrel should be administered to aspirin-intolerant patients acutely with an STEMI
   c. Aspirin is FDA approved for primary prevention of coronary disease in high risk patients
   d. Aspirin is indicated in acute thrombotic stroke
   e. Late coronary stent thrombosis in both bare-metal and DESs is strongly linked to cessation of aspirin therapy

76. Which of the following is **not** a recognized adverse effect of the listed drug?

    a. HMG-CoA reductase inhibitors (statins) and pancreatitis
    b. Beta blockers and bronchospasm
    c. Clonidine and sexual dysfunction
    d. Hydralazine and visual disturbances including photophobia
    e. ACE inhibitors and taste disturbances

77. A 64-year-old diabetic man, 2 to 3 days after PCI for an ACS, develops hemoptysis and lung infiltrates. On bronchoscopic lavage there is sequentially blood aliquots with the presence of significant hemosiderin-laden macrophages.

    Which of the following agents is most likely responsible for this complication?

    a. Clopidogrel
    b. Metoprolol
    c. Enoxaparin
    d. Abciximab
    e. NTG

78. Which of the following statements concerning adverse effects of drugs are true?

    a. Mild decreases in platelet counts are uncommon with heparin therapy
    b. Mexiletine is associated with the development of a lupus-like syndrome
    c. Adenosine may provoke VF in a patient with an accessory pathway
    d. HMG-CoA reductase inhibitors (statins) are relatively safe in pregnancy
    e. Amiodarone is not associated with toxic effects on the fetal thyroid

79. Which of the following combinations do **not** have the potential for drug-drug interactions?

    a. NTG and tadalafil
    b. Gemfibrozil and atenolol
    c. Naproxen and loop diuretics
    d. Aspirin and warfarin
    e. Verapamil and atenolol

80. The following agents/treatments are of value in metoprolol overdose **except**:

    a. Isoproterenol
    b. Dobutamine
    c. Pacing
    d. Dialysis
    e. Glucagon

81. A 73-year-old man undergoes coronary angiography and multivessel coronary intervention with a total of 550 cc of iodinated contrast. Six hours later you are called because the patient is unable to see. Examination is otherwise unremarkable. You should recommend:

    a. Reassurance
    b. Mannitol and furosemide
    c. N-acetyl cysteine
    d. Benadryl and corticosteroids
    e. Heparin for presumed thromboembolic stroke

82. Which is **not** a function mediated by adenosine?

    a. Endothelial-independent vasodilation of the microvasculature
    b. Prolongation of the atrial tissue refractory period
    c. Decreased adhesion of activated platelets to one another
    d. Endothelial-independent vasodilation of the macrovasculature
    e. Decreased leukocyte adhesion to damaged endothelium

83. Four hours after PCI in a patient with stable angina the patient's platelet count is 10,000. The most likely cause is:

    a. Heparin-associated thrombocytopenia
    b. Idiopathic thrombocytopenic purpura
    c. Aspirin
    d. Abciximab
    e. Clopidogrel-induced TTP

84. Which of the following agents would give the following hemodynamic effect, illustrated on the diagram of pressure-volume relationship, as moving from the continuous line (baseline) to the dotted line?

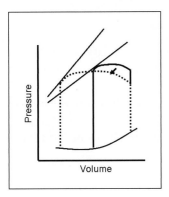

    a. Isoproterenol
    b. Propranolol
    c. Digoxin
    d. NTG
    e. Norepinephrine

85. In a patient on warfarin, amiodarone is initiated for AF. You will need to:

    a. Increase the amiodarone dose by 50%
    b. Increase the warfarin dose by 50%
    c. Follow prothrombin time and adjust warfarin dosage
    d. Switch warfarin to aspirin
    e. Decrease amiodarone dose by 50%

86. Torsades de pointes can result from all **except**:

    a. Erythromycin when taken with cisapride
    b. Dofetilide, a Class III antiarrhythmic, in renal insufficiency
    c. Haloperidol in a patient on quinidine
    d. Propafenone, a Class IC antiarrhythmic
    e. Mutation in sodium and potassium channels

87. Which of the following is true regarding the use of digoxin in patients with heart failure?

    a. Digoxin improves survival in patients with low EF (EF < 35%) heart failure
    b. Digoxin improves survival in patients with normal EF heart failure
    c. Digoxin decreases likelihood of hospitalization in patients with low EF heart failure
    d. Digoxin has no effect on exercise capacity in patients with low EF heart failure
    e. Verapamil is favored over digoxin for AF in the setting of decompensated low EF heart failure

88. Concerning calcium channel blockers, which of the following is **incorrect**?

    a. Nifedipine can cause hypokalemia secondary to a weak diuretic-like action
    b. Diltiazem may slow the development of posttransplant coronary disease irrespective of effects on BP
    c. Digoxin levels are essentially unaltered when coadministered with diltiazem
    d. Unlike metoprolol, diltiazem has no effect on survival in postinfarct patients with preexisting LV dysfunction
    e. Verapamil improves walking distance in patients with intermittent claudication

89. Which of the following is true regarding milrinone?

    a. Milrinone is useful in patients with heart failure secondary to HCM
    b. Milrinone is hepatically cleared and hence the dose should be reduced in patients with severe hepatic congestion
    c. Milrinone increases cardiac contractility through inhibition of the breakdown of cAMP
    d. Unlike dobutamine, milrinone does not increase the incidence of ventricular dysrhythmia
    e. Milrinone is indicated in patients with AMI

90. Which of the following drugs has the effects on the cardiac action potential as demonstrated in this figure as drug X?

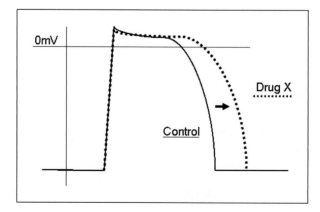

    a. Quinidine
    b. Verapamil
    c. Mexiletine
    d. Flecainide
    e. Sotalol

Answers

1. Answer e.
By accounting for organ function, minimizing or adjusting for drug-drug interactions, and selecting the right dose, the chance for positive outcomes and reduced risk for side effects is optimized. Increasing the frequency of administration rather than increasing the dose reduces the likelihood of excessive peaks in drug concentration and, therefore, dose-dependent side effects.

2. Answer d.
The diagram denotes an increase in preload without an effect on contractility—the answer is saline.

3. Answer a.
Thiazide diuretics (in high doses) and beta blockers both reduce insulin sensitivity. Calcium channel blockers and nitrates have no significant effects. ACE inhibitors, though, do increase insulin sensitivity.

4. Answer d.
The relative decrease in skeletal muscle mass tends to produce a smaller volume of distribution of a drug, which, if unrecognized, adversely affects the frequency of adverse drug events.

5. Answer a.
Despite the elevated INR, this patient should receive heparin, aiming for an activated clotting time of 250 to 300 sec. The onset of action of SQ enoxaparin administered in the catheterization laboratory would be too slow to facilitate emergency PCI.

6. Answer d.
Chronic heparin use is associated with *maternal* osteoporosis; however, heparin does not cross the placenta and hence is not associated with *fetal* osteoporosis. The remainder is all true and is the reason for the absolute or relative contraindications of these medications in pregnancy.

7. Answer e.
Oral doses require much higher doses than IV doses with high first-pass drugs.

8. Answer a.
Drug side effects may be dose-dependent or immunogenically-mediated. Most commonly, they are concentration- or dose-dependent.

9. Answer b.
Metoprolol is predominantly eliminated through the hepatic system and hence is unaffected by renal function. The remainder should all be used with caution in patients with renal insufficiency.

10. Answer c.

HTN is not seen with procainamide. Hypotension, however, can occur, although it is rarely dose-limiting.

11. Answer b.

The risk of myopathy is present with gemfibrozil and pravastatin individually; the risk is enhanced when they are used together, and even greater when the metabolism of pravastatin is inhibited inhibited by a CYP3A4 inhibitor, such as itraconazole.

12. Answer b.

The therapeutic index or window is the most important predictor for the significance of interactions. It is the ratio of a drug's toxic dosage to its maximally effective dosage. The lower the index, the greater the chance is for toxicity.

13. Answer c.

Loop diuretics may cause *hypo*calcemia but not *hyper*calcemia. Early venodilatory effects of loop diuretics are likely prostaglandin-dependent.

14. Answer d.

Unlike other inotropes, levosimendan acts as a calcium sensitizer and does not increase calcium through an increase in intracellular cAMP.

15. Answer d.

Dopamine-mediated tachycardia occurs through action on beta-1 receptors. Beta-1 agonists have little effect on peripheral vessels, as peripheral vasodilatation is mediated through activation of beta-2 receptors. Isoproterenol is a specific beta agonist, having no action on alpha receptors.

16. Answer e.

Grapefruit juice inhibits intestinal CYP3A4 metabolic activity, thereby increasing the oral bioavailability of these medications.

17. Answer b.

In a patient with underlying liver dysfunction, lidocaine is preferred over amiodarone. Given his liver disease, a lower dose of lidocaine will be sufficient.

18. Answer d.

Neutropenia (<0.05%) and a maculopapular pruritic dermatitis (1%) have both been linked with captopril use, likely related to the sulfhydryl group, and are not features associated with other ACE inhibitors. While captopril has been shown to decrease proteinuria in both diabetic and non-diabetic nephropathy, it does cause proteinuria in up to 1% of patients.

19. Answer c.

Amiodarone is favored, given the patient's age and renal dysfunction.

20. Answer d.

Concomitant use of amiodarone has no effect on enalapril.

21. Answer a.

Quinidine is associated with many potential adverse effects, including diarrhea. Constipation is not a feature seen with quinidine.

22. Answer b
Drugs that block sodium channels increase the pacing threshold, whereas potassium channel blockers decrease them.

23. Answer a.
Dofetilide is a pure potassium channel blocker, inhibiting the IK_R.

24. Answer b.
Flumazenil is a potent short-acting antagonist of benzodiazepines; however, it should be used with caution in patients on chronic benzodiazepines.

25. Answer c.
The most serious concern of dofetilide use is QT prolongation and the risk of torsades de pointes.

26. Answer d.
Potency is a measure of the activity of a drug in a biological system.

27. Answer c.
The combination of digoxin with amiodarone, propranolol, or verapamil can lead to AV block.

28. Answer c.
Selective beta blockers are preferred over non-selective agents in patients with peripheral vascular disease.

29. Answer d.
Terfenadine (though not now available in the U.S.) was considered an innocuous antihistamine. However, large doses of terfenadine, or settings in which terfenadine metabolism is impaired (such as concomitant erythromycin), can result in terfenadine-induced torsades de pointes. There is nothing in the case to suggest digoxin toxicity.

30. Answer d.
In the presence of suspected HIT and renal insufficiency, the appropriate step is to stop heparin and start Argatroban. Lepirudin, although indicated in patients with HIT, is excreted renally and hence should be avoided in the presence of significant renal insufficiency. While enoxaparin has a decreased incidence of HIT over unfractionated heparin, it is still contraindicated once HIT has occurred. Warfarin should ultimately be started, although it will be a number of days before warfarin provides adequate anticoagulation. Warfarin should not be started until the thrombocytopenia resolves, as the initial hypercoagulable state induced by a decline in protein C levels would only compound the hypercoagulability of HIT.

31. Answer e.
Digoxin is excreted from the liver and kidney by protein transporters (one of them being P-glycoprotein). Captopril has no effect on the protein transporters.

32. Answer d.
In combination with a Class Ib agent, such as mexiletine, the effect of disopyramide can be enhanced while avoiding further prolongation of the QT interval. Disopyramide has been effective in treating neurally mediated syncope in patients refractory to beta blockers.

33. Answer d.

The figure demonstrates an isolated increase in afterload.

34. Answer d.

Torsades de pointes is usually associated with high drug dosages or plasma concentrations of CV drugs (such as sotalol and ibutilide) and "non-CV drugs" (terfenadine, cisapride, haloperidol, and thioridazine). An exception to this rule is quinidine, where the reaction can occur with the first dose and at "subtherapeutic" plasma concentrations.

35. Answer c.

Patients treated with an initial bolus of lidocaine followed by a maintenance infusion may experience transient subtherapeutic plasma concentrations at 30 to 120 minutes after therapy is begun and may require a subsequent bolus.

36. Answer b.

ACE increases the degradation of bradykinin, hence ACE inhibitors decreased this degradation. ARBs have no effect on bradykinin metabolism.

37. Answer e.

Two-half lives of the drug will reduce the plasma level by a quarter.

38. Answer c.

Chronic infusion of dobutamine has not been shown to have a survival benefit in heart failure.

39. Answer b.

Endothelin is the most potent vasoconstrictor. Adenosine is a potent vasodilator.

40. Answer b.

NTG is active on arteries $>100 \, \mu m$ and the venous system.

41. Answer c.

Acetylcholine causes endothelial-dependent vasodilation. In the absence of endothelial function, acetylcholine causes paradoxical vasodilation. Adenosine causes endothelial-independent vasodilation.

42. Answer b.

IV administration of a drug bypasses all first-pass metabolism and gives complete bioavailability.

43. Answer c.

Methemoglobinemia is a rare complication of nitrites including those seen from environmental exposure. It has not been associated with sildenafil use.

44. Answer c.

Digoxin effects are increased with low muscle mass due to less skeletal binding. Hemodialysis is not helpful in digoxin toxicity due to the large volume of distribution. Digoxin decreases the pacing threshold.

45. Answer d.

Due to potential negative inotropic actions, calcium channel blockers have no therapeutic role in right-sided heart failure and should be avoided or used with extreme caution in patients with right-sided heart failure.

46. Answer c.

This question focuses on disease states that alter first-pass metabolism and, hence, bioavailability of a drug. The question asks in which condition will the oral bioavailability be highest, ie, in which state will first-pass metabolism be lowest. Liver cirrhosis impairs hepatic metabolism, here leading to an increased oral bioavailability of metoprolol.

47. Answer d.

Due to the presence of more heparin-binding proteins, a greater plasma volume, increased renal clearance, coagulation factors, and heparin degradation in the placenta, heparin dosing is unpredictable in pregnancy, with patients invariably requiring higher doses. Hyperthyroidism is associated with an increased catabolism of vitamin K. Lepirudin is renally excreted and patients with HIT in the setting of renal failure should receive argatroban. While contraindicated with thrombi in left-sided chambers, slow infusions of thrombolytics are frequently used in the presence of right-sided thrombi.

48. Answer a.

The efficacy of a drug is best described by the maximal effect of the drug, regardless of dose.

49. Answer d.

Sodium lactate is an effective agent for procainamide toxicity by increasing the sodium current and reducing drug-receptor binding by alkalizing the tissue. Hyperkalemia predisposes to procainamide toxicity.

50. Answer a.

The combination of reducing phase 0 (sodium channel inhibition) and prolongation of action potential duration (I_{KR} inhibition) is classical for class 1A antiarrhythmic agents, eg, quinidine.

51. Answer d.

Loop diuretics such as ethacrynic acid decrease serum potassium.

52. Answer b.

Methyldopa is rarely associated with Coombs positive hemolytic anemia. Minoxidil is used topically to promote hair growth due to its side effect of hirsutism. Cyanide toxicity is a potential side effect of nitrites.

53. Answer c.

The combination of increased cGMP from nitrates and impaired cGMP degradation from sildenafil potentially may lead to exaggerated hypotension and organ malperfusion due to hypotension. Hence the combination should be avoided.

54. Answer d.

Despite vasodilatory actions, the reflex tachycardia with hydralazine can exacerbate angina in the absence of HR control.

55. Answer c.

The curve shift to the left denotes a decrease in afterload without a change in contractility, mediated here by enalaprilat.

56. Answer c.

While antiarrhythmics, amiodarone and quinidine may both potentially exacerbate arrhythmias caused by digitalis toxicity.

57. Answer e.

Digoxin is the only listed therapy without proven effect on survival in patients with low EF heart failure.

58. Answer a.

Sotalol is cleared renally and hence should be used with extreme caution when there is the potential for renal insufficiency.

59. Answer c.

Potency of a drug denotes the effect per unit mass. It does not describe the magnitude of its maximal effect (efficacy).

60. Answer a.

Metoprolol is not beta-2 selective.

61. Answer c.

A proportion of patients lack significant cytochrome CYP2D6 activity and, hence, are poor metabolizers of propafenone. This leads to relative increases in propafenone plasma levels that are associated with greater beta blocker effects than the metabolite 5-hydroxypropafaone.

62. Answer e.

*Hyper*calcemia is a potential complication of thiazide diuretics.

63. Answer c.

Amiodarone is the only agent that will convert the rhythm from AF to sinus. The other agents are useful agents for rate control.

64. Answer e.

The nonspecific ET-A and ET-B receptor antagonist bosentan is highly teratogenic, decreases the efficacy of estrogen contraceptive, and causes significant liver dysfunction in up to 10% of patients.

65. Answer e.

Heart failure by reducing hepatic blood flow may decrease the clearance of drugs metabolized in the liver. Cigarette smoke induces the CYP1A2 enzyme and may increase drug metabolism.

66. Answer c.

Niacin should be avoided in patients with gout due to the potential for exacerbating it. Bumetanide is a loop diuretic and, unlike thiazide diuretics, does not affect gout.

67. Answer c.

Methylene blue is the treatment of methemoglobinemia seen rarely as a complication of benzocaine administration for TEE or with sodium nitroprusside treatment. Cyanide toxicity, however, is treated with amyl nitrate, sodium nitrite, and then sodium thiosulfate.

68. Answer c.

Bleomycin, while potentially toxic to the lungs (interstitial fibrosis), is not directly cardiac toxic.

69. Answer b.

Class 1B agents, such as mexiletine, inhibit sodium channels and shorten action potential duration.

70. Answer c.

Niacin acts by reducing VLDL secretion by the liver. Fibrates act by inhibiting lipid hydrolysis by lipoprotein lipase.

71. Answer d.

All the answer choices have potential drug-drug interactions except sildenafil and dobutamine. (The combination of sildenafil and nitrates should be avoided.)

72. Answer a.

Distribution of a drug to a specific tissue is directly dependent on the concentration gradient between that drug and the tissue and the blood flow to that tissue.

73. Answer b.

A pharmacologic antagonist is a drug that competitively blocks a drug's receptor without activating it.

74. Answer d.

Isoproterenol has beta-specific action leading to tachycardia and an increase in pulse pressure due to reductions in diastolic BP.

75. Answer c.

While recommended in patients with a >10% 10-year risk of coronary disease, aspirin is not FDA approved for primary prevention.

76. Answer d.

Adverse effects of hydralazine therapy include hepatitis, neuropathy, flushing, and, rarely, a lupus-like syndrome. Photophobia, a potential sign of digoxin toxicity, is not a feature seen with hydralazine therapy.

77. Answer d.

Alveolar hemorrhage is a recognized, albeit rare, complication of abciximab therapy.

78. Answer c.

Mild reductions in platelet counts (HIT type 1) occur commonly with heparin therapy. Mexiletine, unlike procainamide, is not associated with a lupus-like syndrome. Statins are contraindicated in pregnancy due to a high rate of teratogenic effects.

79. Answer b.

Gemfibrozil and atenolol do not interact. NTG and phosphodiesterase inhibitors, such as tadalafil or sildenafil, should be avoided.

80. Answer d.

Metoprolol is not dialyzable. Isoproterenol, dobutamine or glucagon are all reasonable agents in patients with an overdose of beta blockers. Temporary pacing maybe required for certain cases.

81. Answer a.

Acute cortical blindness following a large contrast exposure is due to osmolar disruption of the blood-brain barrier. If clinical examination including funduscopy is normal, the treatment involves fluids and reassurance. Symptoms typically resolve within 12 to 24 hours.

82. Answer b.

Adenosine is an endothelial-independent vasodilator of both the micro- and macrovasculature. It does not prolong the refractory period in atrial tissue. However, it does shorten the atrial action potential and hyperpolarizes the membrane. This results in depression of the sinus node rate and gives transient AV block.

83. Answer d.

The fall in platelet count is too quick and too low for HIT and is most consistent with an acute fall secondary to abciximab use.

84. Answer a.

The diagram illustrates an increase in contractility and a decrease in afterload, with a mild decrease in pressure—characteristics of the beta agonist isoproterenol.

85. Answer c.

Typically, warfarin doses need to be decreased between 25% and 50% after starting amiodarone, although the response is variable.

86. Answer d.

Class 1C agents have no significant effect on prolongation of the action potential and, hence, do not predispose to torsades de pointes.

87. Answer c.

Digoxin is safe and well tolerated in CHF, improving exercise capacity and reducing hospitalization rates without affecting mortality. In decompensated CHF calcium channel blockers, particularly those which are negatively inotropic, eg, verapamil, should be used with caution. Digoxin and beta blockers tend to be preferred for AF in patients with (particularly decompensated) CHF.

88. Answer d.

Diltiazem increases mortality in patients post-MI with preexisting LV systolic dysfunction and should be avoided. The other statements are all true.

89. Answer c.

Milrinone leads to the inhibition of cAMP breakdown, through inhibition of phosphodiesterase-III.

90. Answer e.

All class III drugs act by reducing the outward potassium current (phase 3 – I_{KR}) to prolong action potential duration. Class 1A agents, such as quinidine, in addition to prolongation of action potential duration also reduce inward sodium current affecting phase 0. Class 1B agents, eg, mexiletine, shorten action potential duration.